Praise for *Whole*

"After reading *The China Study* and drastically changing my diet toward the more whole food, plant-based diet recommended by Dr. Campbell, my career numbers shot up when they were supposed to be declining. I thought to myself, 'Why doesn't everyone eat this way?!' This new book, *Whole*, answers that question with great clarity. Never again be confused about diet and nutrition."

—Tony Gonzalez, Atlanta Falcons, 16-year National Football
League player, Record-Setting Tight End

"*Whole* makes a convincing case that modern nutrition's focus on single nutrients has led to mass confusion with tragic health consequences. Dr. Campbell's new paradigm will change the way we think about food and, in doing so, could improve the lives of millions of people and save billions of dollars in health care costs."

— Brian Wendel, Creator and Executive Producer of *Forks Over
Knives.*

"America's premier nutritionist, T. Colin Campbell, with courage and conviction, articulates how the self-serving reductionist paradigm permeates science, medicine, media, big pharma and philanthropic groups blocking the public from the nutritional truth for optimal health."

—Caldwell Esselstyn, Jr., MD; Bestselling Author,
Prevent and Reverse Heart Disease

"In this provocative book, T. Colin Campbell, based on his long career in experimental research and health policy making, uncovers how and why there is so much confusion about food and health and what can be done about it. *The China Study* revealed *what we* should eat; *Whole* answers *why*. Read and enjoy; there's something here to inspire and offend just about everyone."

—Dean Ornish, MD, Founder and President, Preventive Medicine Research Institute in Sausalito, California; Clinical Professor of Medicine, University of California, San Francisco; and Bestselling Author, *Dr. Dean Ornish's Program for Reversing Heart Disease*

"T. Colin Campbell, PhD, has been the most influential nutritional scientist of the past century. His work has already saved hundreds of thousands of lives."

—John McDougall, MD, Founder and Medical Director of the McDougall Program

"There are very few material game-changers in life, but this book is truly one of them. The information herein—backed up by extraordinary peer-reviewed science—has the power to halt and reverse disease, give you energy you've never known, and put you on a path of transformation in just about every positive way. Read it and get ready to soar."

—Kathy Freston, *New York Times* Bestselling Author, *The Lean* and *Quantum Wellness*

"Dr. Colin Campbell opened our eyes with *The China Study*. In *Whole*, Dr. Campbell boldly shows exactly how our understanding of nutrition and health has gone off track and how to get It right. Beautifully and clearly written, this empowering book will forever change the way you think about health, food and science."

—Neal Barnard, Founder and President, Physicians Committee for Responsible Medicine

"Dr. Campbell succeeds in taking a fresh, honest look at the science of nutrition, as he unveils the startling truth behind sickness and reveals a sure-fire way to achieve the excellent health you deserve."

—Chef AJ, Author of *Unprocessed*

"This book is the key to understanding how to increase our natural longevity and health, it is key to slowing global warming, and all of this at no cost, rather, at immeasurable savings to society."

—Mike Fremont, World Record Holder for Marathons for 88 and 90
    year olds

"*Whole: Rethinking the Science of Nutrition* should be required reading for anyone interested in health. Dr. Campbell's ability to take complex topics and make them understandable to the average person is unparalleled. Like *The China Study*, I predict that this book will be the catalyst for millions of people to not only change their diets, but how they think about and make decisions concerning health and medicine. The revolution that will reform our broken healthcare system has begun."

—Pamela A. Popper, PhD, ND, Executive Director of
    The Wellness Forum; Coauthor of *Food Over Medicine*

"In *Whole*, Dr. Campbell defines a super-paradigm that elucidates a philosophy—wholism—which medicine needs to aspire to in order to attain an enlightened solution. *Whole* is a masterpiece of intellectual triangulation, outlining the past, the present, and the critical next steps in the future of biochemistry, human nutrition, and healthcare. This book is going to unleash a health revolution!"

—Julieanna Hever, MS, RD, CPT; Bestselling Author,
    The Complete Idiot's Guide to Plant-Based Nutrition; and
    Host of *What Would Julieanna Do?*

"Why is the most expensive health care system in the world not working? This book provides scientific 'big picture' clarity amidst a sea of confusion about how commercially driven 'disease management' is costing us millions of lives—while wasting trillions of dollars. Understanding how this 'health care monster' operates is the first step toward creating a system that truly promotes health."

—J. Morris Hicks, Consultant; Author of *Healthy Eating,
    Healthy World*; International Blogger at hpjmh.com

"The reductionist view of nutrition and medicine deeply threatens our health unlike any disease we have ever battled. Unfortunately, so many of our medical and wellness systems are entrenched in this destructive mentality that people are routinely exposed to 'health care' that does not benefit them, or worse, causes harm. By understanding and helping to spread the revolutionary concepts in this book, *Whole*, you are taking those first pivotal steps to change a failing paradigm while also helping yourself, your loved ones, and our nation recover its lost health."

—Alona Pulde, MD, and Matthew Lederman, MD, Co-Founders of Transition to Health: Medical, Nutrition, and Wellness Center

"In *Whole*, leading nutritionist, Dr. T. Colin Campbell, explains how and why nutrition research and education have gotten so far off course that even the most health-conscious consumers are confused. With our current health and healthcare crises, Dr. Campbell's book is an important guide to understanding how we got here and how we can and must restructure the systems that brought us to this point."

—Jeff Novick, MS, RD, VP of Health Promotion, Executive Health Exams International

"It sometimes seems that the more advanced our knowledge, the more likely it is for us to lose our way. In his latest contribution, Dr. T. Colin Campbell brilliantly guides us back to profound and simple truths. With characteristic clarity and scholarship, he illuminates the path to better health and a better world."

—Douglas J. Lisle, PhD, and Alan Goldhamer, DC, Coauthors of *The Pleasure Trap*

"The *China Study* has helped me enormously in my life, as well as my family and friends in theirs. I continue to believe that obesity is a curse to the world, therefore in my opinion, it is essential for people to read *Whole!*"

—Gary Player, World Golf Hall of Fame Professional Golfer

WHOLE

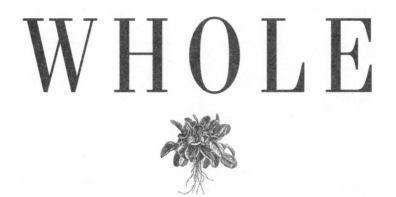

Rethinking the Science of Nutrition

T. COLIN CAMPBELL, PhD
with HOWARD JACOBSON, PhD

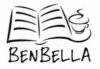

BenBella Books, Inc.
Dallas, Texas

BenBella

BenBella Books, Inc.
10300 N. Central Expressway, Suite 530
Dallas, TX 75231
www.benbellabooks.com
Send feedback to feedback@benbellabooks.com

Printed in the United States of America
10 9 8 7 6 5 4 3 2 1

Library of Congress Cataloging-in-Publication Data has cataloged the hardcover edition as follows:

Campbell, T. Colin, 1934–
    Whole : rethinking the science of nutrition / T. Colin Campbell, PhD with Howard Jacobson, PhD.
        pages cm
    Includes bibliographical references and index.
    ISBN 978-1-937856-25-0 (e-book) — ISBN 978-1-937856-24-3 (hardback)
1. Nutrition. 2. Longevity—Nutritional aspects. 3. Vegetarianism. I. Jacobson, Howard, 1930– II. Title.
    RA784.C23524 2013
    613.2—dc23

                                                    2012051561

Copyediting by James Fraleigh
Proofreading by Gregory Teague and Kimberly Marini
Cover design by Faceout Studio
Text design and composition by Publishers' Design and Production Services, Inc.
Printed by Bang Printing
Figure 7–1 © William L. Elliott
Figures 7–2 and 7–3 © the International Union of Biochemistry and Molecular Biology

Distributed by Perseus Distribution
(www.perseusdistribution.com)
To place orders through Perseus Distribution:
Tel: 800-343-4499
Fax: 800-351-5073
E-mail: orderentry@perseusbooks.com

Significant discounts for bulk sales are available. Please contact Glenn Yeffeth at glenn@benbellabooks.com or 214-750-3628.

To all those who unnecessarily paid the ultimate price of a failed health care system, including my wife's mother, Mary, and my father, Tom.

And, as always, to my wife, Karen, and our children, their spouses, and our grandchildren.

Contents

Introduction   *xi*

PART I   ENSLAVED BY THE SYSTEM

Chapter 1   *The Modern Health-Care Myth*   3

Chapter 2   *The Whole Truth*   14

Chapter 3   *My Heretical Path*   26

PART II   PARADIGM AS PRISON

Chapter 4   *The Triumph of Reductionism*   45

Chapter 5   *Reductionism Invades Nutrition*   58

Chapter 6   *Reductionist Research*   75

Chapter 7   *Reductionist Biology*   88

Chapter 8   *Genetics versus Nutrition, Part One*   107

Chapter 9   *Genetics versus Nutrition, Part Two*   125

Chapter 10   *Reductionist Medicine*   140

Chapter 11   *Reductionist Supplementation*   150

Chapter 12   *Reductionist Social Policy*   164

PART III   SUBTLE POWER AND ITS WIELDERS

Chapter 13   *Understanding the System*   *181*

Chapter 14   *Industry Exploitation and Control*   *196*

Chapter 15   *Research and Profit*   *214*

Chapter 16   *Media Matters*   *231*

Chapter 17   *Government Misinformation*   *247*

Chapter 18   *Blinded by the Light Bringers*   *262*

PART IV   FINAL THOUGHTS

Chapter 19   *Making Ourselves Whole*   *285*

              Acknowledgments   *291*

              About the Authors   *293*

              Notes   *295*

              Index   *313*

Introduction

In 1965, my academic career looked promising. After four years as a research associate at MIT, I was settling into my new office at Virginia Tech's Department of Biochemistry and Nutrition. Finally, I was a real professor! My research agenda couldn't have been more noble: end childhood malnutrition in poor countries by figuring out how to get more high-quality protein into their diets. My arena was the Philippines, thanks to a generous grant from the U.S. State Department's Agency for International Development.

The first challenge was to find a locally produced, inexpensive protein source. (Even though malnutrition is largely an issue of not getting enough calories overall, in the mid-1960s we thought that calories from protein were somehow special.) The second challenge was to develop a series of self-help centers around the country where we could show mothers how to raise their children out of malnutrition by using that protein source. My team and I chose peanuts, which are rich in protein and can grow under lots of different conditions.

At the same time, I was working on another project at the request of my department chair, Dean Charlie Engel. Charlie had secured U.S. Department of Agriculture funding to study aflatoxin, a cancer-causing chemical produced by a fungus *Aspergillus flavus*, and my job was to learn all I could about how the fungus grew so we could prevent it from growing on various food sources. This was clearly an important project, as there was quite a bit of evidence that *Aspergillus flavus* caused liver cancer in lab rats (the mainstream assumption was, and still is to this day, that anything that causes cancer in rats or mice probably also causes cancer in humans).

One of the main foods *Aspergillus flavus* contaminates is peanuts, and so, in one of those cosmic coincidences that appears amazing only years later, I found myself studying peanuts in two completely different contexts simultaneously. And what I found when I looked deeply into these two seemingly unrelated issues (protein deficiency among the poor children of the Philippines and the conditions under which *Aspergillus flavus* grows) started to shake my world and caused me to question many of the bedrock assumptions on which I and most other nutritional scientists had built our careers.

Here's the main finding that turned my worldview—and ultimately, my world—upside down: the children in the Philippines who ate the highest-protein diets were the ones most likely to get liver cancer—even though the children with high-protein diets were significantly wealthier and had better access to all the things we typically associate with childhood health, like medical care and clean water.

I chose to follow this discovery everywhere it led me. As a result, the trajectory of my career veered in unexpected and unsettling directions, many of which are detailed in my first book, *The China Study*. I ultimately became aware of two things: First, nutrition is the master key to human health. Second, what most of us think of as proper nutrition—isn't.

If you want to live free of cancer, heart disease, and diabetes for your entire life, that power is in your hands (and your knife and fork). But, sadly, medical schools, hospitals, and government health agencies continue to treat nutrition as if it plays only a minor role in health. And no wonder: the standard Western diet, along with its trendy "low fat" and "low carb" cousins, is actually the cause, not the cure, of most of what ails us. In a nutshell, the "miracle cure" science has been chasing for the past half century turns out not to be a new wonder drug painstakingly formulated after decades of brilliant and relentless lab work, or a cutting-edge surgical tool, or technique using lasers and nanotechnology, or some transformation of our DNA that will turn us all into immortal Apollos and Venuses. Instead, the secret of health has been in front of us all along, in the guise of a simple and perhaps boring word: nutrition. When it comes to our health, it turns out the trump card is the food we put in our mouths each day. In the process of learning all this, I also learned something else very important: why most people didn't know this already.

The medical and scientific research establishments, far from embracing these findings, have systematically dismissed and even suppressed them.

Few medical professionals are aware that our food choices can be far more effective shields against disease than the pills they prescribe.

Few health journalists report the unambiguous good news about radiant health and disease prevention through diet.

Few scientists are trained to look at the "big picture," and instead specialize in scrutinizing single drops of data instead of comprehending meaningful rivers of wisdom.

And paying the piper and calling the tune for all of them are the pharmaceutical and food industries, which are trying to convince us that salvation can be found in a pill or an enriched snack food made from plant fragments and artificial ingredients.

The truth. How it's been kept from you. And why. That's what this book is all about.

WHY ANOTHER BOOK?

If you've read *The China Study*, you've heard some of this before. You know the truth about nutrition, and you've heard a little bit about the resistance other scientists and I have faced in trying to bring this truth to light.

Since its publication in 2005, millions of people have read or read about *The China Study* and shared its insights with friends, neighbors, colleagues, and loved ones. Not a day goes by that I don't hear grateful testimonials to the healing power of whole, plant-based foods. Anecdotal as each of these stories may be, the overall weight of their combined evidence is substantial. And each of them is more than ample compensation for the troubles and obstacles placed in my way by powerful interests who make money from our collective ignorance.

Also, since 2005, many of my colleagues have conducted varied studies that show even more powerfully the effects of good eating on the various systems of the human body. At this point, any scientist, doctor, journalist, or policy maker who denies or minimizes the importance of a whole food, plant-based diet for individual and societal well-being simply isn't looking clearly at the facts. There's just too much good evidence to ignore anymore.

And yet, in some ways, very little has changed. Most people still don't know that the key to health and longevity is in their hands. Whether maliciously or, as is more often the case, due to ignorance, the mainstream of Western culture is hell-bent on ignoring, disbelieving, and, in some cases, actively twisting the truth about what we should be eating—so much so that it can be hard for us to believe that we've been lied to all these years. It's often easier to simply accept what we've been told, rather than consider the possibility of a conspiracy of control, silence, and misinformation. And the only way to combat this perception is to show you how and why it happened.

That's why this new book felt necessary. *The China Study* focused on the evidence that tells us the whole food, plant-based diet is the healthiest human diet. *Whole* focuses on why it's been so hard to bring that evidence to light—and on what still needs to happen for real change to take place.

WHOLE: THE SUM OF ITS PARTS

This book is split into four parts.

The first, Part I, provides a little more information about my and others' research on the whole food, plant-based diet, my reflections on some of the most prominent criticisms this research has received since the publication of *The China Study*, and more of my own background and journey, as context for understanding where the philosophies in this book have come from.

Part II looks at the reason it's so hard for so many not to just accept, but even notice, the health implications of this research: the mental prison, or paradigm, in which Western science and medicine operate, which makes it impossible to see the obvious facts that lie outside it. For many reasons, we now operate under a paradigm that looks for truth only in the smallest details, while entirely ignoring the big picture. The popular expression "can't see the forest for the trees" makes the point well, except that there's much more at stake here than just trees and forests. Modern science is so detail obsessed that we can't see the forest for the vascular cambium and secondary phloem and so on. There's nothing wrong with looking at details (I spent most of my research career doing just that); the trouble occurs when we start denying that there *is* a big picture, and stubbornly insist that the narrow reality we see, heavily laden with our own biases and experiences, is all there is.

The fancy word for this obsession with minutiae is *reductionism*. And reductionism comes with its own seductive logic, so that people laboring under its spell can't even see that there's another way to look at the world. To reductionists, all other worldviews are unscientific, superstitious, sloppy, and not worthy of attention. All evidence gathered by non-reductionist means—presuming that research can get funding in the first place—is ignored or suppressed.

Part III looks at the other side of this equation: the economic forces that reinforce and exploit this paradigm for their own self-interest as they chase financial success. These forces completely manipulate the public conversation about health and nutrition to suit their bottom line. We'll look at the many ways money affects thousands of small decisions that add up to a big impact on what you, the public, hear (and don't hear) and thus believe about health and nutrition.

Last, in Part IV, we look at the totality of what's at stake here, and what's needed if we want things to change.

THE TRUTH BELONGS TO ALL OF US

I wanted to tell this story because I owe it to you, the public. If you are a U.S. taxpayer, you paid for my career in research, teaching, and policy making. I have known too many people, including friends and family, who suffered ill health unnecessarily, just because they did not know what I have come to know—and they also were taxpayers. You have a right to know what your money bought and a right to benefit from its findings.

My own disclaimer: I have no financial interest in you believing me. I don't sell health products, health seminars, or health coaching. I'm seventy-nine years old, I've had a long and rewarding career, and I'm not writing this book to make a buck. When you start talking about what you've learned from this book with your friends and you encounter passionate disdain for me and my motives (and you will!), just consider the original source of the claims they're citing. Ask yourself: What's their financial interest? What do they have to gain from suppressing the information I share here?

Telling this story has been a challenge. I know well that a diet consisting only of plants sounds like a wacky idea to many folks. But that's starting to change. This idea becomes bigger and bigger with the passing of time. The current system is unsustainable. The only question is, will we free ourselves before it takes us down with it? Or will we continue to pollute our bodies, our minds, and our planet with the slag of that system until it collapses under its own economic weight and biological logic?

In previous generations, how we ate appeared to be a personal and private matter. Our food choices didn't seem to contribute much, one way or the other, to the well-being or suffering of other people, let alone animals, plant life, and the carrying capacity of the entire planet. But even if that were ever true, it no longer is. What we eat, individually and collectively, has repercussions far beyond our waistlines and blood pressure readings. No less than our future as a species hangs in the balance.

The choice is ours. My hope is that this book will encourage you to choose wisely—for your health, for the next generations, and for the entire planet.

T. Colin Campbell
Lansing, New York
November 2012

PART I

Enslaved by
the System

1

The Modern
Health-Care Myth

He who cures a disease may be the skillfullest, but
he that prevents it is the safest physician.

—THOMAS FULLER

What a great time to be alive! Modern medicine promises salvation from scourges that have plagued humanity since time began. Disease, infirmity, aging—all soon to be eradicated thanks to advances in technology, genetics, pharmacology, and food science. The cure for cancer is just around the corner. DNA splicing will replace our self-sabotaging or damaged genes with perfectly healthy ones. New wonder drugs are discovered practically every week. And genetic modification of food, combined with advanced processing techniques, will soon be able to turn a simple tomato, carrot, or cookie into a complete meal. Heck, maybe someday soon we won't have to eat at all—we can just swallow a pill that contains every nutrient we need.

There's only one problem with that rosy picture—it's totally false. None of those lofty promises is anywhere close to being realized. We "race for the cure" by pouring billions of dollars into dangerous and ineffective treatments. We seek new genes, as if the ones we've evolved over millions of years are insufficient for our needs. We medicate ourselves with toxic concoctions, a small number of which treat the disease, while the rest treat the harmful side effects of the primary drugs.

We talk about the health-care system in America, but that's a misnomer; what we really have is a disease-care system.

Fortunately, we have a far better, safer, and cheaper way of achieving good health, one with only positive side effects. Furthermore, this approach prevents most of the diseases and conditions that afflict us before they show up, so we don't need to avail ourselves of the disease-care system in the first place.

THE DISEASE-CARE SYSTEM

The United States spends more money per capita on "health" care than any country on earth, yet when the quality of our health care is compared with other industrialized nations, we rank near the bottom.

As a country, we're quite sick. Despite our high rate of health expenditures, we're not any healthier. In fact, rates of many chronic diseases have only increased over time, and based on health biomarkers like obesity, diabetes, and hypertension, they may be headed for further increases. The prevalence of obese individuals increased from 13 percent of the U.S. population in 1962 to a staggering 34 percent in 2008.[1] The U.S. Centers for Disease Control and Prevention (CDC) report that the age-adjusted Type 2 diabetes rate in the United States has more than doubled from 1980 to 2010, from 2.5 percent to 6.9 percent of the population.[2] Hypertension (high blood pressure) among American adults increased 30 percent between 1997 and 2009.[3]

Drugs and surgical advances are keeping the death rates more or less constant despite the increased risk factors (except for diabetes, whose mortality rate has increased an astounding 29 percent in North America from 2007 to 2010).[4] But the data make it clear that none of our advances in medicine deal with primary prevention, and none are making us fundamentally healthier. They aren't *decreasing* the death rate. And the price we're paying for these advances is steep.

For many years, the cost of medically prescribed drugs has been increasing at a rate faster than inflation. Think we're getting our money's worth? Think again.

Side effects of those very same prescription drugs are the third leading cause of death, behind heart disease and cancer. That's right! Prescription drugs kill more people than traffic accidents. According to Dr. Barbara Starfield, writing in the *Journal of the American Medical Association* in 2000, "adverse effects of medications" (from drugs that were correctly prescribed and taken) kill 106,000 people per year.[5] And that doesn't include accidental overdoses.

Add to that the 7,000 annual deaths from medication errors in hospitals, 20,000 deaths from errors in hospitals not related to medications (like botched surgeries and incorrectly programmed and monitored machines), 80,000 deaths from hospital-caused infections, and 2,000 deaths per year from unnecessary surgery, and the tire-screeching ambulance ride starts to look like the safest part of the whole hospital experience.[6]

Yet when you ask the U.S. government about this, you're met with deafening denial. Look at the CDC web page on the leading causes of death shown in Figure 1-1.

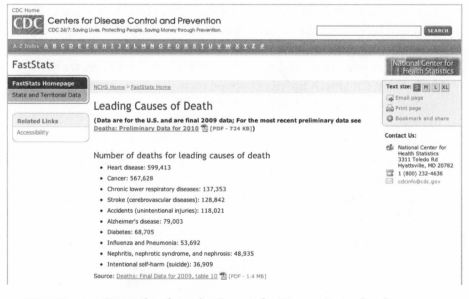

FIGURE 1-1.   Screenshot from the Centers for Disease Control and Prevention website[7]

Notice anything strange? Not a peep about the medical system being the third leading cause of death in the United States. Admitting that would be bad for business, and if the U.S. government cares about one thing here, it's the economic interests of the medical establishment.

But what about when medical care doesn't kill? Surely the benefits to millions outweigh a few hundred thousand deaths each year?

Visit a nursing home or geriatric center to see for yourself how well the system serves those who need it most. You'll feel the physical and emotional pain of once-vibrant people suffering needlessly with ailments and illnesses caused in large part by the pharmaceutical cocktails they take. Who can blame them? Doctors know best, right? And how many daytime TV commercials promoting drugs to decrease their blood cholesterol, drive down their blood sugar, and increase their sex drive have they watched?

I could go on and on. But I think you get the picture: the more we spend on disease care, the sicker and more miserable we seem to become.

THE GOOD NEWS

All our trillions of dollars are not improving our health outcomes. The promised breakthroughs are always a decade away and recede just as fast as we chase them. Genetic research has led to nightmarish anti-privacy scenarios, as well as tragic misunderstandings in which mothers are having their young daughters' breasts chopped off just because some geneticist pricked their daughters' fingers, tested their DNA, and scared them half to death with predictions of possible future breast cancer.

That's all pretty depressing, I admit.

The good news is that we don't need medical breakthroughs or genetic manipulation to achieve, maintain, and restore vibrant health. A half century of research—both mine and that of many others—has convinced me of the following:

- What you eat every day is a far more powerful determinant of your health than your DNA or most of the nasty chemicals lurking in your environment.
- The foods you consume can heal you faster and more profoundly than the most expensive prescription drugs, and more dramatically

than the most extreme surgical interventions, with only positive side effects.

- Those food choices can prevent cancer, heart disease, Type 2 diabetes, stroke, macular degeneration, migraines, erectile dysfunction, and arthritis—and that's only the short list.
- It's never too late to start eating well. A good diet can *reverse* many of those conditions as well.

In short: change the way you eat and you can transform your health for the better.

THE IDEAL HUMAN DIET

For some reason, "health food" has a reputation for being tasteless and joyless. You might be thinking at this point that the miracle diet for human health must be the most grim fare imaginable. Fortunately, that's not the case. Evolution thankfully has programmed us to seek out and enjoy foods that promote our health. All we have to do is get back to our dietary roots—nothing radical or miserable required.

The ideal human diet looks like this: Consume plant-based foods in forms as close to their natural state as possible ("whole" foods). Eat a variety of vegetables, fruits, raw nuts and seeds, beans and legumes, and whole grains. Avoid heavily processed foods and animal products. Stay away from added salt, oil, and sugar. Aim to get 80 percent of your calories from carbohydrates, 10 percent from fat, and 10 percent from protein.

That's it, in 66 words. In this book I call it the whole food, plant-based (WFPB) diet, and sometimes the WFPB lifestyle (I'm not crazy about the word *diet*, which implies a heroic and temporary effort rather than a sustainable and joyful way of eating).

IF THE WFPB WERE A PILL

Just how healthy is the WFPB diet? Let's pretend that all its effects could be achieved through a drug. Imagine a big pharmaceutical company holding a press conference to unveil a new pill called Eunutria. They unveil a list of scientifically proven effects of Eunutria that includes the following:

- Prevents 95 percent of all cancers, including those "caused" by environmental toxins
- Prevents nearly all heart attacks and strokes
- Reverses even severe heart disease
- Prevents and reverses Type 2 diabetes so quickly and profoundly that, after three days on this drug, it's dangerous for users to continue to use insulin

What about side effects, you ask? Of course there are side effects. They include:

- Gets you to your ideal weight in a healthy and sustainable fashion
- Eliminates most migraines, acne, colds and flu, chronic pain, and intestinal distress
- Improves energy
- Cures erectile dysfunction (that makes the pill a blockbuster success all by itself!)

Those are just the side effects for individuals taking the pill. There are also environmental effects:

- Slows and possibly reverses global warming
- Reduces groundwater contamination
- Ends the need for deforestation
- Shuts down factory farms
- Reduces malnutrition and dislocation among the world's poorest citizens

How healthy is the WFPB diet? It's hard to imagine anything healthier—or anything more effective at addressing our biggest health issues. Not only is WFPB the healthiest way of eating that has ever been studied, but it's far more effective in promoting health and preventing disease than prescription drugs, surgery, vitamin and herbal supplementation, and genetic manipulation.

If the WFPB diet were a pill, its inventor would be the wealthiest person on earth. Since it isn't a pill, no market forces conspire to advocate for it. No mass media campaign promotes it. No insurance coverage pays for it. Since it isn't a pill, and nobody has figured out how to get hugely wealthy by showing people how to eat it, the truth has been buried by half-truths, unverified claims, and downright lies. The concerted effort of many powerful interests to ignore, discredit, and hide the truth has worked so far.

WHY THE WFPB DIET MAKES SENSE

I have spent the last few decades studying the effects of the WFPB diet; for me, the diet's results are convincing based solely on the data. But it's still helpful to explore the question of why. Why is the WFPB diet the healthiest way for humans to eat? Based on my training in biochemistry, I have a few conjectures that can be boiled down to one concept: oxidation gone awry.

Oxidation is the process by which atoms and molecules lose electrons as they come into contact with other atoms and molecules; it's one of the most basic chemical reactions in the universe. When you cut an apple and it turns brown in contact with air or when your car fender rusts, you're witnessing oxidation at work. Oxidation happens within our bodies as well. Some of it is natural and good; oxidation facilitates the transfer of energy within the body. Oxidation also gets rid of potentially harmful foreign substances in the body by making them water soluble (and therefore able to be excreted in urine). Excessive uncontrolled oxidation, however, is the enemy of health and longevity in humans, just as excessive oxidation turns your new car into a junker and your apple slice into compost. Oxidation produces something called free radicals, which we know are responsible for encouraging aging, promoting cancer, and rupturing plaques that lead to strokes and heart attacks, among other adverse effects impacting a host of autoimmune and neurologic diseases.

So how might a plant-based diet protect us from the disease-causing effects of free radicals? For one thing, there is some evidence that high-protein diets enhance free radical production, thus encouraging unwanted tissue damage. But it's virtually impossible to eat a high-protein diet if you're consuming mostly whole, plant-based foods. Even if you munched on legumes, beans, and nuts all day, you'd be hard pressed to get more than 12–15 percent or so of your calories from protein.

But there's much more to whole, plant-based foods than the high-protein animal foods they replace. It turns out that plants also produce harmful free radicals—in their case, during photosynthesis. To counteract that free radical production, plants have evolved a defense mechanism: a whole battery of compounds capable of preventing damage by binding to and neutralizing the free radicals. These compounds are known, not particularly poetically, as antioxidants.

When we and other mammals consume plants, we also consume the antioxidants in those plants. And they serve us just as faithfully and effectively as they serve the plants, protecting us from free radicals and slowing down the aging process in our cells. Remarkably, they have no effect on the useful oxidative processes I talked about earlier. They only neutralize the harmful products of excessive oxidation.

It seems reasonable to assume that our bodies never went to the trouble of making antioxidants because they were so readily available in what, for most of our history, was our primary food source: plants. It's only when we shifted to a diet rich in animal-based food and processed food fragments that we tilted the game in favor of oxidation. The excess protein in our diet has promoted excess oxidation, and we no longer consume enough plant-produced antioxidants to contain and neutralize the damage.

It's important to remember, however, that this is just a theory. The most important thing is not *why* the WFPB diet works so much as the fact that it *does* work. The evidence is clear about the WFPB diet's effectiveness—whatever specific reasons there may be.

FREQUENTLY ASKED QUESTIONS

When I lecture publicly, I'm often asked about the numbers. Many people want precise formulas and rules. How many ounces of leafy greens should I eat daily? What proportion of my diet should be fat, protein, or carbohydrate? How much vitamin C and magnesium do I need? Should certain foods be matched with other foods and, if so, in what proportion? And the number one question I'm asked is, "Do I need to eat 100 percent plant-based to obtain the health benefits you talk about?"

If you're asking those questions right now, here's my answer: relax. When it comes to numbers, I am reluctant to be too precise, mostly because (1) we don't yet have scientific evidence that fully answers these questions; (2) virtually nothing in biology is as precise as we try to make it seem; and (3) as far as the evidence suggests at this point, eating the WFPB way eliminates the need to worry about the details. Just eat lots of different plant foods; your body will do all the math for you!

As far as whether one should strive to eat 100 percent plant-based instead of something less—say, 95–98 percent—my answer is that I am not aware of reliable scientific evidence showing that such purity is absolutely necessary, at least in most situations. (Exceptions would include patients with cancer, heart disease, and other potentially fatal ailments, for whom any deviation can lead to worsening or relapse.) I do believe, however, that the closer we get to a WFPB diet, the healthier we will be. I say this not because we have foolproof scientific evidence of this, but because of the effect on our taste buds. When we go the whole way, our taste buds change and remain changed, as we begin to acquire new tastes that are much more compatible with our health. You wouldn't advise a heavy smoker who wants to quit to continue smoking one cigarette per day. It's much easier to go 100 percent than 99 percent, and you're much more likely to succeed in the long run.

I'm also often asked whether I consider the WFPB diet to be vegetarian or vegan. When describing the WFPB diet, I prefer not to use the "V" words. Most vegetarians still consume dairy, eggs, too much added oil, refined carbohydrates, and processed foods. Although vegans eliminate all animal-based foods, they also often continue to consume added fat (including all cooking oils), refined carbohydrates (sugar and refined flour), salt, and processed foods. The phrase *whole food, plant-based* is one I introduced to my colleagues as a member of a National Institutes of Health (NIH) cancer-research grant review panel from 1978 to 1980. Like me, they were reluctant to use the words *vegetarian* and *vegan*, or assign a particular value to the ideology that lies behind much vegetarian and vegan practice. I was interested in describing the remarkable health effects of this diet in reference to the scientific evidence, rather than in reference to personal and philosophical ideologies—however noble they may be.

WHY SHOULD YOU LISTEN TO ME?

Later in this book, I'll share a more personal life and career trajectory, but I do want to recap my research career briefly so you can decide right away whether I have credibility on the subjects I cover here.

For more than fifty years, I have lectured and done experimental research on the complex effects of food and nutrition on health. For approximately forty of those years, I did laboratory experiments with my many students and colleagues. For twenty of those same years, I was a member of expert committees that evaluated and formulated national and international policies on food and health and determined which research ideas should be funded. (Often, my views were in the minority and did not end up having the impact on policy I would have liked—one reason, in fact, that I left academia and started writing "popular" books.) I have published more than 350 research papers, most of which were peer-reviewed, in the very best scientific journals. I have served on the editorial review boards of several top-flight scientific journals. In short, for the last half century I have been deeply immersed in the development of scientific evidence all the way from its experimental origin to the presentation of results in the classroom, food and health policy boardrooms, and the public arena.

WFPB: AN IDEA WHOSE TIME
HAS (ALMOST) COME

In my previous book, *The China Study*, which I coauthored with my son Tom, I shared the research (my own and that of others) that led me to champion the WFPB diet as the optimal human diet. I must admit to some naïveté when that book hit the shelves in early 2005. I was hopeful that the incontrovertible evidence reported in that volume would shake up the American way of eating. I innocently thought that the truth, by itself, could inform government policy, shape business decisions, and change the public debate on food.

To a limited extent, all those things have happened. Some very powerful ex-government officials (including former President Bill Clinton) have touted *The China Study* and plant-based nutrition in general. Progressive and influential companies like Google and Facebook offer many WFPB dishes in their cafeterias. It's much easier to buy WFPB ingredients, meals, and snacks at grocery stores, restaurants, and online outlets than ever before. And the recent "gluten-free" craze (about which the scientific debate is still raging) has pushed many people away from highly processed breads, cookies, and pastas and toward less refined and more natural alternatives.

But the mainstream culture has not embraced plant-based eating. The government still teaches and subsidizes the wrong things. Businesses still cater to the Standard American Diet (aptly abbreviated the "SAD" diet), composed largely of white flour, white sugar, hormone-injected and antibiotic-doused meat and dairy, and artificial colors, flavors, and preservatives. And "low-carb" supporters typically advocate a diet consisting of an unconscionable amount of animal protein and fat. This book is partly my attempt to answer a very troubling question: Why? If the evidence for a WFPB diet is so convincing, why has so little been done? Why do so few people know about it?

Before I share what I believe, based on my decades of work in the nutrition field, are the answers—answers that have implications not only for our food choices and health-care system, but for the vibrancy of our democracy and our future as a species—I want to make sure you are aware of the evidence for the WFPB lifestyle. In the next chapter I'll share that evidence and explain how to evaluate the efficacy of proposed health interventions.

2

The Whole Truth

*History is a race between education and
catastrophe.*

—H. G. WELLS

In the previous chapter I inferred that what we eat can have a bigger impact on our health than just about anything else. The evidence that I and others have amassed over the years points to WFPB as the optimal human diet. I refer you to my last book, *The China Study*, for an in-depth look at the evidence supporting these assertions.

Of course, not everyone in the world believes that a plant-based diet is the best way to eat for our health and for the planet, despite all the evidence. The media is awash with pundits who contradict what I say, often in quite articulate and entertaining ways. The fact is, it's pathetically easy for critics to take individual data points out of context and misapply them to support opposite conclusions from mine. The question is, how can they evaluate the evidence without becoming experts in biochemistry, cardiology, epidemiology, and the dozen other disciplines that would provide the necessary context?

Before we discuss the barriers to more widespread adoption of the WFPB diet, I want to address those critics and those criticisms by sharing with you my model for evaluating diet and health research. My hope is that it will help you make sense of the barrage of nonsense and half-truths that passes not just for legitimate criticism of the WFPB diet, but also for health coverage in the media. Once you're inoculated against "fad of the week" reporting, you'll navigate health claims in general with much more savvy and confidence—and be even better equipped to judge the evidence in favor of the WFPB diet, and criticisms of it, for yourself.

EVALUATING HEALTH RESEARCH

If you watch TV news, you'll see lots of stories each week about promising new drugs, new gene therapies, new high-tech machines, and new health claims about foods, vitamins, enzymes, and other micronutrients. None of these "breakthrough discoveries" come close to the benefits of the WFPB diet, although you wouldn't know it from the hyped-up and ill-informed reporting of the studies upon which these claims are based.

Before I stack up my evidence against theirs, let's talk about how to evaluate research in general. Otherwise we'll be trapped in a "he said, she said" shouting match in which the loudest (or in this case, best-funded) voice wins. When you hear a health claim, ask yourself three questions: Is it true? Is it the whole truth, or just a part of it? Does it matter?

Is it true? The first step in evaluating a health claim is determining whether or not the studies supporting that claim were properly done—in other words, whether they were well-constructed, professionally conducted, and accurately reported enough to uncover some facet of the truth. Unfortunately, some studies are constructed and conducted so poorly that their conclusions are pure nonsense. The likelihood of such a result increases dramatically when the organization funding the research stands to make money from a particular result. Reliable study results are those that, ideally, have been replicated in multiple experiments, preferably by different researchers, and definitely underwritten by different funders.

Is it the whole truth? It's also important to look at what "they" aren't telling you about potential side effects and other unintended consequences of a particular course of action. In nature (and our bodies ideally are products of nature), pretty much everything is connected to everything else. If you have a headache and take a pill, you can be certain that the pill is doing a lot more in your body than just relieving your headache. Likewise, if you're on a WFPB diet to prevent heart disease, that way of eating will have effects that reach far beyond your arteries. When you hear about a wonder pill that lowers blood pressure, always get curious about the additional ("side") effects of the pill. In reality, there are no side effects, just effects. What is this health intervention doing beyond its stated goal?

Does it matter? As we'll see throughout this book, a lot of so-called health breakthroughs are not nearly as impressive as their marketing makes them appear. While it may be good business to spin the numbers to increase sales, it isn't good science. One of the ways to do this (without outright lying) is to cherry-pick details, report them out of context, and imply a much greater significance than they actually possess. For example, a drug may be shown to reduce cholesterol, but to have absolutely no effect on the rate of heart attacks and strokes. Given that the public assumes that lower cholesterol leads to better heart health, the ads for this drug may make a big deal about the drop in cholesterol, and even state accurately that lower cholesterol is typically associated with lower risk of cardiovascular disease. They just conveniently leave out the fact that this particular drug doesn't seem to lead to that same lower risk. The drug's ability to reduce cholesterol doesn't really matter, at least when it comes to its users' length and quality of life.

Realistically, you need to have a working knowledge of the scientific method to assess a health claim according to the first two tests (is it true and is it the whole truth?), along with access to the details of how the study was constructed. If you're not a scientist, however, don't despair. If you're looking at a drug ad in a magazine, you can just turn the page to read the voluminous fine print about its side effects and warnings. Or you can consult peer-reviewed journals. Peer review is a process in which research findings are reviewed and critiqued by qualified professionals before publication. This strategy affords the scientific community an opportunity to challenge study results in a way that is open to professional and public scrutiny—it is a chance to replicate and verify research observations or to demonstrate that the findings are false. This may not be a perfect system, but I know of nothing better. At a minimum, it encourages objectivity and integrity. And it provides readers of peer-reviewed journals with a level of confidence about the findings published in its pages.

However, when it comes to the third question—whether a new health claim's implications matter—that's something just about everyone can evaluate for themselves. It just requires a little common sense.

HOW TO TELL IF A HEALTH INTERVENTION MATTERS

When I think about whether a health intervention matters—in other words, whether it is worth pursuing for an individual, business, or researcher—I use three basic criteria, listed here in reverse order of importance:

- How quickly does it work? (Rapidity)
- How many health problems does it help solve? (Breadth)
- How much will my health improve due to the intervention? (Depth)

Let's look at each of these in turn.

Rapidity

How long does it take for a nutrient, drug, genetic modification, or whatever to actually function within the body? I'm not talking about how long it takes for a substance to be absorbed in the bloodstream and transported to tissue cells. Instead, I'm asking, "How long before there's a meaningful effect, like an energy boost or reduction of disease symptoms?"

The speed at which most nutritional benefits appear when switching to a WFPB diet is jaw-dropping. Diabetics must be monitored from the very first day they adopt the diet, so their meds can be reduced as the diet takes effect. Otherwise, they're in real danger of having their blood sugar drop low enough to send them into hypoglycemic shock.

Nonnutritious food also works really quickly, but in the opposite direction. Within one to four hours of consuming, for example, a high-fat McDonald's meal (Egg McMuffin®, Sausage McMuffin®, two hash brown patties, non-caffeinated beverage), serum triglycerides shoot up (increasing the risk of heart disease and diabetes, as well as many other conditions) and arteries stiffen (raising blood pressure). Recovery to normal fluidity takes several hours. None of this occurs following a low-fat meal consisting of cereal and fruit.[1]

When my friend and colleague, Caldwell Esselstyn, Jr., MD, used a mostly WFPB diet to reverse advanced heart disease in a study that began in 1985, he found that chronic chest pain (also known as angina) typically disappeared within one to two weeks. Compare that to an angina drug such as ranolazine (marketed under the trade name Ranexa), which was approved by the Food and Drug Administration (FDA) in 2006.[2] One clinical trial undertaken to establish its effectiveness randomly assigned 565 patients to a Ranexa group or a placebo group. The Ranexa group experienced a "statistically significant reduction" in angina episodes over six weeks. Sounds great, right? What it means is that the Ranexa group went from 4.5 to 3.5 angina episodes per week. Not exactly the speedy solution anyone really wants, is it? Add to that the common side effects reported by the manufacturer, including "dizziness, head-ache, constipation, and nausea" (the study didn't say how rapidly those showed up), and you have Western medicine's best answer to a WFPB diet: expensive interventions with limited positive effect and a host of potential side effects.

Some may think it's unfair to compare pharmaceuticals to WFPB, since the drugs are meant to treat symptoms rather than root causes of disease. But if there is one thing these prescription meds *should* have going for them, it is rapidity of effect. Indeed, the one useful function they can perform is "buying time" for a patient for whom a lifestyle and dietary intervention otherwise might be too late. When someone is wheeled into the ER after suffering a heart attack or stroke, it's a better idea to administer a thrombolytic drug to dissolve the blood clot than to give them an intravenous kale smoothie. But aside from true emergencies, the rapidity of response of WFPB is superior to any drug—without the negative side effects.

Breadth

How widespread are the intervention's effects throughout the body? Does the intervention improve a wide range of functions, or just one specific measure of biological functioning, like blood pressure or lipid profile? You might think that a one-size-fits-all approach, where one strategy could resolve a wide variety of medical conditions, would be exactly what the doctor ordered. But medical science is deeply suspicious of anything claiming to be a panacea (from the Greek words *pan*, meaning "all," and *akos*, meaning "remedy").

In contrast, the most highly prized Chinese medicines are the ones that treat the widest variety of ailments. In the early 1980s, senior medical people in China introduced me to their centuries-old tradition of using herbs medicinally. Often, these herbs are used in their whole form, typically steeped in water and often as one of several ingredients. The "king" of these Chinese herbs, the one most prescribed and consumed, is ginseng. Carl Linnaeus, who pioneered the scientific system for naming plants and animals, dubbed ginseng "Panax" based on his awareness of the plant's multiple uses in traditional Chinese medicine.

Remember Daniel Boone, that famed American frontiersman? Do you know what he was doing out there in the wilderness with his coonskin cap and rifle? Hunting and trapping, right? Sure, Boone did his share of harvesting animal parts. But when he faced financial ruin because of some bad real estate deals in the 1780s, he went where the money was: American ginseng (scientific name *Panax quinquefolius*). Boone paid Native Americans to harvest the roots, which he shipped to China for a fortune. He wasn't the only one making money on the herb; we know that John Jacob Astor earned $55,000 for his first shipment of ginseng to China, equivalent to more than $1 million today.

The reason the Chinese were willing to pay so much for ginseng, and why the Native Americans knew exactly where to harvest it, is because the plant works to promote health in so many different ways. The Cherokee used ginseng to ease colic, convulsions, dysentery, and headaches. Other Native American tribes found the roots helpful in treating indigestion, weak appetite, exhaustion, croup, menstrual cramps, and shock.[3] Now that's breadth!

The WFPB diet deals with so many diseases and conditions that you begin to wonder if there isn't just one basic disease cause—poor nutrition—that manifests through thousands of different symptoms. Rather than focus on the underlying cause, Western medicine has decided to focus on the individual symptoms and call each of them a disease. And admittedly, it's good business to identify thousands of different diseases, then make and sell treatments for each of them, rather than to look at the big picture and prescribe one simple intervention that helps them all. But it's not good medicine.

If you're impressed with the range of effects of the ginseng root alone, you'll be blown away by the breadth of results from a WFPB diet. While ginseng can relieve a wide variety of symptoms, good nutrition deals with the root causes of disease—including those as different as cancer, cardiovascular disease (e.g., cardiac arrest, stroke, and atherosclerosis), obesity, neurological disorders, diabetes, a wide variety of autoimmune diseases, and bone diseases. Since *The China Study*'s publication, I have heard from readers about other illnesses, mostly nonfatal, that have also been alleviated or resolved by a WFPB diet—illnesses like headaches (including migraines), intestinal distresses, eye and ear disorders, stress disorders, colds and flu, acne, erectile dysfunction, and chronic pain. This is an exceptionally broad scope of nutritionally controlled diseases, although for each of these diseases or disease groups, more professional research would be helpful to document mechanisms for these effects. My impressions of the impact of this diet on a few of these illnesses (e.g., colds and flu, headaches, various aches and chronic pain conditions) are based more on anecdotal evidence than on empirical, peer-reviewed, and published evidence. Still, the number of times I've heard individuals and physicians say that adopting a WFPB diet simultaneously resolves these health problems has begun to convince me that it works for the vast majority of people most of the time. In earlier years I had my own problem with migraine headaches and arthritic-type pain. These problems disappeared when I fully adopted the WFPB diet.

Let's try a thought experiment. Someone you care about tells you they have a chronic disease (take your pick from the list above) and their doctor gave them a choice of two treatments. Treatment #1 would slightly reduce the severity of a single symptom of that disease, but would not improve their chances of being cured of it (or even living longer), and would threaten a wide array of nasty side effects. (Of course, their doctor would prescribe additional meds to deal with those side effects, and then still more meds to deal with the side effects of all the interactions of the other meds, and so on.)

Treatment #2 would typically resolve the root cause of the disease fairly quickly, thus ending all symptoms and increasing their life expectancy and the quality of that life. Side effects would include achieving their ideal weight, having more energy, looking and feeling better, and even helping to preserve the environment and slow global warming.

Which treatment would you suggest to them?

To the medical establishment this thought experiment is totally nonsensical. The vast majority of medical research looks only at the very specific effects of one element (whether a drug, vitamin, mineral, or procedure such as an operation) on a single symptom or system. Anything else—such as looking at macro differences like lifestyle and diet—is just considered too messy to be reliable.

Depth

Okay, so far we've looked at how quickly nutrition affects bodily functioning (rapidity) and how many systems it influences (breadth). There's one last crucial factor in evaluating the power of a health intervention: the size, or significance, of the effect. Another word for this is *profundity*. All things being equal, would you rather undergo a therapy that made a slight improvement to your well-being, or an enormous one?

Plant-based nutrition tends to elicit enormous effect sizes. I first saw this in a set of experiments in India that I read about and then replicated with my graduate students at Cornell, in which researchers exposed laboratory animals (rats) to a powerful carcinogen (cancer-causing agent), then fed one group a diet of 20 percent animal protein and the other a diet of 5 percent animal protein. Every single animal in the 20 percent group developed cancer or cancer precursor lesions, while not one of the 5 percenters did. One hundred percent to zero percent. That kind of result is rarely seen in biological studies that have so many confounding variables. Yet that's what we found. We repeated this experiment in several different ways because it was hard to believe at first, but that result held, experiment after experiment. You don't get more profound than that.

Maybe you're thinking, *Hold on. Just because diet has this kind of effect on rat cancer doesn't mean it can improve human health on the same scale.* Animal studies are one thing. What about a study that looked at really sick people and changed their diet drastically? Could a nutritional intervention produce as profound an effect?

Two cardiologists, Lester Morrison and John Gofman, undertook studies in the 1940s and 1950s (almost 70 years ago!) to determine the effect of diet on heart disease in people who had already had a heart attack.[4] The doctors put these patients on a diet with less fat, cholesterol, and animal-based foods—a regimen that dramatically reduced subsequent recurrence of heart disease. Nathan Pritikin did the same thing in the 1960s and 1970s.[5] Then Drs. Esselstyn[6] and Dean Ornish[7] set out to learn more in the 1980s and 1990s. Working separately, they both showed that a plant-based, high-carbohydrate diet controlled and even reversed advanced heart disease. We touched on Esselstyn's remarkable study in the section on rapidity above, and you can read more about his and all these researchers' work in *The China Study*. But let's talk a little more now about Esselstyn's findings in terms of depth of effect.

ESSELSTYN'S HEART DISEASE REVERSAL STUDY

In 1985, Esselstyn recruited patients with advanced but not immediately life-threatening heart disease for a clinical trial to explore whether heart disease might be reversed using diet.[8] He confirmed the severity of the coronary artery disease with angiograms to be sure that their disease progression was advanced. The only other requirement for admission into the study was a willingness to attempt the dietary changes he proposed: effectively, a WFPB diet.

Dr. Esselstyn formally reported his findings at five and twelve years.[9] In the eight years prior to the study, his eighteen subjects had had forty-nine coronary episodes (e.g., heart attacks, angioplasty, bypass surgery), but during the twelve years after adopting a WFPB diet, there was only one event, involving a patient who strayed from his diet. He has casually followed his subjects since then, and all but five are still alive today, twenty-six years later. The five who passed away did not die of cardiac failure, but from other causes. (The average age of his subjects in 1985 was 56; someone who was 56 in 1985 would be 83 in 2012, so that's really not unexpected.) And the ones who are still alive are cardiac symptom free. The subjects had forty-nine cardiovascular events in the ninety-six months prior to the intervention, and zero cardiovascular events in the roughly 312 months since the intervention began. This life-and-death finding is about as profound as any health benefit I have ever known. Nothing else in medicine comes close.

Compare these findings to the drug Ranexa, which we looked at earlier in this chapter, in terms of reducing deaths from heart disease and other causes. A giant follow-up study of 6,500 Ranexa patients found a few trivial improvements in certain numbers, but the overall verdict, as reported in the *Journal of the American Medical Association*, was: "No difference in total mortality was observed with ranolazine compared with placebo."[10]

STATISTICAL SIGNIFICANCE VERSUS MEANINGFUL SIGNIFICANCE

The depth of an effect is important not just to the person who experiences that effect. The depth of effect you expect to see in an experimental study determines the number of subjects you need for that study in order to assess with any degree of confidence whether the results are real or just a meaningless blip. In other words, the smaller the difference between two conditions (say, experiment and control group, or Treatment A and Treatment B), the more experimental subjects you need in order to show that the difference is real, and not simply due to chance. In a case like Ranexa, where episodes of angina were reduced from 4.5 to 3.5 per week, you'd need several hundred study participants to show that the result is unlikely to have occurred randomly—or, in scientific jargon, to be "statistically significant."

You may be wondering about the size of Esselstyn's study, since his experimental group was so small. Is eighteen a large enough sample size to prove statistical significance? To answer that question, let's imagine a different outcome to the experiment above. Let's say Group B, the control group, still gets four to five attacks per week on average. Group A, the group getting the new treatment, gets no more attacks at all. None. Zero. Hundreds of data points are no longer required when the effect is so large. The likelihood that such profound, consistent results are the result of chance is nearly zero.[11]

When you spend time poring through scientific research, you come across the concept of statistical significance a lot. The concept is very useful; it prevents people from drawing conclusions based on not enough data. If you flip a coin once and it lands heads, for example, you can't announce that it's a fixed coin that will always land on heads. You can't distinguish a pattern from the noise of randomness inherent in coin tosses from a single toss, or even five or six. The problem is, many researchers worship statistical significance at the expense of something equally important: actual significance, as in, "Who cares? Why does this result matter?" Are we really that excited about reducing angina attacks from 4.5 to 3.5 per week? Not to minimize the suffering of patients with heart disease, but shouldn't we spend our time and money seeking and evaluating treatments that significantly improve lives, as opposed to just maintaining and managing a disease state?

TOWARD A BETTER HEALTH SOLUTION

Given the evidence I've shared with you in this chapter, you would think that the top med schools in the country would make plant-based nutrition the premier "medical" science of the future. The majority of medical school training and NIH funding should be for training and research in nutrition to discover the best ways to counsel patients to improve their diets and create environments where eating well is easier than eating poorly. Nothing of the sort is happening.

Sure, healthy eating (a purposefully vague term that means nothing in the public discussion) is given lip service by the medical establishment. But that establishment doesn't really take diet seriously as the first and primary means of treating and preventing disease. The importance of eating a diet of whole, plant-based foods (especially high-antioxidant, high-fiber vegetables) has really only been accepted by the alternative, preventive medicine community, while within the medical establishment, the idea that nutrition might impact diseases as serious as cancer is considered just plain "wacko"—despite the fact that almost none of those professionals who systematically reject nutrition's potential have any training in this field.

Research shows this way of eating is actually our best means of treating disease. Better than prescription drugs. Better than surgery. Better than anything the current medical establishment has in its arsenal in the various "wars" on cancer, stroke, heart disease, MS, and so forth. Perhaps it's time to stop declaring war on ourselves through toxic drugs and dangerous surgeries, and instead treat ourselves with kindness by feeding ourselves the sorts of foods shown to grow and sustain healthy, vibrant people and cultures.

We need a new way of relating to words like *health* and *medicine*. Health is more than a few superficial expressions like "eat a good diet" or "use alcohol in moderation" or "use the stairs, not the elevator." Of course, there is merit in these statements, but for the most part they dismiss the possibility of real change. They are politically correct statements lacking specificity and substance.

Instead of feel-good pabulum that accomplishes nothing, we need to make nutrition the central element of our health-care system. Furthermore, we must get away from the "diet" mentality that promotes heroic and unsustainable spurts of healthy eating. Instead of "dieting," we must change our lifestyle to include a diet that promotes health. People who adopt a WFPB diet find that most of their health problems were caused or significantly worsened by their old diets and resolve naturally and quickly once the body starts getting the proper fuel. It's like someone who hits their head with a hammer three times a day and finds that nothing cures their headaches. It just makes sense to put down the hammer!

I naïvely believed that everyone in the research and medical communities would be able to see the common sense wisdom in this approach once they saw the findings I had. But when I began to state my conviction that nutrition should be the centerpiece of our medical system, I saw how wrong I was. One of the most eye-opening phenomena has been the ferocity with which I've been attacked for sharing my research findings and their implications—sometimes even by fellow medical practice and research professionals.

As foolish as it appears to me now, I had no idea when I started on this path that the ideas in this chapter would brand me as a heretic and threaten my funding and career. Fortunately for me, those effects have proved to be far more unsuccessful than successful. But before we jump into the big issues driving those attacks, I'd like to share my heretical path with you. After all, I've had a fifty-year head start on some of these ideas. Let's bring you up to date before we jump into the fray.

3

My Heretical Path

*When we live in a system, we absorb a system and
think in a system.*

—JAMES W. DOUGLASS

When I began my research career in nutritional science, I was naïve
to a fault. My childhood environment of hay fields and milking
barns did not prepare me for the dark side of "science" as it is currently done: the greed, the small-mindedness, and the outright dishonesty
and cynicism of some of its practitioners. Not to mention the shocking
examples of how public officials closed their eyes to important findings
that got in the way of their reelection.

I entered the academy eager to participate in my idealized version of
scientific inquiry. I couldn't imagine anything better: learning new things,
choosing which questions to research, then sharing and debating ideas
with students and colleagues. I loved the transparency and integrity of the
scientific method—how personal opinions and biases faded away before
the majesty of real evidence. How a well-conceived experiment was like
setting the table beautifully and inviting Truth to dinner. How honest
questioning could banish ignorance and create a better world.

What I discovered is that science was, is, and can be just like that—as long as the researcher is careful not to pursue politically incorrect ideas outside the boundaries of "normal" science. You can wonder and ask and research anything you like, until you cross the line defined by prejudice and reinforced by the moneyed interests that fund almost all science.

Normal science. That's a strange phrase, isn't it? Normal science means anything that doesn't challenge the prevailing paradigm—the agreed-upon story of how the world is. "Normal" doesn't mean "good" or "better" in any way; it just means that the researcher has refrained from asking questions whose answers are considered already known and no longer subject to debate. For much of my career I've found myself bumping up against the invisible boundaries of the scientific paradigm. In the last few decades, I finally decided to blast through them altogether. That's how I know so much about those boundaries: sometimes you have to cross the line to find out where it is.

One of the most devilish things about paradigms is that they're almost impossible to perceive from the inside. A paradigm can be so all-encompassing that it simply looks like all there is. For example, let's look at an obsolete paradigm that reigned for hundreds of years: the idea that the sun revolved around the earth, and not the other way around. You can't blame people for believing that the earth was the center of the universe; when you go outside, you see the earth standing still while the sun, moon, planets, and stars move across the sky. When Copernicus published *De Revolutionibus* in 1543, asserting that the earth rotated around the sun, he was challenging common sense, a millennium of scientific agreement, and an outraged religious community. The fact that he had evidence—that his theory in fact explained phenomena that were unexplainable under the prevailing earth-centric theory—didn't matter one bit. As philosopher-songwriter Paul Simon put it, "A man hears what he wants to hear and disregards the rest."

I'm not trying to compare myself to Copernicus. His story is just a well-known example of an obsolete paradigm standing in the way of progress and the discovery of truth. In a perfect world (the one I believed in when I began my research career), the scientific method would simply compost inadequate paradigms when the evidence showed their limitations. But people who have built their careers upon these paradigms can act like threatened dictators; they cling to power at all costs, and the more they are challenged, the nastier and more dangerous they become. (This is doubly true when the paradigm supports powerful moneyed interests—but we'll get to that shortly.)

Once I stepped outside the prevailing nutritional paradigm, I discovered something exhilarating: you can learn a lot about the inside of a paradigm from the outside. Think of a fish swimming in the ocean, blissfully unaware of other environments. Once she is caught in a net, hoisted in the air, and then dropped on the deck of a ship, she has no choice but to confront the inadequacy of her old belief that the entire world was water. Suppose she wriggles free of the net and flops back into the water. How can she describe what she has seen to her fellows? What would be their likely reaction, if they were anything like us? "Poor Dori has gone mad. She's babbling and making up lies." What's happened, of course, is that Dori now sees the ocean for what it is: one environment among many. She realizes that it has boundaries, and understands some of the properties of this element called "water." Because she has experienced dry air, she now perceives water as wet and cold. She now knows that water has a certain feel, and responds to tail and fin movements in a particular way that isn't universal. There are other truths out there, and Dori can now place the ocean within that larger context.

My journey "out of the water" has led me to be branded a heretic by many of my colleagues. Unlike Dori, I wasn't thrown out of the paradigm; I just kept swimming in a direction that led me closer and closer to shore until eventually I reached dry land. My heretical path through the research world has been a result of my curiosity about and dogged pursuit of "outlier observations." An outlier is a piece of data that doesn't fit with the rest of the observed results. It's a weird blip, an anomaly, something out of place—an unusual outcome that, if we're honest with ourselves about it, can call into question the integrity of our current understanding.

Often, outlier observations are simply mistakes. The scale was broken. Two test tubes were accidentally switched. That sort of thing. Sometimes outlier observations are the result of deliberate fraud, perpetrated by researchers seeking to make a name (or a fortune) for themselves. So science is rightly skeptical of data that seems to contradict prevailing wisdom. After all, we don't want our understanding of the universe to lurch and sway with every random measurement.

The scientific method, at its best, looks at outliers and says, "Prove it! Show us that wasn't a fluke, a mistake, or a lie." In other words, reproduce that result under laboratory conditions. Describe the experiment in enough detail that others can repeat it and see if they get the same outlier result. If an outlier can withstand that kind of scrutiny, it's supposed to get folded into our knowledge base and change our paradigm.

Unfortunately, scientists are human and don't always represent the very best of the scientific method. When a finding threatens the validity of their life's work, they can become irrationally defensive. And when new evidence threatens their funding, they can get downright nasty. You can tell when this happens because they stop arguing about the evidence and start slinging epithets.

My first step onto the path of heresy occurred when I discovered an outlier observation that called into question one of the most deeply held beliefs in nutrition: the notion that animal protein is good for us.

THE COW AND I

Coming from a dairy farm, I thought my contribution to humanity's well-being would be to figure out how to get more protein from farm animals. After all, millions of people around the world suffer from malnutrition, and one of the principal nutritional problems was protein deficiency. If we could make milk and meat cheaper and more plentiful, we could alleviate untold suffering. As a popular folk song written in 1947 put it, "If each little kid could have fresh milk each day, if each working man had enough time to play, if each homeless soul had a good place to stay, it could be a wonderful world." Fresh milk was right up there with a humane work week and ending homelessness! What could be more noble?

The topic was perfect for me. My entire childhood had been about milking cows and sharing the goodness with our customers. My background in veterinary medicine, biochemistry, and nutrition gave me knowledge and insights I could use to manipulate animal feeds to improve the human food supply. And the beef and dairy industries were—and still are—very generous with grant money to further such research. It would have been hard to find anyone less likely than me to throw all that away when confronted with evidence that animal protein was actually harmful to humans.

What did me in, as I look back, was my insatiable curiosity when it came to outlier observations. I believed that my job was to discover the truth, wherever it led. And my research into protein led me, step by step, to a realization that the entire modern scientific paradigm was badly flawed.

PROTEIN, THE (NOT SO) PERFECT NUTRIENT

My slippery slope to heresy began with that puzzling, even alarming observation I made in the late 1970s, which you'll recall from the introduction: the children in the Philippines who ate the most protein were the ones most likely to get liver cancer. That finding was so strange, and so counter to everything I believed and thought I knew, that I immediately searched the scientific literature to see if anyone else had ever seen such a connection between protein and cancer.

Someone had. A group of Indian researchers had conducted a "gold standard" clinical trial, the kind that isolates one variable and performs a controlled experiment on it.[1] The researchers had fed aflatoxin, a powerful carcinogen, to two groups of rats. One group was fed a 20 percent animal protein (casein) diet. The other group was protein deprived, ingesting only 5 percent of their calories from casein. The results? Every single 20 percent protein rat developed liver cancer or cancer precursor lesions. Not a single 5 percent protein rat did. (You may recall this study from chapter two's discussion of depth of effect.)

Looking back, the wise career move would have been to imbibe several stiff drinks, go to bed, and never think about it again. Tackling such a controversial topic so early in my career was a lot more dangerous than I knew. And despite my growing awareness that the actual practice of science was not all about the selfless discovery of truth, I was still naïve enough to think that the world might appreciate (and reward) information that could eradicate the scourge of cancer.

I will say that I proceeded cautiously, and so managed to fly under the radar of potential critics for many years. I set up research labs, first at Virginia Tech, then for many more years at Cornell, to investigate the role of nutrition in preventing or causing cancer. We conducted very conservative experiments that looked at the biochemistry of proteins, enzymes, and cancerous cells, the sort of beaker-and-test-tube, high-powered microscope science that grant reviewers and journal editors like. Except our group of mad scientists was slowly proving, beyond any doubt, that not just excess dietary protein, but a particular *type* of excess dietary protein, promoted cancer formation and growth. And these results, seen in our experiments with rats, were consistent with human population and case-control studies that showed impressive associations between animal-based protein consumption and cancer rates.

When I say "protein," what foods do you think of? Probably not spinach and kale, although those plants have about twice as much protein, per calorie, as a lean cut of beef. No, to most of us in the United States, protein means meat, milk, and eggs. Our love affair with protein has been around for a long time. The word *protein* gives us a clue as to how deeply we revere our protein: its Greek root, *proteios*, means "of prime importance." And the "really good kind" of protein has long been the kind found in animal-based foods. Shortly after protein was discovered by Gerardus Mulder in 1839,[2] a famous chemist, Justus von Liebig, then went on to exclaim that animal-based ("high quality") protein "was the stuff of life itself." The high-quality label even made sense from a biochemical perspective—our bodies, themselves made up of animal protein, can metabolize animal protein much more efficiently than they can plant protein.

So imagine our shock when animal protein, but not vegetable protein, was the culprit in turning on cancer in our studies. The most significant carcinogen, the substance that almost invariably led to cancer at 20 percent of the rats' diet, was casein, or milk protein. Plant proteins, such as those from wheat and soy, had no effect on cancer development, even at high levels.[3]

In fact, in 1983, my Cornell University research group showed that we could switch early cancer growth on and off in rats simply by changing the amount of protein they consumed. Equally amazing, when cancer was switched off for a relatively long time by feeding a low-protein diet, it could be turned on again by switching to a high-protein diet.[4] The effect was striking. When turned on, cancer growth was vigorous and robust. When turned off, it was totally shut down. Major changes in cancer development, both positive and negative, were triggered by only modest changes in protein intake.

Boy, did we have outlier research on our hands! Part of the significance of our findings was the relatively low animal protein levels needed to trigger cancer. Most carcinogen studies (for example, the ones on food dyes and nitrates in hot dogs and environmental toxins like dioxin) dose the lab animals with hundreds or thousands of times the amount they would ever encounter in nature. The extremely powerful carcinogenic effect we saw was occurring at levels of animal protein that humans routinely consumed, and were encouraged to consume.

At this point I knew we had a provocative finding on our hands. We needed airtight experimental design, rigorous documentation, and as much transparency as we could provide to back up the protein–cancer connection. We approached our continuing research from different perspectives and published our results in the most critical peer-reviewed scientific research journals. We had to do our studies very carefully according to the accepted criteria for research in order to survive and secure the necessary but very competitive funding.

Because we followed those research criteria so rigorously, we were able to get funding despite the incendiary nature of the topic. We received funding from the National Institutes of Health (NIH) for twenty-seven years in a row, money that allowed us to learn an incredible amount about the nature of animal protein and its biochemical effects within the body. We learned how protein, once consumed, works within the cell to turn on the cancer process. As with the similar Indian research on rats, our results were lopsidedly convincing. Something quite dramatic and provocative was going on.

During these early days of our research, I was invited to give a lecture at the Fels Institute of the Temple University School of Medicine by Peter Magee, the editor in chief of the leading journal in the field of oncology research, *Cancer Research*. At dinner after my lecture, I told him of a new experiment that we were planning, one that might prove to be quite provocative. I wanted to compare this remarkable protein effect on cancer growth with the well-accepted effect produced by a really potent chemical carcinogen. I told him that I suspected that the animal protein effect would be of far more concern. He was highly skeptical, as the editor of a prestigious journal should be. When a scientific paradigm comes under attack, the burden of proof falls squarely and rightfully at the feet of the attacker.

Part of our current paradigm is that bad stuff in the environment causes cancer, and the more enlightened elements involved in the war on cancer seek to reduce our exposure to that bad stuff. *Not* part of our current paradigm is that the food we eat is a much more powerful determinant of cancer than just about any environmental toxin. And I suggested that a relatively modest change in nutrient consumption might be even more relevant for cancer development than consuming a potent carcinogen. I asked the journal's editor whether he would consider highlighting our findings on the cover of his prestigious journal if we actually got such results. To his credit, he agreed to consider it despite his well-entrenched skepticism. He "knew," as did almost all cancer specialists back then, that cancer occurs because of chemical carcinogens and viruses and genes, not because of modest changes in nutrient consumption. But he agreed that if I could prove my heretical statement to his satisfaction, he would accept the findings and publish our research.

When we actually did these new experiments, it supported our previous findings even more clearly than I had expected.[5] Animal protein intake determined cancer development far more than the dose of the chemical carcinogen. But my hope for having these exciting results featured on the cover of our association's journal was dashed. My editor in chief colleague was now retired, and his replacement and the Editorial Review Board were changing policy. They were inclined to dismiss nutritional effects on cancer. Instead, they referred manuscripts on the connection between cancer and nutrition to a new, untested journal, *Cancer Epidemiology, Biomarkers & Prevention*, a good way of relegating such nutrition-related research to second-class status. They wanted papers that were more "intellectually stimulating"—ones with aims like figuring out how cancer works in molecular terms, especially if the answer concerned chemicals and genes and viruses. They considered investigating nutritional effects on cancer growth, as we were doing, to be almost akin to nonscience.

At about this same time, when we had even more convincing evidence of this remarkable protein effect, I gave a keynote presentation at the World Congress of Nutrition in Seoul, South Korea. A good-sized audience of researchers was in attendance, and during a question-and-answer period, a former colleague of mine in the audience—and a well-known advocate for consuming more, not less, protein—arose and lamented, "Colin, you're talking about good food! Don't take it away from us!" He did not question the validity of our research results; he was concerned that I was trying to undermine his personal love for animal protein.

I knew then that our research was becoming a lightning rod for people's strong feelings about their food habits. Even rational, data-driven scientists could be sent into prolonged states of hysteria when presented with evidence that their favorite foods might be killing them. Talk about hitting a sensitive nerve! The sad part of this story is that my questioner has since traveled to greener pastures, at an age much too young. He suffered from a kind of heart problem that is promoted by animal-based protein.

Our research continued to pose a series of very provocative heresies focusing on the idea that so-called high-quality protein might not be as high in quality as always thought. Associating a valued nutrient like protein with increased growth of a feared disease like cancer was heresy squared. Our most revered nutrient promoted our most feared disease. (Other heresies to come!)

THE CANCER MINEFIELD

During the late 1980s, I accepted an invitation to give a Grand Rounds lecture to the McGill Faculty of Medicine in Montreal, the top-ranked medical education program in Canada. Because it was before the publication of the results of our nationwide study in China (the one I discuss in depth in *The China Study*), I spoke only of the potential relationship between cancer and imbalanced nutrition, based on our own findings on protein, along with a few observations of other research groups. I showed in some detail the remarkable results that we were getting on cancer reversal when dietary protein was decreased. I went on to speculate about someday using a nutritional strategy to treat cancer in humans. I could say no more than that, however, because at that time, I did not know what specific strategy might be used.

Later that evening, I was taken to dinner by the chairs of the Big Three departments involved in cancer treatment: surgery, chemotherapy, and radiotherapy. During our conversation, Surgery Chair asked me what I meant by my remark on the possibility of nutrition affecting cancer development after patients had learned of their cancer. I pointed out that we had enough preliminary evidence to justify the testing of this hypothesis. We had a lot more evidence than is generally available for risky commercial treatments, such as new forms of chemotherapy and radiotherapy. Really, it was no comparison. Potential upside of nutritional therapy: turning off cancer development completely. Likelihood based on experimental data: very high. Potential downside of nutritional therapy from a health perspective: none. We all know about the side effects of chemo and radiation, as well as their far-from-stellar success rates. Surely it made sense to give nutrition a try?

Surgery Chair quickly responded to say that he would never allow any of his patients to try a nutritional approach as a substitute for the surgery that he knew well. He went on to give as an example: the superior ability of surgery to treat breast cancer. But Chemotherapy Chair took issue with Surgery Chair's opinion, saying that chemotherapy was more effective than surgery. While Surgery Chair on my left was contesting Chemotherapy Chair on my right, Radiotherapy Chair, sitting across the table from me, found fault with the opinions of both of his colleagues. On the case under discussion, he insisted, radiotherapy could offer the best treatment. I was in no position to know who might have the better argument and merely listened. Looking back, it was really quite funny, except when you consider all the death and suffering these attitudes have caused.

At the time, I took note of three interesting things. First, these medical luminaries could not agree on which treatment—surgery, chemotherapy, or radiotherapy—was best for treating breast cancer. Second, they had no tolerance for nutritional therapy, because according to them, and me at that time, it hadn't yet been shown to be effective for humans. Third and far more important, they clearly had no interest even in discussing ways in which research might be conducted to explore the possibility of using nutrition as a means of treatment. Now, more than twenty years later, the discussion remains the same. It was clear that there was a serious disconnect between these gentlemen and me as to what the emerging evidence of nutrition on cancer was showing. The majority of oncologists still worship one of the three "traditional" treatments and have no patience for or understanding of nutritional treatment options.

I since have presented two recent talks, one to an audience of cancer researchers and specialists in Chicago sponsored by two highly reputable medical schools, and the other to a U.S. National Cancer Institute venue in Sacramento, California, in which I recalled this twenty-year-old story.

I did so simply to make that point that while the clock is still ticking, the conversation is barely shifting. If it isn't a new surgery, chemo cocktail, or radiation protocol, the cancer industry isn't buying.

HERESIES AND MORE HERESIES

I don't mean to say that everyone who disagrees with me is some sort of dogmatic, narrow-minded caveman. I'm a scientist, and I expect (and hope) that my findings will be challenged by other researchers. Given the importance of what I believe I and others have discovered, it's critical that we put it to the test to make sure it's correct, and that it's not the result of sloppily and poorly executed studies. I welcome those who critique my statistical methods. I'm thrilled when someone attempts to replicate one of my findings, even if their goal is to prove me wrong. Over the years, many of my critics have been responsible for pointing out the next phase of my research, or helping me tighten up a study design, or helping me imagine new ways to approach a thorny issue. That's the scientific method at its best: all of us competing not for personal glory and wealth, but to serve the highest truth and the highest good.

The attacks on and dismissals of my findings are more than the normal scientific discovery process, however. The real issue in many cases is that I am asking questions that threaten the reigning research and medical paradigms. The questions I and others have asked over the years have produced answers that are outside the rigid mental boundaries that small-minded science enforces.

We've discovered that cow's milk protein at reasonable levels of intake markedly promotes experimental cancer growth, which is outside of the nutrition paradigm.

We've discovered that experimental cancer growth can be turned on and off by altering practical levels of nutrient intake, and can be treated by nutritional means, which is outside of the cancer treatment paradigm.

We've observed that these effects are driven by multiple mechanisms acting in concert, which is outside of the medical paradigm.

We've found that cancer growth is controlled far more by nutrition than by genes, which is outside of the scientific paradigm.

We've shown that the nutrient composition of foods is more a determinant of cancer occurrence than chemical carcinogens, which is outside of the cancer-testing and regulatory agency paradigms.

We've found that saturated fat (and, for that matter, total fat and cholesterol) is not the chief cause of heart disease (there's animal-based proteins as well), which is outside of the cardiology paradigm.

I could go on and on. I'm just thankful I don't live in a past era, when heretics were sentenced to house arrest or burned at the stake for their views!

These findings may not be that striking to readers outside of the world of scientific research, but be assured that they clearly are unexpected, even unbelievable phenomena (heresies?) for virtually anyone inside the medical research community. Most of these findings—and many more that I could cite—arose partly by luck, but after making that first unlikely observation (high casein "causing" cancer growth), I became more and more aware that I had strayed beyond the paradigm of normal science.

Once I had tasted the forbidden fruit, I was hooked. Having accidentally strayed from the straight and narrow, I was becoming more and more curious about what else might be hiding in plain sight outside of the existing paradigms. I then began to see, through my public policy work, why paradigms exist and how they function. I especially became aware that the ideas inside of a paradigm are often strikingly opposed to ideas outside of it, thus making the boundaries clearer.

You may be thinking that all this talk about what's inside and what's outside of paradigms seems abstract and even academic. Why does this argument really matter? Actually, deciding whether an observation is or is not heretical has real consequences. In the medical research world, unexpected observations are oftentimes ignored. Researchers dismiss them, saying something like, "That can't be right." Such observations therefore may never see the light of day (or come to rest on the page of a professional publication). In reality, they might be gems, either pointing out flaws in what we consider to be normal or suggesting a new dimension to our thinking.

Much philosophy has been written through the ages on the research done to discover elusive truths. We make rules to guide our thinking, but we fail to see that these same rules, although helpful in articulating and sharing our current understanding of the world—within science and elsewhere—also may be constraining. We formulate hypotheses, then create or search for evidence to "prove" them.

Another way to pursue truth, proposed by the famous science philosopher Karl Popper, is to try to *falsify* our hypotheses—in effect, to seek out the boundaries of our mental paradigms and push against them, to see if they can withstand scrutiny. Can we find evidence to disprove our hypotheses, and are we able to take seriously such evidence? At times, I cannot help but wonder how much and how often our rules and strategies keep us from straying from the status quo.

I have always liked exploring outlier observations in my research. They make me think. During my career, I obtained (or at least noticed) more than my share of observations that were not considered normal. After collecting enough of these heresies, however, I began to see an emerging pattern of them that suggested a substantially different worldview—at which point, it seemed to make sense to call them not heresies but "principles." Here are a few examples.

In the China Study, we discovered that blood cholesterol for rural Chinese adults averaged 127 mg/dL, with individual village averages ranging 88–165 mg/dL.[6] At that time (the mid-1980s), 127 mg/dL was considered dangerously low. The "normal" range for serum cholesterol in the United States at that time was 155–274 mg/dL (with an average of 212 mg/dL), and there was some surprising evidence among Western subjects that incidences of suicides, accidents, and violence,[7] as well as colon cancer,[8] were higher when total cholesterol levels were below 160 mg/dL. Should I therefore have assumed that virtually all rural Chinese were at high risk range for suicides, accidents, violence, and colon cancer? Of course, we found nothing of the sort. Instead, we discovered that the Chinese villagers averaging 127 mg/dL were actually far healthier than Americans with so-called normal cholesterol levels.

My first thought was that perhaps our cholesterol assay method (how we collected and analyzed the blood samples) might be faulty. Following Popper's principle of trying to disprove my own hypothesis, I tried to discredit my own finding by using another assay method and repeating these analyses at laboratories in three different locations (Cornell, Beijing, and London). All the analyses showed the same low cholesterol levels. Now we had to make sense of the apparent paradox that the healthiest

Chinese people had cholesterol levels that would have been considered dangerously low in the United States.

Further examination revealed that, for this Chinese range of 88–165 mg/dL, like the U.S. range of 155–274 mg/dL, lower levels of cholesterol were associated with increased protection from several cancers and serious related diseases. The Chinese population showed correlations between low cholesterol and health that could not be observed in the United States because almost no Americans had cholesterol that low. The Chinese range showed us that cholesterol of 88 mg/dL could be healthier than cholesterol of 155 mg/dL, a finding that simply could not have been gleaned from a study of a U.S. population.

Another example of an outlier that led me away from "accepted wisdom" was our finding that casein, which for decades had been the most highly rated and respected protein, dramatically and convincingly promoted cancer. Even today, it is so heretical that no one wants to say the obvious—that casein is the most relevant chemical carcinogen ever identified. The implications of this heretical finding, like the implications of the exceedingly low blood cholesterol level in rural China, have been among the many hinges on which new doors of understanding opened on the relationship between nutrition and health.

Interestingly, this effect of casein on cancer proved so heretical that even the researchers in India who first showed this effect in a far more limited study never wanted to acknowledge their finding for what it was.[9] They preferred to focus not on casein's long-term effect on initiating cancer, but on the seemingly opposite effect casein had in quickly reducing the toxic effects of huge single doses of carcinogens.[10] (We'll discuss these two effects in greater depth in Part II.) In other words, they ran away from the immense implications of their discovery by focusing on an insignificant detail.

I'm glad I didn't run because I have observed that giving some attention to unexpected observations that might otherwise be discounted or discarded can be unusually rewarding, especially if these observations are pursued to an explanation. My career began when I followed some outlier observations into murky territory, risking (and ultimately parting with) the pro-animal-protein beliefs of my childhood and early research career. When enough of these heresies accumulated, interconnected patterns began to emerge. Those patterns morphed into principles and then into full-blown theories, alternate paradigms that changed the way I saw the world. The rewards of living with heresies can be an exhilarating experience, well worth the costs of being considered a heretic.

True, my social and professional collegialities changed when I began to speak of research findings that lay outside the norm. Skepticism and silence, to put it gently, became more common. Yet the rewards have been numerous, and I do not hesitate to encourage young people to follow the same path that I trod. (When they ask me, as many have, how they might be able to do what I do, I tell them very simply to never be afraid to ask questions, even ones everyone tells you are stupid. Just be prepared to use good science and logic when defending your perspective.)

The view from the outside of a paradigm can be especially rewarding, and also meaningful, when it is considered within the context of everyday life. As time has passed, the odd and unexpected research observations collectively began to shape a new worldview for me. They seemed to be more and more connected. If this worldview touched on matters of life and death, that's when personal passions arose, both pro and con. That's when the boundaries of these paradigms sharpened and came into view.

THE FINAL (PARADIGM) FRONTIER: REDUCTIONISM

Now that you have a taste of my encounters with rigid paradigms, it's time to share what I've learned, from all this questioning, about the prevailing scientific and medical paradigm.

From those initial outliers came heretical questions. From the questions flowed heretical answers, which led to a heretical set of principles. But for a long time I was trying to apply these principles inside a paradigm so big that even I couldn't see it. It was only when I started questioning the mechanisms of the scientific method itself that I stepped outside the biggest, most restrictive, and most insidious paradigm of all: reductionism.

PART II

Paradigm
as Prison

In Part I, I introduced the idea that important information about our health is being withheld from us, and that the lack of this information has contributed to our expensive and tragically ineffective health-care system. In Part II, we'll take on the first of two things responsible for that withholding: the current reductionist paradigm.

We'll begin in chapter four by introducing reductionism and its opposing worldview, wholism, in a philosophical and historical context. In some ways these two lenses represent a more fundamental division in consciousness than any other in modern society, including political and social views and religious affinities.

In chapters five through twelve, we'll examine exactly how reductionism has affected the way we think about nutrition and health. We'll consider how it influences not just how we interpret research results, but also what kind of research is done in the first place. We'll look at its role in the ascendency of genetics in the scientific community—and the limitations of genetics for addressing disease—and at how reductionism influences the way we think about the connection between environmental toxins and cancer. We'll see how reductionism has infected the most fundamental tenets of research, as well as the development of health products and services, turning powerful institutions into veritable zombies: seemingly animate, yet devoid of any compassion or desire to make us well. Last, we'll broaden our view to the repercussions of reductionism in our eating habits far beyond our individual and collective health, in areas as diverse as human poverty, animal cruelty, and environmental degradation.

By the time we're done, you'll discover that "conclusive proof" can look very different depending on which paradigm you embrace. You'll discover why most research into diet and health is contradictory and confusing. And you'll see why it's so important for us to rescue nutrition from the rustic backwaters of science and social policy to which it has been relegated.

4

The Triumph of
Reductionism

We do not see things as they are. We see them as we are.

—TALMUD

An old story: Six blind men are asked to describe an elephant. Each feels a different body part: leg, tusk, trunk, tail, ear, and belly. Predictably, each offers a vastly different assessment: pillar, pipe, tree branch, rope, fan, and wall. They argue vigorously, each sure that their experience alone is the correct one.

I can't think of a better metaphor to highlight the big problem with scientific research today. Except that instead of six blind men, modern science tasks 60,000 researchers to examine the elephant, each through a different lens.

Now, there's nothing wrong with that, in and of itself. You could argue that the six men, each focused on an individual part, together produce a richer and more detailed description of an elephant than could be generated by one person just walking around looking at the creature in its entirety. Similarly, think of the level of detailed understanding that 60,000 scientists can glean when they are empowered to focus on such granular component parts.

The problem arises only when, as in the parable, the individual points of view are mistakenly seen as describing the whole truth. When a laser-like focus is misunderstood as a global overview. When the six men or 60,000 researchers don't talk to one another or acknowledge that the overall goal of the exploration is to perceive and appreciate the whole elephant. When they assume that any view that questions their own is simply wrong.

In this chapter, we'll look at the two competing paradigms in science and medicine: reductionism and wholism. We'll see that the triumph of reductionism over wholism over the past several hundred years—rather than reductionism being used as a tool in the service of wholistic understanding—has seriously impaired our ability to make sense of the world.

THE LIMITS OF PARADIGMS

In a 2005 commencement address, the late novelist David Foster Wallace told a story that gets to the heart of how paradigms work: "There are these two young fish swimming along and they happen to meet an older fish swimming the other way, who nods at them and says, 'Morning, boys. How's the water?' And the two young fish swim on for a bit, and then eventually one of them looks over at the other and goes, 'What the hell is water?'"[1]

We talked about paradigms in chapter three to help explain the way many of my colleagues reacted to our research findings about animal protein and the health benefits of a WFPB diet. I compared my experience to that of a fish who leaves the water and encounters air for the first time: because I found myself outside the predominant scientific paradigm, I was therefore able to better understand where the limitations of that paradigm were.

What we didn't look at in that chapter was the purpose of paradigms, along with their benefits and weaknesses. Paradigms start out as useful ways to frame knowledge and test theories. In fact, I would argue, we can't really live without them. We certainly can't advance our knowledge of the universe without them.

In its broadest sense, a paradigm is a mental filter that restricts what you are able to see at any one time. Mental filters are essential; without your brain's reticular activating system, you would be overwhelmed by stimuli and therefore unable to respond to the important ones. Without the ability to focus on one thing and shut out distractions, you wouldn't be able to get much done. And in science, without the literal filters of microscopes and telescopes, we would know precious little about inner and outer space.

Filters—mental and literal—become problematic only when we forget about them and think that what we're seeing is the whole of reality, instead of a very narrow slice of it. Paradigms become prisons only when we stop recognizing them as paradigms—when we think that water is all there is, so we don't even have a name for it anymore. In a world shaped by the paradigm of water, anyone who suggests the existence of "not water" is automatically a heretic, a lunatic, or a clown.

So first, let's dive into some troubling philosophical waters and try to pin down those two competing paradigms I introduced a few pages ago: reductionism and wholism.

REDUCTIONISM VERSUS WHOLISM

If you are a reductionist, you believe that everything in the world can be understood if you understand all its component parts. A wholist, on the other hand, believes that the whole can be greater than the sum of its parts. That's it: the entire debate in a nutshell. But the debate is one that has been raging among philosophers, theologians, and scientists since antiquity. Is this just academic philosophy, the equivalent of arguing about how many angels can dance on the head of a pin? Hardly. As we'll see, choosing one paradigm or the other leads to very different approaches to science, medicine, commerce, politics, and life itself.

I'll show how these approaches influence our understanding of nutrition in chapter five. For now, let's look more broadly at the battle between wholism and reductionism, and explore how the latter got the upper hand.

I must begin by saying that it's a battle that isn't actually necessary; there's no inherent conflict between the reductionist techniques of science and an overarching wholistic outlook. Reductionism is not, in itself, a bad thing. Indeed, reductionist research has been responsible for some of the most profound breakthroughs of the past several centuries. From anatomy to physics to astronomy to biology to geology, we have gained a greater appreciation of—and ability to interact positively with—the universe through scientific advances brought about by the focused, controlled experimentation of reductionism.

Wholism does not oppose reductionism; rather, wholism *encompasses* reductionism, just as each whole encompasses its parts. I don't think we need to reverse two millennia of scientific progress and go back to a time where humans worshipped nature without desiring to understand its workings. I think it's great that we've got six blind men working on the elephant problem. I just wish someone would clue them in about the whole elephant.

You may be puzzled by my spelling of the word *wholism* with a "w." The more common spelling is *holism*, which I think is part of the problem. Holism reminds scientists of the word *holy*, which smacks of religion. And many scientists are as hostile to religion as religious fundamentalists are to science. When they encounter the word *holistic*, they think of sloppy, "fairy-tale" belief systems that have no place in a serious exploration of the "real world." Ironically, this dismissal of wholism by scientists is the height of dogmatism, a fundamentalist stance that denies the possibility of any truth other than that granted by reductionism. I can just see my science colleagues recoiling at the suggestion that we might be raging fundamentalists without knowing it!

REDUCTIONISM: A HISTORY

From the beginning of our existence, humans have had an insatiable desire to know more about our world and ourselves. Where did we come from? What are human emotions, and how do we come to grips with them? Where are we going? What is the meaning of life?

In ancient Greece—the birthplace of much of Western thought—the philosophies of science and theology were closely intertwined, with much common ground. Both dealt with the all-time great questions concerning the meaning of human existence and the mystery of nature's secrets. They worked hand in hand, with science providing the raw materials—the observations—and theology working those raw materials into overarching theories, or big stories about the universe.

Science and theology are both lenses through which to interact with and interpret reality, sort of like a microscope and a pair of binoculars. Both sets of lenses tell us more about the world than we could see with the naked eye, but the information we get from each can diverge considerably. Greek scientist/theologians such as Pythagoras, Socrates, Aristotle, or Plato would have chafed at the suggestion that they choose one instrument and abandon the other. These philosophers (literally, "lovers of wisdom") wrote and spoke about food and health, justice, women's rights, literature, and theology as easily and with as much passion and conviction as they wrote about geology, physics, and mathematics.

Somewhere along the line—and I don't claim to be a historian, so I'll leave the details to them—science and theology diverged, to the impoverishment of both. Church officials attached rigid dogmas to certain understandings of the universe, with the result that any questioning of those understandings constituted heresy. Science went into retreat in the West. What had been perfectly logical scientific assumptions based on observable facts (such as the earth being the center of the universe, as in Ptolemaic astronomy) were distorted into immutable principles of faith. Firsthand observation of reality was now rightly viewed as a dangerous activity—for what if you observed something that contradicted current theology?

It was not until the thirteenth century or so that science began to reemerge, thus defining a new era, the Renaissance, that led to a clash between the faith-based and rationalist viewpoints. Scholars rediscovered the writings of the classical Greeks and were inspired to pursue their methods of observation instead of clinging to faith-based conclusions. Copernicus (1473–1543) challenged theological dogma by offering that the sun, not the earth, occupied center stage of our known universe. Galileo (1564–1642) invented the telescope and showed that Copernicus was right.

For the next 300 years (1600–1900), many notable and courageous scholars and scientists made observations that continued to build a foundation for the supremacy of scientific facts over theological faith—at least in the minds of many. Human-based, reasoned observations and thought—humanism—flourished, and it proved itself both enlightening and useful.

But this new humanism, having clawed its way to respectability against a doctrinaire Church, became far less tolerant of theology than its classical Greek ancestor. Rather than seeking partnership with theologians, scientists increasingly sought to distance themselves and their endeavors from "superstitions" not grounded in observable fact. This included not just religion, but any idea that did not adhere to scientific views, in which truth was found only through breaking down the observable world into as many smaller parts as possible. In short: reductionism. Although what we humans can observe has changed and grown over time, that fundamental belief about truth has not. Each new advancement in technology only allows us to break the world into smaller and smaller pieces.

The history of the last 200 years has been the inexorable march of reductionism in all aspects of our lives, from science, to nutrition, to education (think of all the "subjects" taught in isolation from one another), to economics (think of microeconomics versus macroeconomics), and even the human soul (think of how it has been reduced to a map of nerves and networks in the brain).

THINGS REDUCTIONISM CAN'T EXPLAIN

Looking at our approach to understanding today, it would appear that reductionism, wearing the guise of science, has won—but at great cost to our understanding of the world. In rejecting religious control of science, we also are rejecting the useful perspectives theology offers: a way of looking at the world as a fundamentally connected whole. A willingness to accept that there are things we may not ever be able to fully understand, and instead can only observe.

Mere "scientific" facts cannot fully explain more than a minuscule part of the far-reaching and complex personal emotions we feel when we experience special moments of our lives or stand before the great wonders of the world. Could facts ever fully explain the inspiration and awe we feel when listening to great music, wondering about the beginning and end of the universe, or admiring other people's talents and emotions? Could describing an enzyme activity, nerve transmission, or hormonal burst really capture what it is like to experience that admiration or those emotions? These things are unimaginably complex and therefore beyond the tools of objective material inquiry. The Austrian mathematician Kurt Gödel demonstrated through his incompleteness theorem (published in 1931) the futility of using reductionist techniques to model a complex system. He proved mathematically that no complex system could be known in its entirety, and that any system that could be known in its entirety was merely a subset of a larger one. In other words, science can never fully describe the universe. No matter how strong the lens or how powerful the computer, we will never be able to model with complete accuracy the chemical reactions that occur when we do something as simple and mundane as watch a sunset. It's not just a technical matter of better tools and more computing power. It's as if reality itself defies the attempt.

At the same time that Gödel was discovering the limits of math to describe numerical reality, particle physicists were realizing that their enhanced tools of perception were inadequate to nail down physical reality as well. Light was either a particle or a wave, depending on how you observed it. Quantum physics dispensed with objectivity altogether, describing subatomic particles in terms of probabilities rather than realities. Werner Heisenberg showed that we could at any moment observe either the position or the speed of an electron, but not both.

Reductionism—in effect, the quest for this kind of full disclosure—is incredibly useful, but the more we learn, the more clear it is that reductionism is insufficient to the task of understanding the universe.

THE DA VINCI MODE

The way we practice science today is the result, then, of a post-Renaissance rejection of a more (w)holistic way of looking at the world along with religion itself. But returning to the pre-Renaissance division of labor between scientists and theologians isn't the answer either. To find a useful model for us today—a model of a scientist who deploys reductionist methods within a wholistic framework—we have to go back to the Renaissance itself.

There may be no individual whose accomplishments were more symbolic of the integration of science and wholism than the ultimate Renaissance man, Leonardo da Vinci (1452–1519). Da Vinci's exceptional significance and reputation was not only due to his brilliant talents in art (e.g., *Mona Lisa*, *The Last Supper*), but also because he was an exceptional scientist. His interests in science were unusually broad, ranging from the biological (anatomy, zoology, and botany) to the physical (geology, optics, aerodynamics, and hydrodynamics). Da Vinci's accomplishments were extraordinary even by modern measures, and, lest we forget, they were achieved over 500 years ago!

Da Vinci had a keen interest in the reality and the wonders of nature as a broad and dynamic whole. The subject matter of his inspired paintings was almost more wondrous than reality, reflecting to me, at least, his understanding of what it means to be human—also a very large and dynamic whole. Da Vinci was also deeply curious about the small details that might be able to explain the human-perceived wonders he painted. This can be readily seen both in his drawings of anatomical structures in biology and his refined representations of mechanical structures in physics. He published amazingly detailed drawings of human anatomy, where, as one biographer noted, he paid "attention to the forms of even very small organs, capillaries and hidden parts of the skeleton." Da Vinci is even credited with being the first in the modern world to introduce the idea of controlled experimentation—the core concept of science—and, for this, he has been considered by some writers to be the Father of Science. Probably more than any other scholastic luminary of that time, he recognized the relationship between the whole and its parts.

Da Vinci was what we call a *polymath*, a term that refers to his exceptional range of artistic, humanistic, and scientific talents. But more relevant than his specific achievements for the purposes of this book is Da Vinci's scholarship, which advanced and supported a new way of thinking: a synthesis of the whole and its parts. He embraced both breadth and depth of thinking both by paying attention to emerging facts and details as they were made available by science, and by apprehending the rapture of human emotion when all parts, known and unknown, acted in symphony to become the whole.

Da Vinci's contributions to our understanding of the universe are profound and enduring precisely because of this integration. He understood that wholism needed reductionism to advance, and reductionism needed wholism to remain relevant. He realized that when you take something out of context to study it more closely or measure it more exactly, you risk losing more wisdom than you gain.

THE "WHOLE" IN WHOLISM

The South African statesman and philosopher Jan Smuts, who is credited with coining the term *holism* (without the "w"), wrote that reality consists of a "great whole" that comprises "small natural center[s] of wholeness." In my work, the body is the great whole and the process by which the body digests food is a smaller center of wholeness within the body. (Nutrition is one perspective on the wholeness of the body.) You can apply this concept to refer also to a human being as a small center of wholeness within the great whole of the biosphere of planet Earth, or to a single human cell as a great whole, of which the mitochondria, DNA, and other blobs you studied in high school biology are small, natural centers that are also whole unto themselves. In either direction, you can continue as far as observation and then your imagination can take you. From the macrocosmic universe to the microcosmic ones, there is, philosophically speaking, a hierarchy of wholes, with each whole having parts that themselves are wholes.

In this book I will be discussing only a few selected parts of biology: genetic expression, intracellular metabolism, and nutrition. Each of these is, in and of itself, an incomprehensibly complex system. But I am somewhat uncomfortable dividing biology into systems at all, because this infers boundaries that are, in reality, vague and arbitrary. Although an organ in the body certainly has physical boundaries, it still communicates with other organs within the body via nerve transmission and hormonal communication, among other means. Every entity within the body, whether physical or metabolic, is both a whole and a part. We have to divide wholes into their component parts so we can talk about them effectively, but even as we do so, we need to remain aware that such divisions are somewhat arbitrary.

Indeed, thinking that our classification system is a perfect mapping of reality is a limiting and potentially dangerous stance. For example, Western medicine views the body geographically; it treats the liver, the kidney, the heart, the left patella, and so on. Chinese medicine, by contrast, sees the body as an energetic network. It might diagnose a patient with a Western label of "liver cancer" as suffering from "too much yang in the triple burner meridian"—a description of an energetic imbalance affecting the so-called burning regions of the body, centered around the head, the chest, and the pelvis. When Western doctors first encountered this system, the vast majority of them dismissed the talk of chi energy and meridians as superstition, as opposed to the "objective reality" of organs, bones, fluids, and muscles. But the documented efficacy of acupuncture, which moves energy along meridians to treat many ailments, testifies to the usefulness of the Chinese paradigm.

Some of you may argue that our limited understanding of biology is a failure of technology, not of paradigm—that, sure, the biological system is beyond our ability to comprehend it *now*, but at some point, we will have a reductionist lens powerful enough to understand even its complexity. To return to our elephant metaphor, we might increase the number of blind men well into the millions, make each one responsible for understanding a microscopic part of the elephant, and then employ advanced computational methods and a massive supercomputer to put it all together. That, in effect, is the thesis of the famed futurist, Ray Kurzweil, Google's Director of Engineering, who imagines our being able to create, from scratch, a human body, once we know all the parts and develop supercomputers sufficiently powerful to enable us to do so.

But I submit that this viewpoint is naïve—at least for biological systems like a whole body. As an example, let's take the enzyme, a protein that is instrumental to the various chemical reactions necessary for the proper function of the human body, like the digestion of food and the construction of cells. Through experimentation and observation, we can discern the chemical composition, size, shape, and some of the functionality of the enzyme. Is a summation of these things the enzyme? According to modern science, the answer is yes. Modern science sees the enzyme as a discrete entity, with discernable edges, and its goal is to discern these edges.

If the world was, indeed, an accumulation of parts, each defined by discernable edges, then perhaps at some future point the technologists could understand the human body through a reductionist lens powered by supercomputers, complex computational models, and other technologies. But the world is far more complex than this. The enzyme is not, in fact, a discrete unit that stands alone; it is an *integral* element of a larger system. It exists in service to the system, as does every other element of that system. If an element ever ceases to act in service to its system, as with uncontrolled cancer growth, the system breaks down, and may even fail entirely. Because each part is an integral element of the same system, all the parts are connected to one another; no one part stands alone. And this means each part affects and is affected by the other parts. Removing or modifying a part changes the whole, just as changing the whole, as we will see in later discussions, impacts the parts—that is, when one part is altered, all the other parts are forced to adapt to try and keep the system running.

In this scenario, the discrete boundaries we assign to individual parts melt away. Put simply, there are no fixed "edges" within the human body that separate any one part from all the other parts. In their place are infinite connection and unending change, and it is this continual cascade of causes and effects that renders reductionist prediction models useless.

This lack of boundaries is important because it means that each "part" of the body involves more than what can be seen when the part is viewed, as it is in reductionism, in isolation from the larger system it serves. What the enzyme is made of, what it looks like, what it does, and why it does it—all of this is a function of the larger system that is the human body. Better, more powerful technology doesn't alter that fundamental reality. No matter how many blind men you employ to observe parts of the elephant, and no matter how much technology is available to support them, you can never generate the understanding required to see the full elephant.

When I lament the idea of taking a part out of context of the whole—whether that part is a nutrient, biological mechanism, or something else—this is what I am lamenting: how, in studying parts out of context, we blind ourselves to wholistic interpretations as well as the real-life solutions to human health those interpretations would provide.

THE INTELLECTUAL COST OF
REDUCTIONIST VICTORY

I hope I'm being clear that I'm not advocating a return to faith-based dogmatic acceptance of any authority's views on reality. To the contrary, I'm asserting that we need less dogma and more open-mindedness in the scientific community when it comes to observing and describing our world. One of the core principles of science—the key element that distinguishes it from every other way of looking at the world—is the idea of falsifiability. Basically, if a theory is falsifiable, that means that evidence can be offered to disprove it. The opposite stance, dogma, is, by definition, anything that is considered unfalsifiable.

Let's say you believe that the bus from New York City to Ithaca always arrives on time. You would agree, I assume, that if it pulled into the station twenty minutes late one day, that would prove your theory false. You might then amend your theory to "95 percent of the time," or to "within half an hour of its scheduled arrival time," and we could agree on observations and experiments that might support or contradict those new theories. But the key point is, you accept in advance that some configuration of observable facts could partially or completely invalidate your theory.

Contrast that with belief in an afterlife in which the good are rewarded and the evil are punished. If you ask those who believe in this brand of an afterlife what evidence would cause them to reconsider that belief, they are most likely to stare at you in confusion. Such faith is not open to factual contradiction. Even if you don't believe in such an afterlife, can you think of any facts that we could gather that might invalidate it? I'm not saying such a belief is right or wrong, just that it's not science because it can't be disproved, or falsified, by observation or experimentation.

The reductionist paradigm is dogma, an article of faith; it rejects, beforehand, the idea that it may not always be the best or only way to apprehend and measure reality. And modern science (and the biological and health sciences in particular) has embraced the dogma of reductionism to the exclusion of common sense and fairness. The most respected and learned individuals in our society are trained to operate exclusively within the confines of this dogma. To return to an earlier metaphor: these individuals spend their time studying and writing about the minutiae of elephants without a single one of them being aware that there is such a thing as an elephant. The tragedy is, this is the system we have entrusted with the search for truth, whose findings determine our public policy and influence our private choices.

5

Reductionism
Invades Nutrition

*The first problem for all of us, men and women, is
not to learn but to unlearn.*

—GLORIA STEINEM

N ow that we understand the fundamental flaws of the reductionist
paradigm in general, it's time to explore how this paradigm has
distorted and degraded nutrition and human health.

I know food and nutrition aren't considered to be very important
outside my little world. The newspapers I read have sections on politics,
business, sports, and entertainment, but none of them devotes a daily
section to food policy. Food writers are restaurant critics or purveyors of
recipes, relegated to the same pages of the newspaper devoted to hairstyles,
fashion, and home decor. But food is pretty much the most important topic
there is. No food, no civilization. Crop failures, outbreaks of mad cow
disease, and contaminated produce could bring our society to its knees
very quickly. We assume we're immune to such catastrophes because

most of us think about food as the stuff we buy at the supermarket. And every time we go to the supermarket, guess what? It's overflowing with food. We aren't going hungry, so everything must be fine.

But just because we don't think about our food all the time doesn't mean it's not critically important. Most of us don't obsess over our oxygen supply, but people who find themselves submerged in water or trapped in a smoky building can think of nothing else. Food is as fundamental to our survival as oxygen. But while we all breathe the same air, we have lots of choices when it comes to food, and those choices determine not just how we eat, but also how we utilize our agricultural land, what our government subsidizes, what we teach our children, and what sort of society we create.

In the same supermarket, we can choose to fill our carts from the produce section, the dairy case, the meat freezer, the canned goods aisle, or the packaged-goods aisle. We can get our produce from local growers or from giant factory farms in South America. We can eat out at fast-food restaurants or cook in our own kitchens. And when our choices cause us to gain unacceptable amounts of weight, we can adopt any one of a thousand different diet plans, from Atkins to Paleo to Weight Watchers to macrobiotic. All these individual choices add up to affect our national food "system," just as the food system itself strongly influences those individual choices. Both the system and our personal choices have been heavily driven by our beliefs about nutrition.

If they weren't, would such a large percentage of food packaging be taken up by nutritional labels? Why else would the federal government spend so much money and time creating food groups, food pyramids, recommended daily allowances, and daily minimum requirements? Why else would the FDA create and enforce rules about what food, drug, and supplement manufacturers are allowed to claim as health benefits?

So although it doesn't make the news very often, food, and our national policies about it, determine a great deal about our society. And nearly everything our society believes about nutrition has reductionist fingerprints all over it. In this chapter, we'll explore how the reductionist paradigm has led to poor nutritional policy and confused consumers, as well as how and why nutrition resists the reductionist model our society works hard to put it in.

REDUCTIONIST NUTRITIONAL SCIENCE

The definition of the word *nutrition* is something I've thought about a lot: every so often during my fifty years in academia, our nutrition faculty would have a retreat and spend some of the time trying to figure out what the word really means. These could not have been very productive, because the same discussion had a way of reappearing at every retreat.

Each time, we'd eventually conclude with some default definition, something resembling the ones found in standard dictionaries. Something like "a process of providing or obtaining food necessary for health and growth" (*Oxford English Dictionary*) or "the act or process of nourishing or being nourished; specifically the sum of the processes by which an animal or plant takes in and utilizes food substances" (*Webster's*).

I don't like either definition. *Webster's* definition fails partly on technical grounds because it uses the word *nourished*, which is a derivative of the word *nutrition*. You can't define a word by referring to itself! That *Webster's* resorts to this sleight of hand shows how troublesome the word really is.

The other, more substantial problem with the *Webster's* entry is the word *sum*. I remember sums from grade school math. We added two numbers and got a third. The third, which we called the sum, was nothing more or less than what you got by adding the first two numbers. That's the very soul of reductionism, remember: the sum (total) can be completely known if you know each individual part.

Both *Oxford* and *Webster's* use the word *process*, which points to something important but, on its own, is inexcusably vague. The *Oxford* definition focuses entirely on the process of nutrition as something that occurs outside the body: food is either provided or obtained. This leaves no room for nutrition as an internal, biological process, nor a complex one. To reductionists, nutrition is just the arithmetic summation of the effects of individual nutrients. These misleading definitions in two of the most respected and frequently used English dictionaries show how profoundly the reductionist concept is embedded in our culture.

If you were taught statements like, "Calcium grows strong bones," "Vitamin A is necessary for good eyesight," and "Vitamin E is a cancer-fighting antioxidant," you learned nutrition the same way. The same is true if you count calories, or pay attention to percentages on the nutritional labels on packaged foods, or wonder if you get enough protein, or start slathering your fries in catsup because you hear tomatoes are a good source of lycopene.

These beliefs make sense only in a reductionist paradigm that identifies the component parts of food—the individual nutrients—and figures out exactly what each one does in the body and how much of it we need. And this is precisely what we scientists are trained to do. I was taught nutrition in this way and I taught it the same way to my students. This included an upper-level course in biochemistry at Virginia Tech, an upper-level course in nutritional biochemistry at Cornell, and two new graduate-level courses in biochemical toxicology and molecular toxicology for a new graduate field of toxicology, also at Cornell. Like other faculty in these fields, I followed the typical textbook model of lecturing, mostly focusing on individual nutrients, individual toxic chemicals, individual mechanisms of action (i.e., biochemical explanations), and individual effects, as if there were, for each nutrient or chemical, one main mechanism that explains and perhaps controls the relationship between cause and effect.

When I taught nutrition in this traditional, reductionist way, here's how it went. We began by considering the chemical structure of the nutrient. Then we discussed how it functions in the body: its absorption across the intestinal wall into the blood; its transport through the body; its storage; its excretion; and the amounts needed for good health. We talked about each nutrient on its own, as if it acted alone in a totally mechanical fashion. In other words, teaching nutrition meant getting students to memorize facts and figures and chemical pathways to pass tests without asking them to think about the context for these discrete bits of information.

We do the same thing in research as we do in education. The gold standard of nutritional research—the type that receives preference for funding and gets published in top-line journals—focuses on one nutrient and one explanation of its effect. My experimental research program focused on the effects of discrete causes, reactions, enzymes, and effects, oftentimes outside of the context of the body as a whole—in part because, as I mentioned, I, too, was taught to think this way,[1] but also because, in order to get research funding, we scientists are forced to focus our hypotheses and experimental objectives on outcomes that can be measured.

Let me give you a specific example from the initial stages of my own research on cancer formation initiated by aflatoxin (AF), a chemical known to cause liver cancer. (As you may recall from the introduction,

AF was the carcinogen produced by the peanut fungus I was looking at in the Philippines.) Figure 5-1 summarizes the process we were studying (using a diet of 20 percent casein, or milk protein).

My lab research at this early stage was completely acceptable according to the reductionist rules. We focused on one kind of carcinogen (AF) that caused one kind of cancer (hepatocellular liver cancer) that depended on one kind of enzyme (mixed-function oxidase) that metabolized AF to produce one kind of highly reactive product (AF epoxide) that produced one biochemical effect (the very tight chemical bonding of the epoxide to DNA that causes genetic damage), each stage of which seemed internally consistent and biologically plausible. And we discovered that the more the carcinogen bound itself to the DNA, the greater the amount of cancer occurred.[2] Aha! This was *the* mechanism that "explained" the effect of protein on cancer!

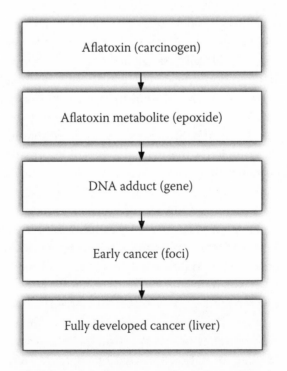

FIGURE 5-1.   A linear model of cancer causation from aflatoxin

A couple of thoughts about the previous paragraph: first, I don't expect you to understand everything I wrote. I'm describing complex biological and chemical reactions in the kind of specialized language used by scientists everywhere to communicate with precision. All you need to know is that, according to this model, A causes B, which causes C, which leads to D. So the more A (cancer-causing chemical) you start with, the more D (cancer) you end up with.

Second, it probably sounds pretty convincing, even if you don't really understand it. Research like this seems airtight because it deals with objective facts—reactions, genetic mutations, and carcinogenesis—as opposed to messy things like human behavior and lifestyle. Only by excluding messy and complex reality can we make linear, causal statements about biological chain reactions.

Although we worked diligently on this series of studies for many years, obtained very impressive results, and published lots of professional papers, we were still left with a major unanswered question: did this finding—that higher dietary casein intake produced more cancer in rats—tell us anything about other proteins, chemical carcinogens, cancers, diseases, and species (e.g., humans)?

In other words, did this startling outlier result about dietary protein suggest that our love affair with animal protein was misguided and dangerous? Did cow's milk in modest quantities promote cancer in humans? What about other diseases? Did other animal proteins have the same effect? While I tried for decades to answer these questions using reductionist tools, it gradually dawned on me that these questions often strayed beyond what reductionist science could answer. Not because you couldn't set up experiments to compare the effects of a diet high in animal protein with other factors typically found in a WFPB diet. Those have been done, and the results are jaw-dropping (particularly the research and clinical experiences of Esselstyn, McDougall, Goldhamer, Barnard, and Ornish, some of which we touch on elsewhere in this book).

No, the problem with reductionist research is that it's too easy to run experiments that show what appears to be just the opposite effect: that milk prevents cancer. That fish oil protects the brain. That lots of animal protein and fat stabilizes blood sugar and prevents obesity and diabetes. Because when you're looking through a microscope, either literally or metaphorically, you can't see the big picture. All you can see is a tiny bit of the far larger truth, completely out of context. And whoever has the loudest megaphone—in this case, the ones shouting that milk and meat are necessary for optimal human health, whose megaphones are thoughtfully provided by the meat and dairy industries—has the most influence.

I'm sure that given enough time and money, I could conduct reductionist-style experiments that show health benefits for Coke, deep-fried Snickers bars (these are very popular at the North Carolina State Fair), and even AF (we actually showed such effects once in our lab[3]). I'd have to manipulate the sample (say, studying the effects of Coke on people dying of thirst in the Sahara, or the effects of a Snickers bar on the mortality rate of tired drivers at 2 A.M.). I could also measure hundreds of different biomarkers and report only on the outcomes that support my bias. Or, like the elephant examiners we met in chapter four, I could perform honest research and still end up with conclusions that are incomplete and misleading because of the limited scope of my vision.

This is why we so frequently see conflicting research results in the media: the predominant research framework actually *encourages* such conflicts. This same reductionist framework is also why our society's beliefs about nutrition often seem so contradictory and confusing, whether we get them from textbooks, food packaging, or government messaging.

REDUCTIONIST NUTRITION IN THE
SUPERMARKET AND THE HOME

Though reductionism originates in the lab, it pervades the public imagination as much as it does the thinking of academics. Because we scientists and researchers are considered "experts," our worldview permeates our culture's understanding of nutrition at every level.

Pick up an elementary or high school nutrition textbook and you will inevitably find a list of known nutrients. There are about a dozen vitamins and minerals, perhaps as many as twenty to twenty-two amino acids, and three macronutrients (fat, carbohydrate, and protein). These chemicals and their effects are treated as the essence of nutrition: just get enough (but not too much) of each kind and you're fine. It's been that way for a long time. We're brought up thinking of food in terms of the individual elements that we need. We eat carrots for vitamin A and oranges for vitamin C, and drink milk for calcium and vitamin D.

If we like the particular food, we're happy to get our nutrients from it. But if we don't like that food—spinach, or Brussels sprouts, or sweet potatoes—we think it's fine to skip it as long as we take a supplement with the same amounts of these nutrients. But even recent reductionist research has shown that supplementation doesn't work. As it turns out, an apple does a lot more inside our bodies than all the known apple nutrients ingested in pill form. The whole apple is far more than the sum of its parts. Thanks to the reductionist worldview, however, we don't really believe the food itself is important. Only the nutrients contained in the food matter.

This belief is reinforced every time we read the labels on food packages. Sometimes these lists are quite extensive; the typical food label lists a lot of individual nutrients, with precise amounts per serving shown for each component (see Figure 5-2).

I was a member of the 1990 National Academy of Sciences (NAS) expert panel assigned by the FDA to standardize and simplify the food-labeling program. Two schools of thought existed on our panel. One view favored using the label to tell customers how much of each of the

Nutrition Facts

Serving Size: 2 fl. oz. (60 ml)
Servings Per Container: about 13

Amount Per Serving

Calories 45	Calories from Fat 10
	% Daily Value*
Total Fat 1g	2%
Sodium 30 mg	1%
Potassium 110 mg	3%
Total Carbohydrate 8 g	3%
Dietary Fiber 2 g	8%
Sugars 7 g	
Protein <1g	

Vitamin A 10%	•	Vitamin C 50%
Iron 2%	•	Vitamin E 50%
Vitamin K 10%	•	Niacin 20%
Vitamin B$_6$ 20%	•	Vitamin B$_{12}$ 20%
Pantothenic Acid 20%		

Not a significant source of saturated fat, trans fat, cholesterol, or calcium.
*Percent Daily Values based on a 2,000 calorie diet.

FIGURE 5-2.   A typical example of a food label[4]

many nutrients is inside. The other, to which I subscribed, intended to minimize quantitative information on the label. I believed that we would serve the public best by providing some general information, like a list of ingredients, while staying away from the finer details. (My school of thought lost, although our report did end up proposing a labeling model that was more focused than the original.)

Ingredients are important, and not just for avoiding ones to which you might be allergic. You probably don't want to eat foods with long lists of unpronounceable words, and I assume you'd like to know if your breakfast cereal contains large quantities of high-fructose corn syrup. But including fine-print details like the number of micrograms of niacin performs two disservices to the public that can lead to poor eating choices. First, it overwhelms consumers and causes most of them to ignore the labels entirely. Second, it implies that the nutrients included on the label (a minuscule percentage of the total known nutrients) are the only important ones—indeed, perhaps the only ones that exist.

This isn't the only way the government supports and furthers reductionist nutritional philosophy. A very public example is the effort expended for many years to develop a nutrient composition database that includes all known foods. Since the early 1960s, the U.S. Department of Agriculture has been working on an enormous database in which each food is accompanied by an extensive list of the nutrients it contains and their amounts. This database is now available on the Internet for the public's use, at http://ndb.nal.usda.gov.

Government scientists have also promoted reductionist nutritional policy through their nutrient recommendations, which focus on the quantities of each nutrient deemed important for good health—and these nutrient recommendations have a much further reach than an online database. Every five years, the NAS's Food and Nutrition Board reviews the latest science to update these recommendations. Generally known as recommended daily allowances (RDAs), they were revised in a 2002 report to provide not single-number RDAs, but ranges of intake to maximize health and minimize disease (now called recommended daily intakes, RDIs). Trouble is, RDIs still focus on individual nutrients. And these recommendations, expressed as numbers, now serve as quality control criteria for public nutrition initiatives like school lunch programs, hospital food guidelines, and other government-subsidized food service programs.

Armed with both these government recommendations and that vast nutritional database, consumers can now look up their RDIs and then cross-check them against the database to determine what foods to add or subtract in order to achieve proper nutrient intake. The RDI creators must wonder how our ancestors, without access to computers, were able to eat well enough to survive and reproduce!

Of course, nobody chooses their diet based on databases and RDIs. But quantifying foods this way reinforces the impression that this is the best way to understand nutrition, and the fear engendered by those reductionist tools leads many people to worry about not getting their daily nutrient allowances. Hence Americans spend $25–$30 billion or so each year (as of 2007) on nutrient supplements.[5] Many consider the use of these products to be the essence of modern nutrition. Similarly, foods have long been fortified with specific nutrients like iron, selenium, calcium, vitamin D, and iodine, because certain areas of the world or groups of people suffer from deficiencies of them. In the case of serious nutritional deficiencies, like nineteenth-century British sailors suffering from scurvy due to the lack of vitamin C, or impoverished Third World villagers dying from protein deficiency, attention to individual nutrients makes some sense. In the case of malnutrition, a supplement can save lives in the short run by buying time to set up longer-term systems that provide sufficient and balanced nutrition from real food. But for most Americans who suffer from too much food and too much granular information about that food, this approach is misguided. It overwhelms us and keeps us, in motivational speaker Jim Rohn's memorable phrase, "majoring in minor things."

WRENCHES IN THE
REDUCTIONIST MODEL

In short, virtually all of us, professionals and laypeople alike, talk about nutrition, study nutrition, sell nutrition, and practice nutrition in reference to specific nutrients and, oftentimes, to specific quantities. We fixate on the *amounts*. Vitamins. Minerals. Fatty acids. And of course, the biggest obsession of them all: calories.

We've seen where this obsession comes from, and it's easy enough to understand. After all, most people want to be healthy and feel good, and we're taught that our health partially depends on getting precisely the right amount of these things into our bodies. So whether it's the obsessive calorie counting of Weight Watchers or the 40/40/30 absurdity of the Zone diet, we believe that the more accurately we track our inputs, the more control we have over the output: our health.

Unfortunately, that just isn't true. Nutrition is not a mathematical equation in which two plus two is four. The food we put in our mouths doesn't control our nutrition—not entirely. What our bodies do with that food does.

Wrench #1: The Wisdom of Our Bodies

Are you sitting down? Because I need to explain something that almost no one acknowledges about nutrition: there is almost no direct relationship between the amount of a nutrient consumed at a meal and the amount that actually reaches its main site of action in the body—what is called its *bioavailability*. If, for example, I consume 100 milligrams of vitamin C at one meal, and 500 milligrams at a second meal, this does not mean that the second meal leads to five times as much vitamin C reaching the tissue where it works.

Does this sound like bad news? To reductionists, it certainly does. It means that we can never know exactly how much of a nutrient to ingest, because we can't predict how much of it will be utilized. Uncertainty: a reductionist's worst nightmare!

Actually, this is very good news. The reason we can't predict how much of a nutrient will be absorbed and utilized by the body is that, within limits, it depends on what the body needs at that moment. Isn't that amazing? In more scientific language, the proportion of a nutrient that is digested, absorbed, and provided to various tissues and the cells in those tissues is mostly dependent on the body's need for that nutrient at that moment in time. This need is constantly "sensed" by the body and controlled by a variety of mechanisms that operate at various stages of the "pathway," from nutrient ingestion to nutrient utilization. The body reigns supreme in choosing which nutrients it uses and which it discards unmetabolized. The pathway taken by a nutrient often branches, and branches further, and branches further again, leading the nutrient through a maze of reactions that is far more complex and unpredictable than the simple linear model of reductionism would suggest.

The proportion of ingested beta-carotene that is actually converted into its most common metabolite, retinol (vitamin A), can vary as much as eight-fold. The proportion converted also decreases with increasing doses of beta-carotene, thus keeping the absolute amounts that are absorbed about the same. The percentage of calcium absorbed can vary by at least two-fold; the higher the calcium intake, the lower the proportion absorbed into the blood, ensuring adequate calcium for the body and no more. Iron bioavailability can vary anywhere from three-fold to as much as nineteen-fold. The same holds true for virtually every nutrient and related chemical.

In brief, the relationship between amount consumed and amount used for virtually all nutrients is not a linear relationship. Although many professionals know this, few fully appreciate the significance of this complexity. It means nutrient databases are not nearly as useful as one might think. It also means reductionist supplementation with large doses of discrete nutrients does not guarantee the utilization of those nutrients. (In fact, our digestive processes are so complex and dynamic that super-dosing with a single nutrient all but guarantees an imbalance of some other nutrients, as we'll see in Wrench #3 later in this chapter.)

Wrench #2: The Variability of Foods

Not knowing how much of a given nutrient will be used by the body is only part of our uncertainty. The nutrient content of the foods we eat themselves varies far more than most of us realize. Look at the research just on one antioxidant vitamin, beta-carotene (and/or its related carotenoids). Beta-carotene content in different samples of the same food is known to vary three- to nineteen-fold, although it may be up to forty-fold or more, as was reported for peaches. That's right—you could hold a peach in each hand, and the one in your right hand could easily contain forty times more beta-carotene than the one in your left, depending on things like season, soil, storage, processing, and even the original location of the fruit on the tree. And beta-carotene is far from the only example. The "relatively stable" calcium content of four kinds of cooked mature beans (black, kidney, navy, pinto) ranges 2.7-fold—from 46 to 126 mg—per cup.

The variation in food nutrient content and the variation in nutrient absorption and utilization by the body compound each other. A simple exercise might help to make the point. Suppose the amount of beta-carotene in a carrot varies about four-fold, and the amount of this uncertain proportion that is then absorbed across the intestinal wall into the bloodstream varies another two-fold. This means that the amount of beta-carotene theoretically delivered to the bloodstream from any given carrot on any given day might range as much as eight-fold.

These are huge but uncertain variations, and whether these ranges are two- or forty-fold, the ultimate message is the same: With the consumption of any particular food at any particular moment, we cannot know with any precision how much of any nutrient is actually available to our bodies, or how much our bodies actually use.

Wrench #3: The Complexity of Nutrient Interactions

But wait—there's more uncertainty! You may be surprised to learn that the three nutrients mentioned above can modify one another's activities. Calcium decreases iron bioavailability by as much as 400 percent, while carotenoids (like beta-carotene) increase iron absorption by as much as 300 percent. Theoretically, in comparing a high-calcium, low-carotenoid diet with a low-calcium, high-carotenoid diet, we might see an 800–1,200 percent difference in iron absorption. But even if this theoretical variation were only 100–200 percent, this is still huge; for some nutrients, tissue concentrations varying by more than 10–20 percent can mean serious bad news.

Interactions among individual nutrients in food are substantial and dynamic—and have major practical implications. An outstanding review by researchers Karen Kubena and David McMurray at Texas A&M University summarized the published effects of a large number of nutrients on the exceptionally complex immune system.[6] Nutrient pairs that were found to influence each other and in turn, to influence components of the immune system include vitamin E–selenium, vitamin E–vitamin C, vitamin E–vitamin A, and vitamin A–vitamin D. The mineral magnesium influences the effects of iron, manganese, vitamin E, potassium, calcium, phosphorus, and sodium, and through them the activities of hundreds of enzymes that process them; copper interacts with iron, zinc, molybdenum, and selenium to affect the immune system; dietary protein exerts different effects on zinc; and vitamin A and dietary fat affect each other's ability to influence the development of experimentally created cancer.

Even closely related chemicals within the same chemical class can greatly influence each other. For example, various fatty acids affect the immune system activities of other fatty acids. The effect of polyunsaturated fats (found in plant oils) on breast cancer, for example, is greatly modified by the amount of total and saturated fat in the diet.

The fact that magnesium has already been shown to be an essential part of the function of more than 300 enzymes speaks volumes about the possibilities for the almost unlimited nutrient interactions. The effects of these interactions on drug-metabolizing enzymes and on the immune system also apply to other complex systems, such as the hormonal, acid–base balance, and neurological systems.[7]

The evidence cited here represents only an infinitesimally small fraction of the total number of interactions operating every moment in our bodies. Clearly, the common belief that we can investigate the effects of a single nutrient or drug, unmindful of the potential modifications by other chemical factors, is foolhardy. This evidence should also make us extremely hesitant to "mega-dose" on nutrients isolated from whole foods. Our bodies have evolved to eat whole foods, and can therefore deal with the combinations and interactions of nutrients contained in those foods. Give a body 10,000 mg of vitamin C, however, and all bets are off.

THE POINTLESSNESS OF
REDUCTIONIST PRECISION

Even in this discussion of the variability of nutrient absorption, you may have noticed, I've still toed a fairly reductionist line. I've examined variability in terms of single nutrients and how much their quantities vary in food and at their site of action in the body. As we've seen, consuming two nutrients simultaneously typically affects the utilization of both. This variation becomes orders of magnitude more complex and uncertain when combinations of a large number of nutrients are simultaneously consumed (also known as "eating food"). Now we're talking not just about three or so different nutrients affecting each other and the various systems of the body; we're talking about all the active elements of a whole food. We simply cannot know how many kinds of chemicals are consumed in a single morsel of food or at a single meal or during the course of a day. Hundreds of thousands? Millions? The complexity increases virtually without limit.

If we had to rely on our brains to figure out what to eat, in what quantities, and in which combinations, or risk malnutrition or disease, the human race would have died out long ago. Luckily, our task is considerably simpler. When we eat the right foods, in amounts that satisfy but don't stuff us silly, our bodies naturally metabolize the nutrients in those foods to give us exactly what we need at any given moment.

Our bodies control concentrations of nutrients and their metabolites very carefully, so that the amounts available to particular sites of action in the body often rest within very narrow ranges. For some nutrients, concentrations must stay within these limits for us to avoid serious health problems and even death. In short, the body is able to reduce the highly variable concentrations of nutrients in food into much more stable concentrations in our tissues by sorting out what's necessary and what's excessive.

One way to gain perspective on this discussion is to consider the "reference" ranges of a few nutrients in our blood plasma, as illustrated in Figure 5-3. You may have seen these ranges on your clinical lab report at

Nutrient	Reference Range	Fold Difference
Sodium	135–145 mmol/L	1.07
Potassium	3.5–5.0 mmol/L	1.43
Chloride	340–370 mg/dL	1.09
Calcium (ionized)	1.03 mmol/L	1.23
Iron	9–21 µmol/L	2.33
Copper	11–24 µmol/L	2.18
Magnesium	0.6–0.8 mmol/L	1.33
Total protein	60–78 g/L	1.30
Vitamin A (retinol)	30–65 µg/dL	2.17

FIGURE 5-3.   Reference ranges for blood tests[8]

the doctor's office. Based on analyses of the blood of presumably healthy people, these ranges are generally considered "normal." But notice how narrow these ranges vary—only 1.1–2.3-fold, compared with the five- to ten-fold (or more) nutrient variation in food.

In short, your body is constantly monitoring and adjusting the concentrations of nutrients in the food you consume in order to turn massive variability into the narrower ranges it requires to be healthy.

CATCHING A BALL

This sounds like a lot of work for the body to be doing, I know. But that's what it's built for. That's what it does best. And it does it without requiring any amount of conscious intervention in the process.

Think about the simple act of catching a ball that someone has tossed to you. Do you have any idea how complicated that process is? First, your eyes have to notice the object and identify it as a ball and not, say, a swarm of hornets or a balloon filled with petroleum jelly. Then your eyes, working in binocular fashion, begin sending a dizzying array of data to your brain to help determine the size and velocity of the ball. Even if you failed high school geometry, your brain calculates its parabolic path. Even if you flunked physics, your brain calculates the mass, acceleration, and force of the ball. And while your brain is processing all this information, it's also communicating with the nerves that control your arm and hand, the stabilizing muscles of your back, neck, and legs, and the parasympathetic nervous system that may need to calm you down following the initial sight of an incoming projectile.

Your body is amazing at juggling all these myriad inputs and orchestrating a perfectly timed response: your arm reaches and your hand closes around the ball. But imagine if someone insisted that the right way to learn how to do this was to do all the math and physics. To measure and calculate the velocity, parabolic arc, wind speed, and everything else. School curricula around "catching" would proliferate; educators would argue about which methods work best. About 1 percent of students would excel at this methodology, while the vast majority of us would walk around getting pelted by balls that we couldn't catch if our lives depended on it. Whenever we came across cultures where everybody could catch, we scientists would study their physiology and the materials used in making their balls and their public policy around the topic of catching, hoping to unravel the mystery and find the "cure" for ball dropping.

Focusing on individual nutrients, their identities, their contents in food, their tissue concentrations, and their biological mechanisms, is like using math and physics to catch balls. It's not the way nature evolved, and it makes proper nutrition far more difficult than it needs to be. Our bodies use countless mechanisms, strategically placed throughout our digestion, absorption, and transport and metabolic pathways, to effortlessly ensure tissue concentrations consistent with good health—no database consultation required. But as long as we let reductionism guide our research and our understanding of nutrition, good health will remain unattainable.

6

Reductionist
Research

*Don't be afraid to take a big step. You can't cross a
chasm in two small jumps.*

—DAVID LLOYD GEORGE

So far we've looked at how the scientific and governmental understanding of nutrition is firmly rooted in the reductionist paradigm, and how that affects the way the public views nutrition. We've also seen how, when you look at it carefully, nutrition is a wholistic phenomenon that can never be fully comprehended within a reductionist framework. It's too complex, with too many variables.

In this chapter I'd like to look a little closer at the differences between reductionist and wholistic scientific research, to show the various ways that the reductionist worldview inevitably fails us when it tries to comprehend and manipulate the amazingly complex system that is the human body.

REDUCTIONIST SCIENCE
AND CAUSALITY

As we saw in chapter five, reductionism treats science like a math equation. It searches for cause and effect, and the more focused that search, the better. The holy grail of research is the ability to state with confidence that A causes B. Once you know this, if you want to reduce or eliminate B (liver cancer, for example), you simply look for ways to reduce or eliminate A (say, aflatoxin) or to block the process by which A causes B.

Baked into reductionist science is the assumption that the world operates in a linear way—that it operates on simple causality. What exactly do I mean by this? The classic conditions for proving that A causes B are three-fold:

1. A always precedes B.
2. B always follows A.
3. There is no C that could also cause B.

Not much wiggle room there. Certainly no room for messy, unpredictable, and complex interactions. No room for acknowledging systems that are too complicated to map out. No room for uncertainty of any kind. That's why tobacco companies were able to get scientists to say that smoking doesn't cause lung cancer: not all smokers develop lung cancer and not all lung cancers are attributable to smoking. In a reductionist universe, the statement "Smoking doesn't cause lung cancer" is perfectly accurate. But it's woefully inadequate when it comes to the practical issue of understanding the profound effect of tobacco on lung cancer, thus convincing people to stop smoking.

In the simple-causality reductionist view, the universe, ultimately, is as mechanical as a clock. Some reductionist philosophers of science have gone so far as to claim there's no such thing as free will, since our very thoughts, emotions, and impulses are simply the result of chemical reactions that themselves were triggered by other chemical reactions, going back to the Big Bang itself.

As psychologist Abraham Maslow wisely observed, "If you only have a hammer, you tend to see every problem as a nail." And if your only way of seeing assumes that the world operates on simple causality, you'll see simple causality everywhere, even where it doesn't exist; we see the world, not as it is, but as we expect it to be. Reductionist research naturally produces reductionist findings. It can be no other way. The flip side is also true: since reductionist research assumes that simple causality is the way the world works, if we can't find simple causality in our research subject it just means we must not be looking at it the right way, or we don't have sufficient observational or computing power to reveal it. The only way to see the miraculous complexity of nature is to allow ourselves to do so.

But looking for complexity is a much harder task. Single-factor causality is much easier to measure, and gives much more satisfying (if ineffective) answers, since no matter how complex the system and its interactions are in reality, a good reductionist scientist still assumes that just one factor among the hundreds, thousands, or billions in the system is necessary and sufficient to cause the end result under study. Smokers get more cancer? That proves nothing to reductionists until you can isolate the single chemical in the cigarette that invariably causes cancer. When the effects of smoking are mitigated by lifestyle, nutrition, or whether the cigarette is a pleasurable interlude or a guilt-raising addiction, reductionist research must steadfastly ignore these complexities.

In one way, though, looking for complexity is actually easier than seeking rigid causality. Reductionism may work from simple models of causation, but those models often provide unexpected and unexplained findings, eventually suggesting complex and confusing (and sometimes totally implausible) solutions. Wholism, on the other hand, presumes complex models of causation in a way that suggests simple solutions. (You can't get much simpler than, "Solve most of our health problems by eating more whole, plant-based foods"!)

In other words, reductionist research often requires the invention of *new* complexities—especially more complicated methods of study and explanation. There's an old joke about a dairy farmer who could not get his cows to produce enough milk. He asked the local university for advice, and they sent a team of professors, headed by a theoretical physicist. After weeks of intensive study, the team returned to the university, where they pondered potential solutions. Finally the physicist returned to the farm with an answer to the production issue. But he prefaced his presentation with a caveat: "This solution assumes spherical cows in a vacuum." The physicists' work, like that of reductionist nutritionists, is a whole lot of academic labor for a solution that doesn't work in the real world. (No wonder one definition of the word *academic* is "moot"!)

Because I grew up on a real dairy farm, the study of spherical cows in a vacuum never occurred to me. When I entered academia, I tried to embrace the staggering complexity of biochemistry as the point and the challenge of my research. What could possibly be gained by trying to simplify it just to fit a theoretical framework?

I don't want you to think that all of science is mired in reductionism. Particle physics, for example, chased and ultimately abandoned the reductionist dream of finding the "monad," the elementary particle that could not be divided into anything smaller.

First physicists discovered atoms. Then the big subatomic particles that we learned about in school: protons, electrons, and neutrons. Then things started getting weird. Neutrinos, quarks, muons, bosons, fermions—each was anointed the elementary particle until theory or observation pointed toward yet another division. The closer the physicists looked, the more solid matter looked like mostly empty space with a tiny particle at its core. Now cutting-edge physicists see matter as simply a dense form of energy. It's no accident that the recently discovered Higgs boson is nicknamed the "God particle." Particle physicists realize that a comprehensive wholism underpins even the most reductionist mode of observation.

Many physicists point out in wonder the self-similarity between atoms, cells, planets, galaxies, and the universe as a whole (self-similarity among different levels is one of the hallmarks of a wholistic system). And the emergence of quantum theory in the twentieth century dealt a body blow to the reductionist paradigm by inserting uncertainty into what were supposed to be purely mechanical events. Theoretical physicist and popular author Stephen Hawking has written about subatomic particles that travel backward in time. The effect, known as retrocausality, suggests that certain effects can precede their causes. Talk about putting a nail in the coffin of cause-and-effect reductionism!

Yet many scientists still operate with both feet firmly planted in a seventeenth-century Newtonian universe—especially the ones (like nutritional scientists) responsible for studying human health and disease.

HOW DO WE KNOW WHAT WE KNOW?

Scientists can argue philosophy all day long, but what really counts is evidence. This begs the question: What counts as evidence? What ways of looking for answers are considered good or bad science? Which methods are appropriate for what subjects of exploration?

The answers to these questions are themselves quite subjective, even if science believes itself to be an objective, value-free pursuit. They depend heavily on the questions being asked, and also on how the answers are sought. Epidemiologists, those scientists who study the causes of human health and disease, refer to the ways we explore scientific questions more formally as "study designs." Let's look at a few of the points on that continuum of study design, from highly wholistic to deeply reductionist. We'll take a closer look at the difference between the two and the types of evidence they collect, as well as how they affect the kind of conclusions we draw from the resulting research—especially when it comes to nutrition.

Wholistic Evidence Source #1: Ecological (or Observational) Research

One way to identify the optimal human diet, pretty obvious to all but fundamentalist reductionists, is to survey and compare populations as they already exist, and see what they eat and how healthy they are. Epidemiologists refer to this kind of study as ecological or observational. Its main characteristics include observation without intervention and looking at certain observable facts, like food intake and rates of disease, without trying to prove that one caused the other. Instead, researchers simply record the diet and disease characteristics of the populations as they are. If an ecological survey looks at those diet and disease rates in a group of people at more or less the same time, like a snapshot, it is called cross-sectional. The population under study can range in size from a small community of a few hundred people to a large country.

The results that ecological studies produce show associations between variables rather than proof that a particular input caused a particular output. These associations are often presented as correlations between input and output, the biological relevance and probable significance of which are determined statistically. Hence a study like this is also known as correlational.

Since the data collected in these studies are averages for entire populations, it is not possible to conclude causality for individuals. If we try to read causality into the data, we make a mistake known as an ecological fallacy. We might observe for various populations, for example, that a higher concentration of cars, indicative of a richer society, is correlated with a higher risk of breast cancer, also present in richer societies. It doesn't make sense to conclude that cars cause breast cancer, or to tell women fearful of breast cancer to avoid driving cars. Instead, it suggests that the two have something in common that warrants further study; the strength of an ecological study is its ability to highlight significant patterns and to compare the relative successes of different lifestyles. But because conclusions about specific causes cannot be made in this type of study, it is considered by reductionists to be a weak study design.

Our project in China (the main study highlighted in *The China Study*) was just such a cross-sectional, ecological study design. Using various kinds of evidence, we found that the higher the consumption of animal products in different regions of China, the greater the incidence of and mortality from a whole host of diseases, including various types of cancer, heart disease, stroke, and many others. Yet critics trumpeted that we could not claim that a plant-based diet had any effect on lowering disease rates based on that correlation, because our study design was not discriminating enough to make such a claim.

They're right in one way, but they're wrong in another. According to reductionist philosophy, it's technically correct to say that we cannot claim that a WFPB diet reduces disease risk, any more than we could say that driving cars causes breast cancer. But on close examination, the analogy breaks down. We weren't comparing one input (driving) with one output (breast cancer). Rather, we were looking at nutrition, which as we've seen is a staggeringly complex set of processes and interactions. There's really no meaningful way to reduce nutrition to a single input. I constructed the China project on the hypothesis that the effects of nutrition on health are wholistic, not reductionist. In other words, I wasn't interested in whether more vitamin C prevents the common cold; I wanted to determine, from a wholistic perspective, whether a particular diet led to markedly better health outcomes than other diets. One way to do that was to study the people in an entire ecosystem—the rural population of China—who ate in a way markedly different from populations in the West. Using the rural population of China allowed us to consider a large-enough number and variety of lifestyle factors and health and disease conditions to see the big picture—the elephant, not just the trunk or tusk. We were able to investigate hypotheses that certain groups of foods are associated with certain diseases that share similar biochemical bases. That then let us assess whether there was something about those groups of foods that might be causing or preventing and remediating those diseases.

Wholistic Evidence Source #2: Biomimicry

Another wholistic way of gaining insight into our "ideal" diet is to look at our nearest animal relatives—gorillas and chimps—and see what they eat, a strategy known as biomimicry. Primates' diets haven't changed much in tens of thousands of years, unlike those of humans. So we would expect a primate's instinctual food choices to produce sustainably healthy outcomes. As well, primates in the wild haven't been influenced by fast food commercials and government propaganda, so perhaps their instincts are more trustworthy than ours. Furthermore, wild primates don't take drugs or undergo surgeries to deal with the effects of poor diets, so if a group of primates did eat unhealthy food, they probably would become too sick and obese to survive and reproduce.

According to Janine Benyus, author of *Biomimicry*, early humans probably used this wholistic research strategy to determine which plants were safe and which were toxic. After all, it makes evolutionary sense to let someone else serve as your taster!

While not conclusive, animal observation can give us a starting point for our own dietary explorations. For example, just noticing that chimps and gorillas have strong bones and muscles while eating WFPB undercuts the notion that humans need lots of animal protein to grow and maintain muscle mass. And of course we can point to the largest land animals in the world, elephants and hippos, whose 100 percent plant-based diets don't seem to render them weak or scrawny.

In short, biomimicry reframes the issue of nutrition as one in which humans are seen as one species among many. Observing animals that resemble us can provide insight into diet in a way that observing human eating habits, which have been affected by human technologies from agriculture to refrigeration to processing, can't. It also identifies areas of current research where we may be wrong (i.e., by casting doubt) as well as suggesting areas of further reductionist inquiry.

Wholistic Evidence Source #3: Evolutionary Biology

A third wholistic approach is that of evolutionary biology, in which we examine our physiology and determine what our bodies have evolved to ingest and process. For example, we can look at the length of our digestive systems, the numbers and shape of our teeth, our upright postures, the shape of our jaws, and the pH of our stomachs, among many other characteristics, and compare those elements to known carnivores and herbivores. (We see, by the way, that we share almost all the characteristics of herbivores, and have almost nothing in common with carnivores.) By doing so, we can use reverse engineering to discover possibilities for the kinds of foods our bodies are "built" to eat.

Reductionist Study Evidence Type #1: Prospective Experiments

The most well-regarded (and therefore best-funded and most common) form of reductionist study design is prospective, meaning that information is recorded in real time, and effects are observed as they occur. In its simplest form, one group of subjects (the experimental group) is given an intervention, while the other group (the control group) is not. The gold standard of reductionist research is a form of prospective experiment known as the randomized controlled trial. The "random" part of the study refers to the way subjects are assigned to either the experimental or control group. The theory here is that random assignment eliminates the effects of potentially confounding variables by evenly distributing them across all groups. If you're worried about whether being a heavy smoker might influence the results of an intervention, random assignment uses the power of statistics to spread this variable evenly across groups, theoretically making it irrelevant.

Randomly controlled trials often include a double-blind feature, wherein neither the researcher nor the subject knows whether the subject is receiving the intervention being tested. In a drug trial, for instance, neither would know whether the pill the subject is taking is the actual substance or a lookalike placebo. That way, patients don't get better just because they think they're taking a wonder pill,[1] and researchers don't subconsciously treat a placebo subject differently than a subject taking the active compound.

Prospective experiments are seen as a "clean" form of study design, because they nail down the details with more precision, and because they minimize the messiness and "noise" of the real world. This allows researchers to isolate the effects of the intervention in which they're interested. This isolation of a single variable (X) supposedly gives the researcher the right to say, "X causes Y," where Y is an outcome that occurs after X and does not occur when X is not present.

This is most useful in cases where it makes sense to isolate a single factor, as when we need to assess the safety and effectiveness of a new drug. But even in the case of drug tests, there's an inherent trade-off between that kind of certainty within a controlled environment and its applicability in the messy, noisy real world. The more perfectly controlled the experiment, the less it resembles reality.

While studying specific chemicals in isolation provides for pretty findings, these research methods cannot provide predictive models for complex interactions with multiple causes and effects—in other words, *life*.

Reductionist Study Evidence Type #2: Case-Control Study

Another commonly used research design, regarded as less discriminating by reductionist researchers than the prospective experiment, is the case-control study. The cases—individuals who, for example, have a disease—are compared with the controls—individuals of the same sex, age group, and so forth, who do not have the disease, as researchers look for lifestyle differences between the two groups that could have influenced their different outcomes. Case-control studies typically examine influences that cannot practically or ethically be imposed on people: diets, lifestyle practices, and exposure to toxins are common examples. You wouldn't force half of the people in your study to eat all their meals at McDonald's, for example, but you could find people who choose this diet on their own and see what happens to them.

Case-control studies can be retrospective when researchers use previously recorded observations to explain disease outcomes. They can also be prospective, in which cohorts of subjects with different lifestyles and diets are studied to see what will happen to them. Either way, because subjects aren't randomly assigned to these cohorts, it's impossible to prove that the differences caused the outcomes. The problem is, people who are alike on one characteristic are probably alike on many others. It's impossible to tell which characteristic or characteristics were the active agents leading to the varying outcomes. So researchers typically resort to a family of statistical procedures to make this problem go away, called "adjusting for confounding."

Here's how statistical adjustment for confounding works. Suppose you are studying the relationship between breast cancer and dietary fat. You start with two groups, one made up of women who have been diagnosed with breast cancer (the cases), and one made up of women who have not been diagnosed with breast cancer (the controls). You question them about their eating habits to figure out if the cases are eating more dietary fat than the controls. But there's a problem: the women with breast cancer carry a higher percentage of their body weight as fat. Assuming that there is a relationship between dietary fat and body fat to begin with, what's causing what here? Is the dietary fat causing the breast cancer? Or are the women more prone to obesity also more susceptible to breast cancer?

The more questions we allow ourselves to ask, and the more possible interactions we entertain, the further we plunge into a reductionist nightmare. Maybe these women with breast cancer and a higher percentage of body fat have a genetic predisposition both to obesity and to breast cancer, so therefore we may not have to worry about how much fat women without that same genetic predisposition consume. Maybe there's some other variable that we haven't even thought about; perhaps heavier women exercise less, or are more depressed because of societal prejudice, and that's the factor that leads to breast cancer. Or maybe they're heavier because they're depressed, and tend to eat more and exercise less. Or maybe they're heavier because they are less educated about healthy eating, which sometimes correlates with less access to healthcare, which correlates to low income, which correlates to less access to fresh produce, which correlates to living in neighborhoods with higher concentrations of environmental toxins.

To deal with this uncertainty, reductionists use statistics to mathematically "hold constant" all these potential sources of data pollution and make their effects magically disappear—that is, they compare, in effect, small segments of each group whose confounding variables are nearly the same. Of course, you can do this only to those confounding variables you're able to think of and then measure in some way. No study has unlimited time or money, so there will always be potentially confounding variables that don't get neutralized by the statistical magic wand.

But the more we scientists try to disentangle the web of influences around a specific health outcome, the less useful the "results" of a study become. Suppose, in the breast cancer example, we "adjust" for every other influence we can think of, so that the only two variables that remain are rates of breast cancer and obesity. If we then say that obese women seem to get more breast cancer, the prescription to prevent breast cancer immediately collapses into "lose weight." Any method that purports to take off the pounds then becomes a form of breast cancer prevention. Meal-replacement shakes, low-carb regimens, lemon juice fasts, and all manner of craziness would now be tied to a healthy outcome, regardless of the actual mechanism of the relationship between obesity and breast cancer. Suppose that increased rates of breast cancer and obesity are both functions of highly processed diets with lots of animal products and not enough whole-plant products. For many women who follow this weight-loss regimen, the "get thin by any means to prevent breast cancer" message could translate into diet choices that would increase, not decrease, their cancer risk.

It's as if you noticed that happy people tend to smile more than unhappy people, so you invented a device that stretched the human face into a smile as a cure for depression. Yes, the smile is a good marker for happiness. Yes, there's a correlation between smiling and happiness. Yes, it's possible that reminding yourself to smile more can affect your mood. But isolating the smile and ignoring all other factors that might contribute to happiness and depression is patently ridiculous.

Think these examples sound unbelievable? We'll talk more in chapter eleven about a real-world consequence of this kind of narrowly reductionist research when we look at the hype surrounding dietary supplements. In this hype, researchers have used statistical adjustment to conclude that certain nutrients are not just markers of good health, but the cause of it, ignoring clusters of factors surrounding those nutrients as if they didn't matter or even exist. The result of this miscalculation isn't merely a waste of vitamin-takers' money; in some cases, the outcomes have been serious illness and even premature death.

WHOLISTIC VERSUS
REDUCTIONIST RESEARCH

The reason wholistic ways of exploring reality come under fire from many contemporary scientists is that they all smack of fuzziness, of imprecision. They don't narrow cause and effect to the point where everything is airtight, completely repeatable, and measurable to the fifth decimal place, the way reductionist experimental design does.

Reductionism by definition seeks to eliminate all "confounding" factors: any variables that might influence the outcome in addition to the main substance under investigation. But because nutrition is a wholistic phenomenon, it simply doesn't make any sense to study it as if it were a single variable. Studying nutrition as if it were a single-function pill disregards its complex interactions.

The whole point of wholism is that you can't tease out one contribution and ignore the rest. Of course body fat, dietary fat, education level, depression, socioeconomic standing, and so many more characteristics are interrelated and interactive with one another and with our bodies' systems. While statistical adjustments can pretend to wrap up reality into neat little packages, they don't explain the underlying reality at all.

You can't study wholistic phenomena solely through reductionist modes of inquiry without sacrificing reality and truth in the process.

A NEW NUTRITIONAL
RESEARCH PARADIGM

At its best, epidemiology draws conclusions from many different types of study design, just as a group of blind elephant scholars pool their findings to increase their understanding of the whole beast. Sadly, however, only reductionist studies are taken seriously and funded generously, so much so that the entire field of epidemiology is substantially biased in favor of reductionist philosophy. You wouldn't give an electron microscope to someone studying elephants and expect them to tell you anything about the animals' personalities or social structures. The only way to find wholistic answers is to allow for the possibility of seeing them.

Reductionist critics argue that the China Study was experimentally weak because it didn't prove independent effects of single agents or show results applicable for individual people. As I hope I've shown in this chapter, this criticism is misguided. We don't need to know the effects of single agents on health, because this is not the way that nature works. Nutrition has a wholistic effect on health; one that we consistently miss and misinterpret when we focus on isolated nutrients. Our project in China, when evaluated from a wholistic perspective as intended by the study's design, provided unique evidence on cause-and-effect relationships between diet and disease through highly significant patterns of association between food consumption and health outcomes.

For drug trials, the most informative study is the randomized control trial. But for nutrition, the most informative study design is the wholistic study: one that allows us to see how unimaginably complex interactions can be influenced, and how radiant health can be achieved through simple dietary choices.

7

Reductionist
Biology

Explanations always go in one direction, from the
complex to the simple and, in particular, toward
what is less distinctly human.

—T. H. JONES

We've just looked at how reductionist design leads to reductionist answers and excludes the true nature of biological complexity. Now it's time to revel in that mind-boggling complexity, specifically when it comes to nutrition.

In this chapter I want to introduce you to an old friend of mine: an enzyme called mixed function oxidase (MFO), which ultimately converted me from a reductionist to a wholist.[1] Sharing more about the function of enzymes, those amazingly complex and powerful molecules responsible for every chemical reaction that goes on in our bodies, is the best way I can think of to show you the complexity of nutrition's effect on health—and the inadequacy of the reductionist model of scientific inquiry to address it.

MY MFO BACKSTORY: PEANUTS
AND LIVER CANCER

As I mentioned in the book's introduction, my first official research project as a professor at Virginia Tech back in 1965 was to analyze peanut samples for the presence of the cancer-causing chemical aflatoxin (AF).[2] A product of the mold *Aspergillus flavus*,[3] AF had recently been shown to be a very potent liver carcinogen for laboratory rats.[4] On the list of America's most popular foods, peanuts rank somewhere up there with milk and T-bone steaks. They're what help keep hands busy at cocktail parties; they're half of that most beloved of lunchbox sandwiches, the PB&J. So the possibility of a mold-produced carcinogen in peanuts was a dreadful thought. The other troubling aspect of these findings was that the amounts of AF required for liver cancer in rats appeared to be exceptionally low, possibly making AF the most potent chemical carcinogen ever discovered, at least for rats.[5]

My team's task was to learn something about the climatic and geographic conditions that fostered *Aspergillus flavus* growth. We studied several edible plants, but focused specifically on peanuts.

Shortly thereafter, the dean who hired me at Virginia Tech, Charlie Engel, asked me to join him in developing the nationwide childhood nutrition program in the Philippines in collaboration with Manila's Department of Health—a project funded by USAID. One of our main goals was to identify a source of protein for these children that could be grown locally and relatively inexpensively. The obvious answer, at least to us, would have been peanuts. They're high in protein, most kids love them, and they grow like crazy in a wide variety of climates and settings. There was just one problem: AF.

Before we could grow peanuts to solve the protein gap, we had to understand and solve the potential AF contamination problem. Because of my earlier experience with AF, that became my assignment. After setting up and equipping an analytical laboratory in Manila, I then began with my colleagues in the Philippines to explore the chief food sources of AF consumption. Were peanuts the main source of contamination? What about other foods? Did the people eating AF-contaminated foods really get more liver cancer? If so, what could we do to eliminate AF, or neutralize its negative effects, so we could use peanuts as a cost-effective protein source for the poor?

We started by collecting peanut products from the marketplace. Shelled peanuts, the more expensive product purchased by the affluent (our original samples came from a cocktail party at the U.S. Embassy!) were clean, with little or no AF. In contrast, peanut butter, a cheaper product especially consumed in urban centers like Manila, was heavily contaminated. All of the twenty-nine peanut butter samples we initially collected contained AF, with an average of 500 parts per billion (ppb),[6] but with exceptional levels as high as 8,600 ppb.[7] These findings were alarming because, at that time, the U.S. FDA had proposed an upper limit of 30 ppb as a "safe" level in human food (later revised downward because even lower levels were shown to cause serious toxicity and cancer in rats, rainbow trout, and very young ducklings).[8]

To learn the reasons for this huge discrepancy in AF levels between whole cocktail peanuts and peanut butter, I joined the Philippines' FDA Commissioner in a visit to a peanut butter manufacturing plant. The answer was easy to see. In the manufacturing plant, whole peanuts in their shells were placed onto one end of a conveyer belt, which moved past a line of workers; at the end of the moving belt, the peanuts were delivered into a grinder and a big cooking pot. As the peanuts passed by the workers, they handpicked kernels for the cocktail peanuts, leaving the rest to be dumped into the grinder and cook pot to make peanut butter. The good, attractive kernels went into the cocktail jars, the bad into the peanut butter tank. By "bad," I mean the discolored, often shriveled kernels—the ones most likely to be infected with the fungus. These kernels, we learned when we tested them, contained AF in concentrations as high as two million parts per billion, meaning that even a single fungus-contaminated kernel could spoil an entire batch of peanut butter and easily push AF levels over the allowable limit.[9]

With additional funding from the National Health Institute, I then did a quick survey of possible consumers of AF and learned that, just like in the United States, children ate most of the peanut butter in the Philippines. Because I assumed that virtually all commercially sold peanut butter was contaminated, my coworkers and I then visited homes to ask whether they customarily ate peanut butter and, if so, whether we could purchase any partly emptied jars for AF analysis. We also asked the mother in the household for an estimate of when and how much peanut butter had been consumed in the previous twenty-four to forty-eight hours, and from this I estimated actual AF consumption. We also collected urine specimens from each family member so that, for future follow-up studies, we might be able to measure some product of AF in the urine as a reliable marker of AF ingestion.[10]

I therefore had estimates both of AF consumption and excretion and was able to show that AF metabolites only appeared in the urine samples of those individuals consuming the AF-contaminated peanut butter.[11] We also found that consumers of AF-contaminated foods were excreting AF metabolites in their urine that proved carcinogenic[12] to animal test subjects.[13]

MFO, AF, AND CANCER

Throughout this research period, I continued to believe, as other researchers did, that AF might be an important carcinogen for humans. But I also understood that this very potent animal carcinogen had not yet been shown to be a human carcinogen—at least not in an independent manner. We knew at that time, for example, that the mouse, unlike the rat, was not susceptible to AF carcinogenicity,[14] and if these closely related species responded to AF in totally opposite ways, one susceptible and one resistant, it was not unreasonable to assume that humans might also be resistant as well. Clearly we still had a lot to learn about AF's connection to cancer: was it relevant to humans, and if so, what was the causal mechanism?[15]

In exploring these questions, I started with the assumption that the MFO enzyme was involved because evidence suggesting its relationship to AF and cancer already had been published by a research group in England.[16] It showed that MFO was responsible for converting AF into not one but several less carcinogenic products that were excreted in milk and urine. The more efficiently MFO functioned (i.e., the more "active" it was), the more AF was detoxified, suggesting that increasing MFO activity might lower the risk of liver cancer.

At around the same time, researchers were discovering that MFO's activity could be modified—sped up, slowed down, and altered in other ways—by certain agents, like drugs.[17] In my laboratory, we were finding that increasing dietary protein increased MFO activity.[18] Perhaps, we thought, protein could be used to supercharge MFO and stop cancer in its tracks.

Then I stumbled upon that 1968 report from India I mentioned in chapter three that showed what appeared to be the opposite: namely, that higher dietary protein *increased* AF-induced tumor development.[19] That couldn't be! Protein, everyone's favorite nutrient, could cause cancer? And the protein they used was casein, the principal protein in the healthiest drink there was: cow's milk. I needed to learn more about this finding and either reproduce it or refute it as a fluke.

At the same time I was discovering an equally unsettling fact about childhood liver cancer in the Philippines: it occurred with much higher frequency not necessarily in the children who consumed greater quantities of AF, but in children from wealthier families, the ones who ate more protein and more "high quality" animal protein. The Indian protein/tumor study and the Philippine animal protein/cancer connection were starting to shake my world. Did more protein prevent cancer or cause cancer?

The possible key to solving this mystery was MFO, the startling enzyme that was now implicated both in the initiation of liver cancer by AF and in the detoxification and disposal of AF from the body. What was going on? Did dietary protein speed up MFO's conversion of AF into nontoxic water-soluble metabolites? Or did it activate AF into nasty carcinogenic metabolites? Or both? We suspected we were on to something much bigger than just a way to neutralize or promote AF-induced liver cancer. We theorized that MFO might be a key factor in turning cancer on and off not just in the liver, but possibly also in other tissues in the human body.

This paradoxical protein effect hinted at what we eventually found to be the case: MFO responds to the foods that we eat every day. Certain diets turn MFO into a highly efficient cancer-fighting machine; other diets send MFO into a frenzy that produces carcinogenic by-products.

To understand how this is possible, we need to look at nutrition and how it affects enzymes more generally. Not only will we resolve the MFO–AF paradox, we'll also see how reductionist nutritional thinking simply can't handle the question—and thereby misses the most powerful lever we possess in our effort to eradicate cancer.

THE BIOCHEMICAL BASIS OF NUTRITION

If you took high school biology, you probably spent some time memorizing bits of a chart of aerobic respiration known as the Krebs cycle. That chart, if it didn't put you to sleep first, probably gave you the idea that nutrition is a very linear process. From the inputs of carbohydrates, fats, and proteins, the cells in the body predictably extract energy, produce a myriad collection of useful metabolites, and release leftover carbon dioxide and water. The arrows that connect different steps in the process seem authoritative, as if the described step always happens in precisely the same way every place, every time, under every condition. While this model is useful for understanding the basics, it doesn't reliably correspond to reality. Nutrition is far more complex than a static diagram might imply.

Nutrients generally do not follow a single predictable path after they enter the trillions of cells in our bodies. In most cases, the potential route a nutrient can take once it enters the body branches out, directly or indirectly, into multiple pathways of products (metabolites), with each pathway possibly branching out into still more pathways. Furthermore as these pathways develop, they may lead to many different kinds of activities or functions, like mobilization of energy and repair of damaged cells. The dominant pathways end up determining to a great extent whether we enjoy health or suffer disease. Understanding metabolism is not just a matter of following a nutrient down a large number of independent pathways, however. As these pathways branch out, their integration with one another seems endless.

Maps of these metabolic mazes decorate the walls of many research facilities; your high school Krebs cycle chart is just a highly pared-down version of part of one of them. I've been in this research business long enough that I've been able to watch the emergence of one of the most complex of these maps, which began many years ago as the glucose-metabolism network of reactions that produces energy shown in Figure 7-1. (This particular chart, which does an excellent job of displaying the complexity of intermediary metabolism, is the work of Dr. William L. Elliott [HealthBuilding.com].) The earliest version of this map was most helpful as I taught biochemistry during the 1960s and 1970s at Virginia Tech's Department of Biochemistry and Nutrition. It took me at least a dozen lectures in a basic biochemistry course merely to describe the series of

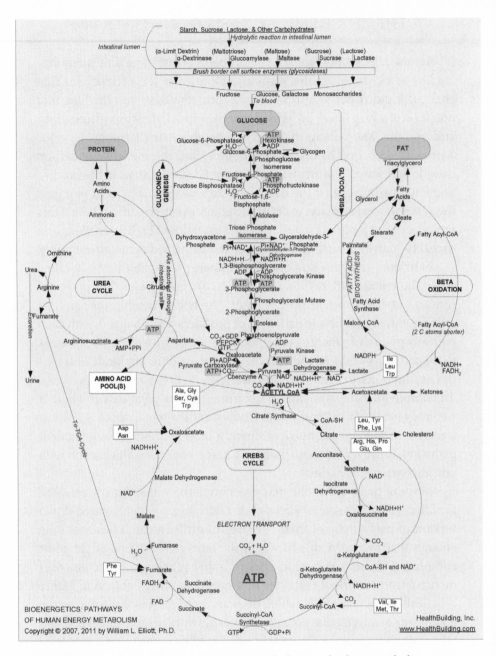

FIGURE 7-1.   Chart mapping glucose metabolism and other metabolic pathways[20]

reactions that lead from glucose to the circular Krebs cycle at the bottom of the chart, primarily representing the extraction of energy from glucose.

Complicated, right? But the map I used in class only scratched the surface of what we know now about glucose's metabolic pathway. Over time, more clusters of metabolic reactions were added to that initial map, including segments on protein, fat, and nucleic acid metabolism. It wasn't long before so many reactions had been added, and the font size had become so small for reasonably sized paper, that it was clear that no more could be added and still be readable by the naked eye. The metabolic cartographers began creating entire atlases of cellular metabolism, with what had once been simple reactions now meriting several pages of diagramming to account for updated discoveries.

These comprehensive maps became more and more specialized and fragmented in a way that graphically symbolizes how reductionism, by pushing for ever smaller and more specific pieces of information, loses sight of the whole. Researchers spent years, even decades, working on just one or two reactions. Gradually, insets of insets of insets emerged on the map, as our probes of knowledge went ever deeper into cellular metabolism and grew ever less able to see the intelligence and power of the whole system.

A phrase with the same root as *reductionism* is "reductio ad absurdum," or following a concept to the point of absurdity. Remember Figure 7-1's complex chart showing glucose metabolism? You can see an updated version in Figure 7-2.

Scientists have gone even deeper than this. Figure 7-3 shows the complexity involved in just a very small section of that map, blown up for visibility.

And the more comprehensive metabolic map in Figure 7-2 is only an infinitesimally small portion of all the reactions in each of our hundred trillion cells.

I emphasize this metabolic complexity so you can see just how impossible it is to fully understand the way our bodies react to the foods we eat and the nutrients they contain. Explaining nutrient function by only one or even a couple of these reactions is not sufficient. Once consumed, nutrients interact with one another and with other food-borne chemicals within an enormous maze of metabolic reactions located in these hundred trillion cells. No single reaction or single mechanism accounts for

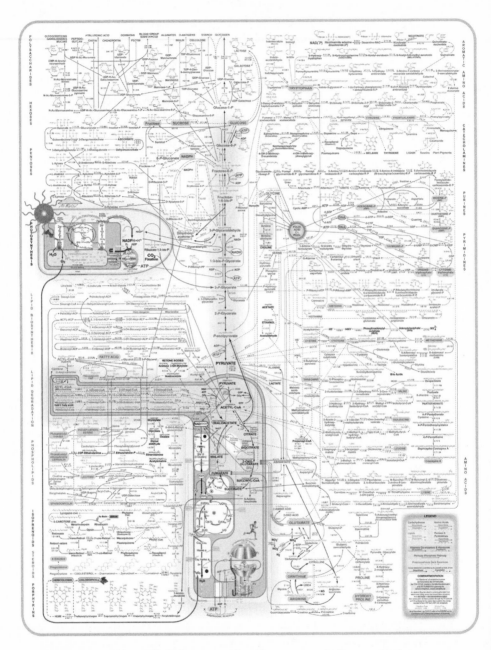

FIGURE 7-2. Expanded chart mapping glucose metabolism and other metabolic pathways

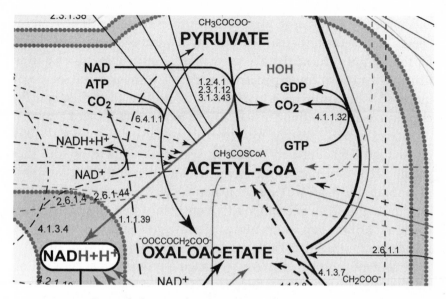

FIGURE 7-3. Expanded inset of Figure 7-2

an individual nutrient's effect. Every nourishing nutrient and related food chemical enters cellular metabolism and gets metabolized into multiple products via highly integrated pathways just as complex as those as shown in Figures 7-1 to 7-3.

The fact that each nutrient passes through such a maze of reaction pathways suggests that each nutrient also is likely to participate in multiple health and disease outcomes. The one nutrient/one disease relationship implied by reductionism, although widely popular, is simply incorrect. Every nutrient-like chemical that enters this complex system of reactions creates a rippling effect that may extend far into the pool of metabolism. And with every bite of food we eat, there are tens and probably hundreds of thousands of food chemicals entering this metabolism pool more or less simultaneously.

METABOLISM AND ENZYMES

Metabolism is the sum total of all the chemical reactions in the body that sustain life. When you think of the billions of reactions that occur all the time, you might wonder how we have enough energy in our bodies to get anything else done. After all, every one of those chemical reactions requires energy. And since one of the main outputs of metabolism is usable energy for the body, it's crucial that the energy produced be greater—by a wide margin—than the energy expended to produce it. Fortunately, we've evolved molecules whose main job is to significantly lower the energy required for chemical reactions within the body. These molecules are called *enzymes.*

I used enzymes, earlier, to help explain why a part cannot be fully understood outside the context of its system as a whole, an idea that should become even more clear as we look further at the role they play in the body. Enzymes are large protein molecules, present in all our cells, that, through a series of reactions, turn one thing (say, a sugar molecule), called a *substrate*, into another (say, a glucose-related chemical the body uses to synthesize fat), called a *product* or *metabolite.* Think of enzymes as large, fully-automated factories. Imagine inserting a small log (the substrate) into one end of a huge factory building and, at the exit end, collecting a nicely designed salad bowl (the product). You could turn the log into a salad bowl by hand, of course, but it would require much more time and labor. The factory dramatically increases the efficiency of the transformation. Enzymes do the same inside cells, converting substrates into products very quickly while using very little energy. The reactions enzymes cause (the word biologists use is that they *catalyze* reactions) rarely, if ever, occur without the assistance of an enzyme. If they do, the rate of reaction—the speed with which the reaction occurs—is a minuscule fraction of what is possible when an enzyme is involved, and the amount of energy required is much higher.

Comparatively speaking, enzymes are very large. An enzyme molecule might be 10,000 to 20,000 times the size of a substrate molecule that it processes—hence the visual of the factory and the log. Figure 7-4 shows a substrate, A, being converted to a product, B. But most reactions do not occur in isolation. They connect with follow-on reactions, like the one in Figure 7-4 where B (now the substrate) is converted to C (the new product). Enzyme 1 converts A to B, while enzyme 2 converts B to C.

A given enzyme can function at different levels of potency based on supply (the amount of substrate available) and demand (the amount of product already in the cell). Just as factory assembly lines can move quickly or slowly based on the supply of raw materials and the demand for finished goods, enzymes adjust the speed at which they convert substrate

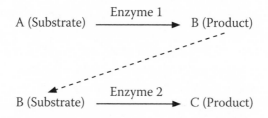

A (Substrate) ⎯⎯ Enzyme 1 ⎯⎯▶ B (Product)

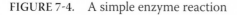

B (Substrate) ⎯⎯ Enzyme 2 ⎯⎯▶ C (Product)

FIGURE 7-4. A simple enzyme reaction

to product (known in the trade as its *activity*). In fact, an enzyme can even reverse reactions to return a product to its substrate. In short, enzymes control whether reactions occur and, if so, how fast and in which direction.

When they initially form, enzymes appear as linear chains of amino acids, carefully arranged in sequences dictated by DNA. But because amino acids have chemical and physical affinities for each other, the chain folds onto itself (as in Figure 7-5), creating a three-dimensional shape the same way a very long string of magnetic beads might.

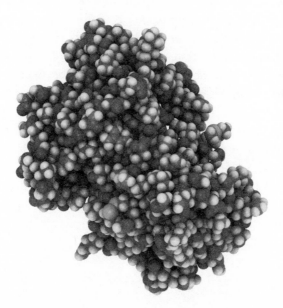

FIGURE 7-5. Computer-developed model of the enzyme cyclic ADP ribose hydrolase (CD38)

This folding gives enzymes one way to vary their activity: they simply change shape. This enzymatic shapeshifting is crucial because it changes the enzyme's chemical and physical properties in ways that alter its ability to modify reaction rates. Many scientists who study enzymes wax poetic about the incomprehensible speed with which enzymes configure themselves to perform their tasks. Here's a typical entry, from the *New World Encyclopedia*:

> For an enzyme to be functional, it must fold into a precise three-dimensional shape. How such a complex folding can take place remains a mystery. A small chain of 150 amino acids making up an enzyme has an extraordinary number of possible folding configurations: if it tested 1,012 different configurations every second, it would take about 1,026 years to find the right one.... Yet, a denatured enzyme can refold within fractions of a second and then precisely react in a chemical reaction.... [I]t demonstrates a stunning complexity and harmony in the universe.[21]

The author cites numbers for a relatively small (by enzyme standards) hypothetical molecule in his attempt to describe the indescribable. The rapidity with which an enzyme responds (from a limp linear chain to a precise glob ready to do its business, in fractions of a second) is phenomenal. The chemical variety of substrates that can be metabolized by a single active enzyme is likewise phenomenal. And the large number of factors capable of modifying enzyme structure, amount, and activity is equally phenomenal.

Inherent in this discussion is the intimate connection between nutrient metabolism and the world of enzymes. Enzyme-catalyzed reactions, infinite in number and infinitely networked, are controlled by nutrients and related compounds, which also are infinite in number. Although nutrients control enzymes, enzymes also act *on* nutrients to manufacture endless products that are then used in the body as well as for the proper functioning of the body.

THE MFO PARADOX

Which brings us, finally, back to MFO and the role it plays in cancer formation.

Unavoidably, I've had to summarize, truncate, and simplify our research and findings here—the topic is just too extensive and too technical to explain in a single chapter. My goal here, after all, is not to turn you into an MFO expert. Rather, in sharing the tale of my fifty-plus-year research journey with MFO, I hope to give you a better understanding of how animal protein affects cancer formation, and a deeper appreciation of how the complexity of MFO eloquently testifies to a wholistic, not reductionist, view of nutrition and health.

MFO is a particularly complex enzyme that metabolizes many chemicals, some normally present in the body and others the body might never have encountered previously. Located largely but not exclusively in the liver, MFO metabolizes steroid-type hormones (e.g., sex hormones like estrogens and androgens, and stress hormones), fatty acids (i.e., precursors to chemicals that support the immune and neurological systems), and cholesterol (involved in cardiovascular disease and the building of cell membranes), among other chemicals, into substances that are closer to the state in which our bodies will ultimately use them. MFO also detoxifies foreign chemicals, rendering them capable of being readily excreted in the urine.

Very early in my research career I was taught that AF (like other carcinogens) is converted by the MFO enzyme to a less toxic metabolite that is excreted in the urine and feces, as is shown in Figure 7-6.

But this model was clearly too simple. For one thing, the Indian researchers I mentioned earlier, who in 1968 published their finding that a high-protein (20 percent) diet increased AF-initiated liver tumors in rats,[22] previously had shown that this same high-protein diet actually decreased the immediate toxicity of AF when it is administered at very high doses.[23] The results were a paradox that the traditional model of AF metabolism didn't account for.

Suspecting MFO as the key to resolving this paradox, my lab started by establishing that the high-protein diet increased MFO enzyme activity in rats,[24] meaning that the more dietary protein the rat consumed, the

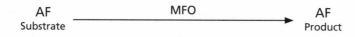

FIGURE 7-6. Presumed model for MFO conversion of AF

faster AF (specifically, the parent substrate, AFB1) was detoxified. This was the finding that made sense, but it ran counter to the Indian researchers' observation[25] that cancer *increased* with a high-protein diet.

One possibility we considered was that the MFO enzyme might be producing two kinds of metabolites: one that was less toxic than AF and safely excreted, and one that was more toxic than AF that gave rise to cancer. But why would an enzyme do such a strange and contradictory thing? Even though it seems strange, it was a real possibility in our minds; for a long time, before this and before the MFO enzyme was discovered, scientists thought that many chemical carcinogens initiated cancer only after they were "activated" by enzymes, and so a chemical like AF producing a more toxic metabolite sounded very possible.

Another key to the puzzle was discovered in the early 1970s, when University of Wisconsin Professors Jim and Betty Miller, both distinguished cancer researchers, working with their younger colleague, Colin Garner, obtained some remarkable evidence: MFO's production of a detoxified metabolite from AF involves forming an extremely reactive intermediate metabolite that initiates cancer.[26] In other words, MFO produces two metabolic products from AF: one that is detoxified and excreted, and one that is activated to initiate cancer. It's as if a tree enters the factory, gets turned into a billy club for a fraction of a second, and only then is transformed into its ultimate shape, a salad bowl.

This intermediate metabolite is known as an *epoxide*, and it's thought to exist only for a few milliseconds. Those milliseconds, unfortunately, appear to be long enough to allow the epoxide to bind very tightly to cell DNA and produce a mutation capable of initiating a series of events that lead to cancer.

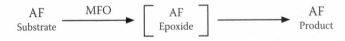

FIGURE 7-7.   MFO conversion of AF, updated with intermediate product

The updated reaction scheme, showing the intermediate epoxide, is shown in Figure 7-7.

This discovery provided us with a new way of understanding how high dietary protein increased cancer but decreased acute AF toxicity, as first reported by the Indian researchers: when a high-protein diet increased

MFO activity, it also increased both the cancer-causing intermediate metabolite and the final, less toxic metabolites.

Another of our key findings that helped explain this paradox: AF, it turns out, is quite toxic in its own right, without requiring activation; it blocks cell respiration, causing cells to die.[27] When a high-protein diet increases MFO activity, it detoxifies the AF that causes cell death—which, out of context, seems like a positive effect. But at the same time, it increases production of the epoxide that can initiate cancer—clearly a negative effect.

Our reaction scheme, one more time, updated to summarize the effects of these AF metabolites (the less toxic metabolite and the carcinogenic epoxide) in the presence of a high-protein diet, is shown in Figure 7-8.

Although we thought this was a reasonably good explanation for our paradox, it left a few questions unanswered. The first is the question of why the body produces a cancer-initiating epoxide in the first place. Or more to the point: how did a process that turns a natural but dangerous mold by-product into an equally dangerous cancer-causing substance evolve in the first place?

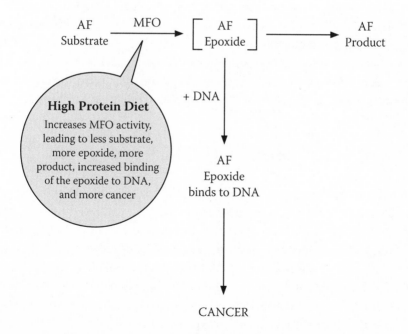

FIGURE 7-8.   Final revised model for MFO conversion of AF

I still don't know the answer to this question. But it does make sense that the body would be willing to tolerate the risk of future cancer in its urgent effort to deal with the immediate threat of cell death posed by AF. Imperfect though it may be, this trade-off clearly proved to be evolutionarily positive, or at least neutral—it couldn't have contributed negatively to human survival and reproduction, or else it wouldn't have survived to the present. This suggests that the body may have a self-correcting mechanism to prevent permanent damage from the epoxide. The epoxide has an unusually short life, existing only for fractions of a millisecond, which does not leave much time for damage to occur. It also turns out that water, aided by another enzyme that is close at hand during this process, epoxide hydrolase, can bind with the epoxide to form harmless products that can be excreted—effectively mopping up epoxide before it can damage DNA.

In addition, we also know that the human body has an amazing capacity to repair damaged DNA. If this ability is supported through proper nutrition, most if not all of the damage can be undone long before cancer is initiated.

The second question is why animal protein increases MFO's activity. A high-animal-protein diet increases a broad array of enzyme activities in the body, of which MFO is only one; animal protein generally puts the body into overdrive. As of this point, we do not yet have an answer for why this occurs. Perhaps in the future we will. In the meantime, the important point is that it does, and that it has a negative effect on our health.

WHAT MFO TAUGHT ME

What you may have noticed about my initial research into AF's connection to liver cancer is that its focus on a single MFO-catalyzed reaction was very reductionist, even though I also took into account other straightforward, reductionist reactions that may or may not have been important to whether liver cancer developed. My focus on a single enzyme (MFO) that presumably catalyzed a single reaction, involving a single substrate (AF) and a single outcome (liver cancer), was naïve to the extreme, and my later search for the mechanism to explain the effect of dietary protein on cancer would prove to be far more complex than a simple MFO-dependent reaction. But it was this period of research with MFO that first forced an awareness of the mind-numbing biological complexity of the body that I had not fully comprehended beforehand.

Consider just a few examples of the complexity MFO presents. First, the MFO enzyme itself is architecturally very complicated. It's comprised of three main components—really a system more than a single protein-based enzyme. In our research, we investigated the contributions of each of these components to the overall enzyme activity by isolating and reconstituting them into different combinations.[28] We also examined these combinations under the influence of dietary protein feeding.[29] Each combination exhibited a different MFO activity—a broad continuum of endless complexity. With just a small chemical nudge here or there, MFO and other enzyme molecules can change their shapes and thereby alter their reaction rates— all within time frames too short to document or estimate.

Second, MFO is only one in a series of enzymes, all more properly understood as systems, and changing the activity of one enzyme in this series almost always influences other enzymes in that same series. When a substrate produces a product, it may, for example, prompt the synthesis of another downstream enzyme to assist in subsequent reactions, and/or send a signal back upstream to the enzyme that initiated the first reaction to slow things down. In AF catalysis, as mentioned, epoxide hydrolase allows the MFO-generated epoxide to bond to water.[30] Further down the line, the detoxified AF metabolite may be bonded to a variety of products to expedite their excretion[31] from the body. Enzymes and their reactions are extensively and unavoidably interdependent.

Third, MFO metabolizes an incredible variety of native and foreign chemicals. Most intriguing, it can rapidly adjust to metabolize even synthetic chemicals never before seen in nature or encountered by the body. It's as if MFO were a factory that can reconfigure itself instantly, turning out salad bowls one second and framing timber the next—a truly remarkable feat.

HOMEOSTASIS: THE BASIS OF HEALTH

We talk in nutritional science about something called *homeostasis*, the body's tendency to always work toward maintaining a stable, functional equilibrium. This is true within bodily systems, from electrolyte balance to body temperature to pH balance, as well as between bodily systems. And this careful balance is what we call health.

Within cells, homeostasis is largely managed by a highly responsive array of enzymes—tens of thousands of them—working together in concert in a hundred trillion cells, all in communication with one another. And the resources they use to maintain homeostasis—to maintain health—are the foods we eat. That's why nutrition, viewed wholistically, is the crucial factor in health. When we eat the right foods, our bodies naturally tend toward homeostasis. Rather than something that needs to be wheedled and coaxed out of countless reductionist interventions, health "just happens" in spite of—or, more likely, because of—the inherent complexity of body chemistry.

MFO catalyzes so many different kinds of chemicals that it is uniquely vulnerable to changes in our diets. Even relatively modest changes lead to measurable differences, as my team witnessed when we tried to pin down its effect on cancer. When we eat the right foods, MFO moves us toward homeostasis. When we don't, MFO may contribute to disease. And MFO is just one of the 100,000 or more enzymes that contribute to the function of the human body; the chemicals we've discussed here are only a few of the substrates, intermediate metabolites, and products—whose total is larger than anyone can estimate—that interact in our body on a daily basis.

My work with MFO helped me see that each of us is an exceptionally dynamic system, one that changes every nanosecond of our lives with incredible rapidity and order in a symphony extraordinaire. This symphony is no less remarkable just because we've discovered and named some of the enzymes and other metabolic "tools" the body uses to manage and control its behavior. And that biological complexity must be acknowledged as the cornerstone of our approach to health. Unfortunately, reductionist science has become so besotted with the growing amount of that complexity it has managed to name, that it all but ignores the relationships between those elements that are the heart of homeostasis and health.

8

Genetics versus
Nutrition, Part One

*Scientists have found the gene for shyness. They
would have found it years ago, but it was hiding
behind a couple of other genes.*

—JONATHAN KATZ

In all things it is better to hope than to despair.

—JOHANN WOLFGANG VON GOETHE

In the last chapter, we saw how reductionism collapses in both theory
and practice in the face of the awe-inspiring complexity of our enzymatic
systems. We also saw how reductionist interventions usually aren't
necessary, providing we consume the right foods, as our biochemistry
naturally moves us toward healthy homeostasis. But instead of turning
their attention to nutrition and acknowledging the futility of efforts to
manipulate enzymatic activity in a way that does more good than harm,
reductionist researchers have focused upstream, on the template that
is used to manufacture those amazing enzymes: deoxyribonucleic acid,
or DNA.

Genetic medicine is the ultimate reductionist fantasy. It sidesteps all the messy big-picture factors that influence health and the development of disease, and focuses on millions and millions of tiny, deterministic elements with no room for fuzziness or randomness. It lets scientists point to a bit of DNA and say, "There, that's why you got pancreatic cancer!" And despite all the evidence calling into question a direct link between genes and cancer (and most other chronic diseases), geneticists are now pointing to bits of DNA and asserting, "There, that's why you're probably going to get pancreatic cancer within the next forty years." They're racing gleefully into a future where they can identify, isolate, and "fix" that faulty gene, to conquer disease once and for all.

For the past fifty years, medical researchers have become increasingly fascinated with understanding, mapping, and manipulating our DNA. This fascination, as we'll see over the next two chapters, has brought with it great cost, both economically and philosophically, to our beliefs about our power to influence health.

AN END TO DISEASE

Despite decades of disappointment, most of us still believe in the Big Promise of modern medicine: a world free from disease and early death, a paradise in which we no longer have to fear scourges like cancer, heart disease, diabetes, and so on.

To understand why we believe this, you need only look at the remarkable advances of twentieth-century medical science. In 1900, medicine could not reliably cure infection, transplant organs, keep people alive on respirators, replace failing kidneys with dialysis, or look deeply into our bodies with MRI and CT scans. The list of recent medical advances leads us to believe that our progress has been staggering. Why wouldn't we assume that future breakthroughs will be even more remarkable? As computers and other technologies advance, it just makes sense that someday soon, all these discoveries and inventions will save us from both our folly and most, if not all, of the diseases that still plague humankind.

The medical establishment has fanned the flames and basked in the glow of our love affair with scientific progress. After all, our collective faith in the Big Promise has funded the War on Cancer, among many others. And popular culture has enshrined the image of the selfless, heroic researcher hot on the trail of the "cure" for cancer.

Trouble is, the medical establishment hasn't had any real wins in a long time. Technology has advanced at a breakneck pace, but technologies that actually improve health outcomes have been hard to find. While death rates in developed countries plummeted in the early part of the twentieth century largely due to an understanding of hygiene,[1] none of the ultra-expensive high-tech advances of the past fifty years have made a dent in overall rates of death and disease in first-world countries. And while medicine is now much better equipped to save someone's life after an acute event like a car crash or a sudden heart attack than it was fifty years ago, we're really no better at preventing chronic degenerative diseases like heart disease and cancer, often called "diseases of affluence," than we were in the 1950s.

Yet we still look for the next medical knight on a white horse to ride to our rescue: the pill, the vaccine, the technology, the intervention that will disease-proof us and save us, not just from the diseases themselves, but from the pervasive fear of diseases that seem to strike randomly in our midst.

It's the (apparent) randomness that scares us the most. I remember the fallout when Jim Fixx, author of the 1977 bestseller *The Complete Book of Running*, died of a heart attack at the age of fifty-two. The media reported his death with an air of ironic fatalism, as proof that death would find us no matter how fervently we pursued a healthy lifestyle.

What we really want from science is an end to randomness. We want to know why diseases strike some people and not others. We want to know how to protect ourselves against the scourges that have our names on them. We want, in short, to banish unpredictability.

In a reductionist universe, you'll recall, unpredictability is not allowed. In a universe that is simply a mechanical expression of physical laws, everything is theoretically knowable. If we can't predict in advance exactly who will get pancreatic cancer or heart disease, it's simply because we haven't collected enough data yet. We don't yet have tools sensitive or powerful enough to lay bare the apparent mystery. But no fear—they're coming! In fact, they're just about here! The problem is, they've been "just about here" for the last forty years or so.

THE GENETIC EARTHQUAKE

In recent years, one discipline has gained prominence over the rest as the one that will solve all our health problems and tell us all those things we don't yet know. I'm speaking, of course, of the genetics revolution that began in the early 1950s and has been gathering steam (and money) ever since. You could argue that we are now living in the Age of Genetics. The mapping of the human genome and individual gene sequencing are the cutting edge of medical technology. DNA is the master code, right? Our entire biography and destiny, mapped out in a fantastically long and complicated blueprint. All the secrets of our development and our nature are contained in that DNA double helix: our physical appearance and function, our personality, our predisposition to various diseases. As computing power and speed increase, we continue to unravel these secrets. Soon, as a March 7, 2012 *New York Times* article trumpeted, the cost of individual gene sequencing will be as modest as that of a simple blood test, with "enormous consequences for human longevity."[2] The scientists at the Silicon Valley start-ups behind this push for fast, affordable sequencing operate from the assumption that the limiting factor in improving human health has been a lack of data. Typical of this faith is the statement of Larry Smarr, director of the California Institute of Telecommunications and Information Technology and a member of the scientific advisory board for Complete Genomics (one of Silicon Valley's gene sequencing pioneers): "For all of human history, humans have not had the readout of the software that makes them alive. Once you make the transition from a data poor to data rich environment, everything changes."[3]

These genetic crusaders view themselves as pioneers in a new age of enlightenment—specifically, reductionist enlightenment. Genes, in the genetic crusaders' view, are simply human software. Just as a good programmer can read code and predict exactly what the program will do, eventually we'll be able to look at genes and predict exactly what diseases we'll develop, perhaps even what emotions we'll experience from moment to moment.

The problem is, we can't. Genes tell us what may happen, but not if or how. The increasing fascination with and funding of genetic technology is simply another medical dead end, another reductionist rabbit hole that will lead us no further toward preventing and reversing chronic illness.

GENETIC COMPLEXITY
VERSUS REDUCTIONISM

As with nutrition, the discipline of genetics is unimaginably complex. This complexity has not filtered down to the public. Most of the population tends to think of genes as relatively fixed entities that cause us to look and function and behave in particular ways. The truth is far more interesting.

When I was on the farm, my brothers, Jack and Ron, and I each had a "self-propelled combine"—a big machine that harvested grain as we drove through the field (our way of helping our father earn money for our college education). In those days, combines were about as mechanically complex as any other machine on the market. I've forgotten how many belts and pulleys there were on my machine, but I remember well the 103 fittings that I had to fill with grease at the start of each and every day. For me it was an engineering marvel of ordered complexity. But these machines were only the beginning of the engineering marvels yet to come: ever-larger airplanes, massive ocean liners, talking radios in color (i.e., TVs), satellites and space stations, communication devices and systems, really fancy laboratory equipment, and now computers everywhere. Marvelous machines, marvelous minds! But as impressive as these engineering and technical feats may be in their complexity and order, they pale into insignificance when compared with the microcosmic universes of molecular genetics.

A SHORT LESSON IN GENETICS

As you may remember from high school biology, DNA is a long thread composed of two parallel strands that are gently twisted together into a double helix shape. Alternating sugar and phosphate molecules link to form the backbones of these adjacent strands (seen as ribbons in Figure 8-1).

Strung along these strands are four precisely arranged, or sequenced, nitrogen-containing bases, each of which is anchored to a deoxyribose unit of the strand. They are named adenine (A), thymine (T), guanine (G), and cytosine (C), and they project perpendicularly from each strand in a way that faces partner bases on the adjacent strand, thus facing inward

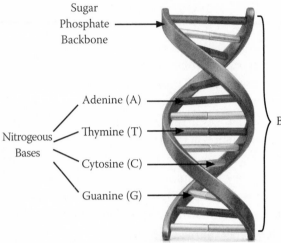

Sugar
Phosphate ———
Backbone

Adenine (A) ———

Nitrogeous — Thymine (T) ———
Bases

Cytosine (C) ———

Guanine (G) ———

Base Pairs (A-T, C-G, T-A, G-C)

FIGURE 8-1.   A DNA molecule

and holding the strands together. The facing As and Ts of each strand have a chemical affinity for each other, thus forming *base pairs*; Gs and Cs form similar pairs.

The DNA molecule is unimaginably long and harbors these four bases in a sequence that is unique for each and every person who ever lived on the planet. Because these bases act like letters of an alphabet that create words, they have the capacity to create an enormous body of information.[4]

This unique DNA chain is clipped and packed into twenty-three pairs of chromosomes located within the nucleus of each of the 100 trillion cells in our bodies (which, individually, are small enough to sit comfortably on the tip of a pin). Our cells use DNA as a blueprint for doing their work. The bases on the twenty-three chromosome pairs (about three billion bases, in total) are grouped into aggregates (around 25,000 of them) called *genes*. And each of these genes, which may contain as few as 100 bases and up to as many as several million, ultimately directs the formation of a unique protein.

However, these genes do not translate into a protein directly. Instead, they do so through the intermediate formation of ribonucleic acid (RNA) (Figure 8-2), a similar strand of bases that mirrors a DNA strand.

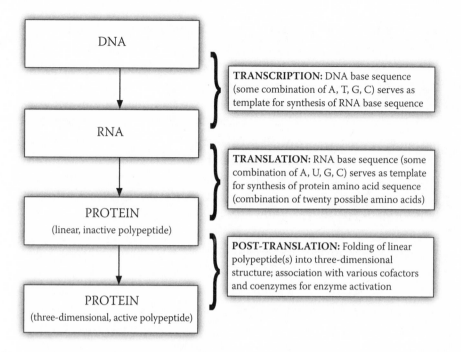

FIGURE 8-2.   The process of DNA expression into active proteins (e.g., enzymes)

The RNA base sequence serves in turn as a code for the selection of amino acids (about twenty amino acids are used in human protein production, each possessing a unique chemical structure) which, when combined into a long strand, form proteins. The bases on the RNA chains don't code for these amino acids on a one-to-one basis, however. Instead, triplet sets of bases are used, each specifying one or more amino acids. With four bases, it is possible to create sixty-four different triplet combinations or *codons* (some amino acids can be specified by more than one triplet codon).

In the early days of genetic research, scientists believed in a "one gene/ one protein" hypothesis, in which each gene was responsible for expressing a single protein. If there were 25,000 genes, then that meant there were 25,000 proteins. However, recent work in the field makes it clear that this hypothesis is too simple. For instance, more than one gene can share in the making of a single protein, because some proteins are made up of more than one strand of amino acids, and each of those amino acid strands is produced by a separate gene. The number of possible proteins and their combinations is impossible to estimate. The complexity at this point is far beyond comprehension by the human mind.

And here's another puzzle. Despite the fact that each of our cells contains the exact same genetic master template as every other cell in our bodies, these cells can do very different things. A liver cell is very different from a nerve cell or a cell on the inner surface of the intestine, both in form and in function. Their structural and functional differences depend solely on which segments of DNA bases are selected for expression within each cell. The act of selecting which bases to use among the three billion bases is an awesome display of nature at work.

To recap: relatively short segments of the DNA base sequence, called genes, are transcribed into comparable RNA sequences, which translate, in turn, into sequences of amino acids that are used to make proteins. These proteins then provide the structure and function of cells, acting as enzymes, hormones, and structural units. It is through the activity of these proteins that DNA manifests its destiny.

That manifestation of destiny—the expression of genes, how they do what they do—operates through a series of enormously complex but very orderly processes. To investigate and understand these processes, researchers like to simplify them by thinking of seemingly discrete stages or events operating one after another, like dominos falling in a row. This simplification is helpful because it allows the details of each stage to be more easily investigated and visualized, but it is not entirely reliable. In reality, these stages or events are highly interconnected and communicative, a virtually seamless and extensively integrated stream of activities.

Every point in this process may be influenced by body biochemistry, diet, physical activity, medication, mood, and just about every other variable you can think of. Not only that: the so-called stages of genetic expression influence one another, too, feeding information backward and forward in an endlessly complex series of loops. These streams of events communicate with one another in many different ways, at every enormously complex stage of the process, as we saw with the series of enzymes (which are themselves one type of protein) in chapter seven. In addition, each change in activity rate can have more than one cause.

The amounts of protein synthesized from DNA, for example, fluctuate according to how much is needed at any moment in time. When there is enough of one protein, its formation is slowed. But slowing the rate of protein synthesis can be controlled in multiple ways. The rate of DNA-to-RNA transcription, and/or the rate of protein synthesis from RNA itself, both can be altered.

This is the system that we are now tampering with, as if it were a human-made machine. Sure, we've mapped the human genome.[5] But that mapping is only the first step. We can label genes with cryptic names all we want; that doesn't mean we'll magically know what those labels mean or how emergent structures like personality, preferences, predispositions—or disease—arise from them . . . assuming it's even possible to do so.

THE GENETICIST'S DREAM

Despite the unimaginable complexity of genetics, geneticists stubbornly persist in advocating and pursuing a genetic research agenda as the future of health care. To reductionists, complexity is simply an invitation to throw more time and money at the problem. All we need is faster processing, or smarter programming, or more research. . . .

Geneticists are sure that we'll crack the genetic basis of disease in a decade or two—if not sooner. And once we do, it will lead to a revolution in health care. Knowing the identity and function of genes involved in disease formation and treatment will let us refine drug development[6] and economize clinical testing of the newly developed products. Drugs will be developed that are targeted either for specific disease-related events or, as recently announced, for individuals whose genes define their likely drug responsiveness. In doing so, drug side effects would be minimized and costs of clinical trials would be lessened. In fact, the Human Genome Program—the ambitious government-led research project that mapped all 20,000 to 25,000 human genes from 1990 to 2003—claims a more streamlined drug development process would have "the potential to dramatically reduce the estimated 100,000 deaths and 2 million hospitalizations that occur each year in the United States as the result of adverse drug response."[7]

But that's only the start of the benefits. Here are a few other verbatim quotations from their website that reflect the U.S. government's "official" enthusiasm:

- "[A]dvance knowledge of a particular disease susceptibility will allow careful monitoring, and treatments can be introduced at the most appropriate stage to maximize their therapy."[8]
- "Vaccines made of genetic material [...] promise all the benefits of existing vaccines without all the risks."[9]
- "The cost and risk of clinical trials will be reduced by targeting only those persons capable of responding to a drug."[10]
- All of these benefits and more "will promote a net decrease in the cost of health care."[11]

NIH Director Dr. Francis Collins, who, with Dr. J. Craig Venter, led the remarkable sequencing of the human genome, and who used to direct NIH's National Human Genome Research Institute, also talks frequently and with extraordinary enthusiasm about the promise of genetics research. He visualizes a time when the identities of individuals' unique DNA profiles will not only establish disease risks but also permit customized programs of prevention and treatment of illness. Because people are unique, he envisions customized prevention and treatment strategies for each individual. One size will not fit all, according to Collins and his colleagues.

These promises all sound inspiring and are said to be ushering in a whole new medical practice paradigm: genetics as the centerpiece of medicine's future! And in fact, many of the promised outcomes of genetics no doubt will be very good. I'm not saying that genetic research is a complete waste of time. I actually find the Human Genome Project to be endlessly fascinating science. There's no way a curious species like ourselves could have left that stone of indeterminate complexity unturned, given sufficient technology. And there's no doubt that genetic interventions will help the 0.01 percent of the population who suffer from rare conditions brought about by faulty genes.

What they won't do, however, is solve the basic problem: our society's failing health. What I object to is our focus on genetics to the near exclusion of everything else. Currently, hundreds of billions of dollars are being spent on genetic testing and sequencing every year in the United States, without getting us any closer to solving our health-care crisis. Our society's multibillion-dollar investment in genetics will help only a very small portion of the population, and even then only at enormous expense.

Once we've eliminated 90 percent of human diseases via nutrition and ended the financial drain of reductionist health care on our economy, then we can avail ourselves of the luxury of genetic testing and sequencing. Right now we have much more urgent things we can do that would benefit a much larger percentage of the population. We're facing a perfect-storm health-care crisis right now. When the hurricane is blowing, you don't redecorate the foyer; you nail plywood over the windows.

Or maybe I'm just jealous. I'll leave that for you to decide. After all, while this new Age of Genetics was rising over the horizon, an Age of Nutrition was sinking below it.

THE DECLINE OF THE AGE OF NUTRITION

In 1955, I was in my first year of veterinary school at the University of Georgia, where my biochemistry professor was enthralled by the recent discovery of the DNA double helix and what it might mean for the future. I, too, was enthralled with this marvelous bit of biochemical and medical research—exactly what I'd envisioned as my cup of tea. When Cornell professor Clive McCay surprised me with an unsolicited offer by telegram for me to drop veterinary medicine and instead come to Cornell and study this new field of "biochemistry" (of which the emerging discipline of genetics was then a part), I jumped at the opportunity. In my graduate research program at Cornell, I formally combined nutrition as a major field of study with biochemistry as a minor. In retrospect, I realize that I was witnessing not only the emergence of a new field, but a tectonic shift in the way science viewed human health.

From the early 1900s to the early 1950s, nutrition researchers were at the forefront of the struggle to improve human health. In the early twentieth century, scientists and medical professionals had begun investigating the causes of such diseases as beriberi, scurvy, pellagra, rickets, and other maladies. These diseases appeared to be linked in some way to food, but the exact mechanism was unclear. Eventually, researchers identified specific nutrients and posed the possibility that inadequate intake of these nutrients might be what leads to these diseases. Around 1912, the word *vitamin* was coined to refer to a substance in food, present in very small quantities, that was thought to be vital for sustaining life.

During the 1920s and 1930s, nutrition researchers identified a number of specific vitamins and other nutrients, including the "letter vitamins," A through K. Amino acids, the building blocks of protein that are assembled from the DNA template, also were being studied to determine how their sequence and arrangement within polypeptide chains affected protein's important, life-giving properties. In 1948, scientists stated with confidence that they had discovered the last vitamin, B_{12}, based on the observation that it was possible to grow laboratory rats on diets composed only of chemically synthesized versions of these newly discovered food nutrients. Now that the elementary particles of nutrition had been found and catalogued, nutrition scientists believed, whole foods need not be eaten. Human beings could get everything they needed from pills, and hunger and malnutrition would be banished to the distant past.

The findings from this impressive period of basic nutrition research filled our lectures as I started my research program at Cornell University in 1956, of course. But news of these exciting nutrient discoveries had filtered down to the popular imagination years earlier. I remember, when I was a child, my mother gave my siblings and me spoonfuls of oil prepared from codfish liver daily because it contained the life-giving nutrient vitamin A (I can still taste that oil—ugh!). I also remember at about that same time my aunt telling my mother with considerable enthusiasm that someday we would not have to eat food because its main ingredients would be in the form of a few pills! Forget about the vegetables grown in my mom's garden. (I remember my mother not taking kindly to that comment.) Protein was another nutrient independently gaining a reputation of epic proportions. On our dairy farm, we were certain that our milk was especially good for mankind (womankind had not yet been invented) because it was a source of high-quality protein that could make muscle and grow strong bones and teeth. Nutrition as a scientific discipline was riding high, although even then it was mostly focused on the discoveries and activities of individual nutrients.

Ironically, it was the reductionist nature of nutrition that provided the opening for the much more reductionist discipline of genetics to replace it as the best answer to the question of Why We Get Sick. All those fortified breakfast cereals and multivitamin pills weren't turning us into a nation of decathletes and vigorous octogenarians. Nutrition as a reductionist science had hit a dead end. And genetics obligingly stepped up to replace it.

THE NATURE–NURTURE DEBATE

The power struggle between nutrition and genetics closely mimics that age-old debate concerning nature versus nurture. Does our initial "nature" at birth—our genes—predetermine which diseases we get later in life? Or are health and disease events a product of our environment, like the food we eat or toxins we're exposed to—our "nurture"? Forms of the nature–nurture debate (or mindless shouting match) have been raging for millennia, at least since Aristotle characterized the human mind as a tabula rasa, or a blank slate to be filled by guidance and experience, in opposition to the prevailing view that humans were born with fixed "essential natures."

Most health researchers agree that neither nature nor nurture acts alone in determining which diseases we get, if any. Both contribute. The debate centers around *how much* each contributes. But the truth is, it's almost impossible to assign meaningful numbers to the relative contributions of genes and lifestyle, let alone the specific contribution of nutrition.

This uncertainty became clear to me many years ago when, from 1980 to 1982, I was on a thirteen-member expert committee of the National Academy of Sciences preparing a special report on diet, nutrition, and cancer,[12] the first reasonably official report of its kind. Among other objectives, we were asked to estimate the proportion of cancers caused by diet versus those caused by everything else, including genetics, environmental toxins, and lifestyle, and through that, suggest how much cancer could be prevented by the food we eat.

Estimating the proportion of cancer prevented by diet was of considerable interest to those of us working on the project because, as had been noted in the media a year or so before, a report[13] developed for the now-abolished Office of Technology Assessment of the U.S. Congress by two very distinguished scientists from the University of Oxford, Sir Richard Doll and Sir Richard Peto, had suggested that 35 percent of all cancers were preventable by diet. This surprisingly high estimate quickly became a politically charged issue, especially as this estimate was even higher than the 30 percent of cancers estimated to be preventable by not smoking. Most people had no idea that diet might be this important.

Our committee's task of creating our own specific estimate of diet-preventable cancers proved to be impossible. I was assigned the task of writing a first draft of this risk assessment, and I quickly saw that this exercise made little or no sense. Any estimate of how much cancer could be prevented by diet that was based on a single number was likely to convey more certainty than it deserved. We also faced the dilemma of how to summarize the combined effects of the various factors that affect cancer risk. What were we to do, for example, if not smoking could prevent 90 percent of lung cancer (our current best guess), a proper diet could prevent 30 percent (there is such evidence), and avoiding air pollution could prevent 15 percent? Did we add these numbers together and conclude that 135 percent of lung cancer could be prevented?

Becoming aware of both of these somewhat contrasting difficulties (i.e., over-precision and inappropriate summation of risk), our committee therefore declined to include a chapter that gave precise estimates of the reduced risk of cancer due to a healthy diet. We also knew that the previous report prepared for the Office of Technology Assessment[14] did not fixate on a precise number for diet-preventable cancers; the 35 percent cited by the media was a result of sloppy reporting. In fact, the report's authors had surveyed relevant professional diet and health communities and found that the estimates ranged broadly, from 10 percent to 70 percent. The seemingly finite figure of 35 percent was anything but conclusive. It was mostly suggested as a reasonable midpoint within this range, because a range of 10 percent to 70 percent would only confuse the public and discourage taking seriously diet's effect on cancer development. It is a generous range within which personal biases can play.

I am convinced that our committee's decision not to go down that path of estimating the size of such an unknowable risk was wise. Even today, writers incorrectly claim with far too much assurance that one-third of all cancers are preventable by dietary means, based on that University of Oxford report. Precise numbers are often over-interpreted, especially by those with a personal or professional agenda. And decades later, diet and health research communities still cannot agree on a precise figure.

The problem is, risk doesn't actually exist as an objective reality. It changes constantly based on how much we know. For example, the television station that broadcast the Washington Nationals' baseball games used to display a statistic they called "odds of winning." If the Nationals were ahead 5-2 in the bottom of the fourth inning, their odds of winning that game might be 79 percent. But if the opposing team then scored a run in the top of the fifth inning, those odds might decline to 65 percent. A grand slam by the Nationals in the eighth inning would raise those odds again, perhaps to 97 percent. But a heroic rally in the top of the ninth could erase that lead and shift the odds yet again. The problem, of course, is that the odds of winning can't be permanently pinned down. Every pitch, every swing of the bat, every change in cloud cover or drop in relative humidity could conceivably affect the final score. Depending on what the statistician who programmed the algorithm chose to include or ignore, the number could change dozens of times each second.

Like a bookmaker seeking precise quantification of risk to set odds on the outcome of a baseball game, individuals who care about their own health and that of their loved ones also seek the reassurance of specific percentages. They want to know with some confidence how to stay healthy and avoid chronic disease. But they don't need misleadingly "accurate" aggregate numbers that predict nothing in any specific instance. The important takeaway from our report wasn't how much cancer was preventable by diet, but that diet was a predominant factor.

What can we do, then, if we can assume neither a specific estimate nor a wide range of possible estimates? Do we just make up stuff? I am convinced that most people simply believe what they want to believe about cancer causation and prevention, according to which way the nature–nurture pendulum swings in their minds. In the absence of a reliable answer to the cancer prevention question, they fall back on personal nature or nurture biases.

HOPE (NUTRITION) VERSUS DESPAIR (GENES)

Where we stand on this continuum, consciously or unconsciously, influences our thinking about health and disease more than we realize. Do we simply accept the cards dealt to us, or do we consider the possibility that we can control our own destiny? If our health trajectory is mostly predetermined by our genes, then there's no point in trying to be healthy. If our choices trump the cards we were dealt at birth, then there's a reason for us to do what we can to achieve and maintain health.

Most medical researchers fall on the nature side of the nature–nurture dichotomy, and affirm the primacy of genetics as the basis of disease. They mistakenly believe that genetics is what will allow us to better diagnose and predict disease risk, through the discovery of faulty genes or gene arrangements in DNA that may be causing disease. Basic to these beliefs is a theory fairly popular in the health sciences called *genetic determinism*. According to this theory, we can draw a more or less straight causal line between genes and their final health- or disease-related outcomes. In other words, genes operate fairly independently, continuing to "do their thing" with little impact from the environment and one's lifestyle. A very simple representation of this process is shown in Figure 8-3.

In contrast, there is an alternative belief system to genetic determinism that I call *nutritional determinism*, wherein nutrition controls the

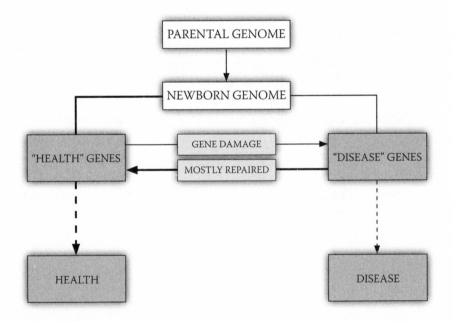

FIGURE 8-3.   Genetic determinism

Health or disease occurrence is primarily determined by "health" and "disease" genes, which arise from the newborn's genome plus damaged but unrepaired genes produced during life.

expression of genes to cause health or disease outcomes, by turning on health genes and suppressing disease genes as shown in Figure 8-4. And this is the belief system to which, based on my years of research and that of others, I subscribe.

Certainly, there also are nonnutrient lifestyle factors that may control gene expression. There are also, of course, relatively rare diseases like Tay-Sachs and others that are entirely genetic in cause, for which nutrition may, at very best, be able to mitigate some of their symptoms—if that. Even nutrition is not a cure-all; there's no diet that can regrow an amputated limb, as far as we know. However, I am suggesting that nutritional inputs are the primary factor in gene expression, and that in the vast majority of cases, the vast majority of the time, good nutrition has a much greater impact than anything else—including the most complicated and expensive genetic intervention.

Genes are the starting point for health and disease events; they are the "nature" part of the equation. But it is nutrition and other lifestyle

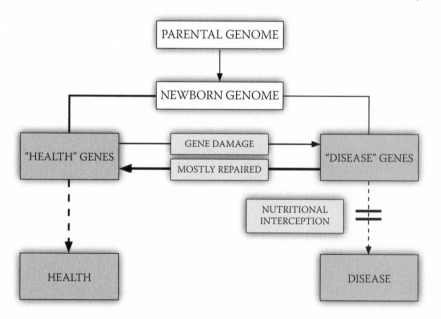

FIGURE 8-4. Nutritional determinism

Health or disease processes begin with "health" and "disease" genes, but nutritional practices control expression of these genes. Good nutrition blocks expression of disease genes, leaving health genes to produce health.

factors, the "nurture" part, that control whether and how these genes are expressed. The influence of nurture (i.e., nutrition) has far more influence on health and disease outcome than nature (i.e., genes).

A belief in genetic determinism suggests that our future health and disease events are already predestined at birth and that, as we age, we simply move from one disease benchmark to another according to the genetic blueprint we inherited at conception. This encourages the impression that there is little or nothing that we can do to prevent serious diseases like cancer. In contrast, the belief that cancer and related diseases are dependent on nutritional practices can encourage a sense of hope and lead to healthier behavior. And as we're about to see, this belief is not just wishful thinking; it's supported by an overwhelming amount of wholistic evidence. Let's now look at how nutrition and genetics compare when it comes to minimizing and repairing our damaged and misbehaving genes, and what our focus on a reductionist approach to disease means for our ability to prevent chronic diseases like cancer.

9

Genetics versus
Nutrition, Part Two

*The saddest aspect of life right now is that science
gathers knowledge faster than society gathers
wisdom.*

—ISAAC ASIMOV

We all get sick. Most of the time it's no big deal. In the memorable
words of physician and writer Lewis Thomas, "The great secret
of doctors, known only to their wives, but still hidden from the
public, is that most things get better by themselves; most things, in fact,
are better in the morning." Our bodies take care of any illness fairly quickly,
no intervention needed (especially if we're eating a WFPB diet). If not,
we go to the doctor or, if it's very serious, to a hospital. These are normal
aspects of modern life that most of us take for granted. Yet most people
don't really understand disease and where it comes from: why we get sick
and what role our DNA plays in letting or making that happen.

WHERE DISEASE COMES FROM

As we discussed briefly in chapter eight, genes are the starting point of both health and disease. They are the source for all our biological reactions that, in effect, lead to bodily form and function—what we call life. Some of our genes start reactions that lead to health. Others lead to disease.

The vast majority of our genes are the health-giving kind—otherwise, we wouldn't last very long. These are the genes that form our cells, our organs, and our bones; that regrow skin after a cut or scrape; that make apples taste sweet and poisonous mountain buckthorn berries bitter. A small number of our genes, however, produce disease.

All disease starts with genes and gene combinations; what we call *diseases* are the end stages of interactions between our genes and elements from our environment, through the medium of our bodies. We get the flu, for example, because our genes produce certain symptoms in response to a particular microbe. We even bleed (and clot) when we get a paper cut because our genes have programmed that response into our physiologies. If our genes have made us hemophiliacs, it means that bleeding, once it's started, is harder to stop. This interaction between genes and environment isn't just the case for short-term illnesses like the flu or conditions like hemophilia. Our genes also trigger chronic diseases like cancer, heart disease, and diabetes in response to environmental stimuli (e.g., our diet, especially over a long period of time).

Our health-producing genes come from our parents. Where do our disease genes come from? There are two main sources. Some come from our parents and their ancestors before them; they are present in our initial germ or embryo. Other disease-causing genes may begin as health-giving genes that become damaged by mutation during our lifetimes.

These mutations are widely thought to be caused mostly by unnatural, synthetic chemicals that pollute our environment; we've already seen how oxidation reactions in our cells can produce such mutations. But these chemicals are not the only agents causing this kind of gene damage. Low levels of certain natural chemicals and other aspects of our environment (e.g., cosmic radiation, excessive sunlight, numerous chemicals in plants and microorganisms) can do the same thing. Together, these natural and unnatural chemicals cause continual low-level genetic damage during our lifetimes.

The good news is, our bodies have learned how to routinely repair such damage. Our cells have a repair capability that works remarkably well right after the damage occurs. They had to have developed such a capability, or our evolutionary ancestors, subject to the same exposure to natural chemicals that we are today (and much less medical care), would not have survived long enough to reproduce. But this process of repair is not perfect. A very small percentage of the genes damaged during our lifetime are not repaired and may spawn successive generations of damaged cells as our tissues are renewed.

Perhaps surprisingly, this small percentage may not be all that bad. Some mutated genes turn out to be beneficial, and contribute to human evolution as their carriers survive and reproduce in greater numbers than the non-mutated population. Mutations are how evolution works. But while that low level of damage is useful for humanity as a whole, it can be less beneficial to individuals, because often these mutated genes are the source of disease.

The aim of health professionals who focus on chronic disease caused by this long-term damage is therefore two-fold: to prevent as much of that damage as possible, and to treat as many of the effects of that damage— what we call disease—as possible. And genetics, at least right now and probably indefinitely, is not a very good place to begin either of these efforts.

As a research discipline, modern-day genetics addresses the consequences of that small percentage of disease-producing genes that we are born with in addition to those damaged genes that we acquire along the way. It operates from the assumption that one day we will be able to locate and identify damaged genes and use that information to more easily diagnose and treat disease. However, it largely fails to consider how to prevent genes from becoming damaged in the first place. And the field's presumption that genetic engineering will be able to prevent disease from occurring by repairing or replacing specific genes that cause disease, is the height of hubris, given the unimaginable complexity of DNA.

CANCER DEVELOPMENT

The explanatory model long used by cancer researchers postulates that cancer begins either with an inherited gene or with a gene that has been damaged by a carcinogen or other factor during a person's lifetime, with different cancer types having different genetic starting points. If the damaged gene or genes are not repaired or removed, the damage will become a permanent part of the cell's genetic code, passed on to each successive generation of cells. This series of cell generations grow into cell masses, then tumor masses, theoretically at a somewhat faster or uninhibited rate. The presumption here is that this process is fixed, with virtually no opportunities for its reversal. If the cell and damaged gene replicate, there is nothing that can be done; the result is cancer. More damaged genes mean more cancer; fewer damaged genes mean less cancer (see Figure 9-1).

However, research has shown that there are other environmental factors involved in whether damaged DNA becomes cancer. During my laboratory work with AF, one line of research showed that even when we had genetically predisposed a mouse or rat to develop liver cancer by

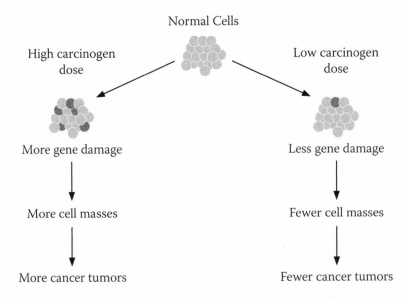

FIGURE 9-1. Traditional explanatory model for cancer development

intentionally damaging its genes through exposure to hepatitis B or to a high dose of AF, the cancer would develop *only in the presence of a high-animal-protein diet.* In other words, nutrition trumped environment, even when the environment was particularly nasty. Although their DNA had been damaged, cancer did not inevitably result (see Figure 9-2).

There's also evidence from human subjects, which you can read in depth in *The China Study*, that supports the idea that the foods we eat and the nutrition they provide is far more important in determining cancer than our genetic backgrounds.[1] Population studies begun forty to fifty years ago show that when people migrate from one country to another, they acquire the cancer rate of the country to which they move, despite the fact their genes remain the same. This strongly indicates that at least 80 percent to 90 percent—and probably closer to 97 percent to 98 percent—of all cancers are related to diet and lifestyle, not to genes.

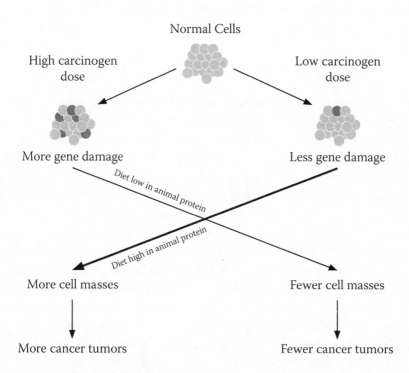

FIGURE 9-2. Revised explanatory model for cancer development

Also, comparisons of cancer rates among identical twins show that even though both members of a twin pair have the same DNA, most of the time they fail to get the same cancers. If genes alone were sufficient for cancer development, you'd expect them to get the same cancer nearly 100 percent of the time. (For those relatively few twins who do get the same cancer, their dietary similarities could be at least partly responsible.)

In short, proper nutrition doesn't just prevent damage; it affects the way our bodies respond to already damaged genes, often mitigating disease symptoms as they arise or even preventing them completely, sometimes with no additional medication or other treatments needed. In experimental animal studies in my own laboratory, cancer progression could even be reversed by nutritional changes. And researchers are now producing evidence that WFPB nutrition can turn cancer-producing genes off altogether.

All this suggests that the way cancer works is a far cry from the way cancer researchers assume it works—and of course, how something works has major implications for the way we go about fighting it.

WEAPONS IN THE WAR ON CANCER

The more work I did with AF and diet, the more I became convinced that AF wasn't the villain most scientists assumed it to be when it came to liver cancer. In fact, I started to see that none of the accepted "causes" of cancer, in the absence of a high-animal-protein diet, mattered that much. Not genetics, not chemical carcinogens like AF, not viruses. But the cancer industry, researchers, policy makers, the media, and the public focus almost exclusively on genes, chemicals, and viruses. Nutrition did not even make the list, even though it was becoming clear from my experiments and those of others that nutrition was cancer's on-off switch.

Our offensive strategy in the War on Cancer primarily involves two main methods of prevention: controlling the expression of cancer-producing genes (by replacing or manipulating them), and getting rid of all environmental substances that might trigger genetic mutations. We saw in chapter eight why focusing on manipulating genes themselves will not be effective. But purging our environments of toxins isn't the answer, either. First, it can't be done. Even if we could remove all the human-made toxins from our environment (an effort I wholeheartedly support), nature still provides us with many mutagenic phenomena that we can't regulate or engineer out of existence, like sunlight and radon. Second, and more to the point, the effect of these environmental mutagens (substances that cause mutations in DNA) is mostly trumped by good nutrition. Yet these findings haven't stopped the government from spending far more time and money chasing after environmental carcinogens that are supposedly causing cancer by creating gene mutations than on promoting WFPB nutrition.

You can't turn around without hearing about another potential source of cancer to avoid: toxic chemicals, viruses, cell phones, the sun... A recent *New York Times* article titled, "Is It Safe to Play Yet?" chronicles the almost paralyzing fears expressed by young parents trying to give their children a healthy start. Many of them purge their homes of makeup, shampoos, detergents, plastic cups and bottles, laminated furniture, and even rubber duckies.[2]

And every so often the media will gravitate toward a terrifying story of a cancer-causing agent in our midst. Alar, a common pesticide used on apples. Microwave ovens. Power lines near homes. Enormous public concern often arises. Then, adding fuel to the fire, we are reminded that an ever-increasing number of chemicals—some intentional, some not— are being added to our personal and public environments (food, water, cosmetics). And finally, we are told that only a tiny fraction (perhaps 2,000) of these chemicals (about 80,000 or so) have been tested for their carcinogenicity.

Social activists speak out, and rightly so, against "cancer clusters": areas where there are abnormally high rates of particular cancers, presumably due to toxic dumping and other nasty practices that befall low-income communities but not their wealthier neighbors. Communities battle each other in NIMBY (not in my backyard) skirmishes that aim to move the toxic output as far away as possible. Movies like *Erin Brockovich* and *A Civil Action* convince us to buy bottled water or install kitchen filters to keep contaminants out of our homes.

The result of this constant onslaught is a pervasive sense of fear that either morphs into passivity ("I give up, there's nothing I can do") or obsessive action ("Let's live in a bubble"). Ultimately, however, neither does much to reduce our cancer risk.

I'm not saying we shouldn't work to block new onslaughts of toxicity. I should know; my speech suffered for decades from my exposure to dioxin, one of the most toxic chemicals known to humans, and one I helped discover when, as a postdoctoral researcher at MIT in the 1960s, I isolated it from oil used in poultry feed.[3] As individuals, we should seek to minimize our exposure to carcinogens. And as a society, we should err on the side of over-caution before approving and disseminating new technologies and substances into our water, air, and soil.

But carcinogenic testing has become a self-perpetuating industry rather than a safeguard of public health. From its origins shortly after the discovery in the 1950s of a harmful chemical agent in a spray used on cranberries, this program has grown to a hundred-million-dollar program today. It is difficult to estimate the total costs for this program because of its secondary effects on regulatory and cancer control programs, but, in my estimation, it surely has amounted in total to tens of billions of wasted dollars. And although the goal of reducing environmental toxins is laudable, the government's approach to this is ineffective and misleading.

The chief arm of the U.S. government's war on "stuff that may cause cancer"—and the poster child for how our current approach wastes time and money—is the carcinogen bioassay program, a multimillion-dollar program that researches hundreds of chemicals in an attempt to figure out which ones cause cancer in humans.

THE CARCINOGEN BIOASSAY PROGRAM

In 1958, the U.S. government added a clause to the Food Additive Amendment of the Food and Drug Act that specified that no chemical should be added to our food supply if it was found to be carcinogenic. One natural outgrowth of the clause was that the government needed a way to determine which chemicals were, in fact, carcinogenic. So a program was set up to do just that. Known popularly as the carcinogen bioassay program (CBP), it seems at first blush like a very good thing: figure out what's harmful and keep it out of our food supply.

The problem is, the reductionist assumptions that underpin the program, from the idea that environmental toxins inevitably lead to cancer, to the ill-considered design of the program's research and testing methods, call its usefulness into question. The CBP distracts us from the significant and easily addressed causes of cancer, and directs us to secondary factors over which we have almost no control, thus accomplishing little and diverting resources from initiatives that could make a significant difference.

PROBLEMS WITH CBP
RESEARCH METHODS

The CBP tests the ability of suspect chemicals to cause cancer in experimental animals (rats and mice) within their lifetimes (about two years). If enough of the lab animals get cancer while being dosed with a particular chemical, it is labeled a carcinogen. If supporting evidence shows a statistically significant (albeit usually contested) association with humans, it is labeled a human carcinogen. Some examples of human carcinogens identified by the CBP include dioxin, formaldehyde, asbestos, DDT (insecticide spray), polycyclic aromatic hydrocarbons (PAHs, in smoked foods and cigarettes), nitrosamines (in bacon and hot dogs), PCBs (used in the manufacture of electrical transformers), benzene (found in solvents, gasoline, and cigarette smoke), and of course the subject of my lab's work, AF.

When the CBP selects a chemical for cancer risk evaluation, it starts with animal trials. First, the researchers select the animal (rat or mouse). Next, the rodents are dosed with levels of the suspected carcinogen about a thousand to ten thousand times higher than the equivalent doses that humans are expected to encounter. If a significant percentage of the animals develop cancer, the substance is classified as a carcinogen.

You may have noticed two gaping holes in this logic. First, there's the assumption that if very high doses of a chemical cause cancer, then much lower doses must also cause cancer. Maybe not as often or as lethally, and maybe not as quickly, but cancer is still assumed to be the end result. In science-speak, this assumption is known as "high-dose to low-dose interpolation." This is a very uncertain procedure because we don't really know if the straight-line relationship seen at these exceptionally high doses continues to be linear all the way down to the much lower doses typically observed for human exposure. What if the high dose is like getting hit by a car, while the low dose is like getting hit by a Matchbox car? The high dose of the nonnutritive sweetener saccharin that caused a very small increase in bladder cancer in laboratory rats was equivalent to the human consumption of 1,200 cans of diet soda in a day. Silly? I think so. And it should be added, as already discussed, that the body is capable of repairing much of the damage that low levels of natural chemicals cause.

Second, this method assumes that a response in one species (e.g., rat) is equivalent to the same kind of response in a second species (e.g., human). This is called "species-to-species extrapolation." And it's a huge leap of faith. Because we have laws that prevent human trials for carcinogens (and a good thing, too!), we can't actually give benzene or PAHs to human subjects and see if they get more cancers. So we have to assume that what's poison for the rat is poison for the human as well. The trouble is, it turns out that some substances that are carcinogenic for rats aren't even necessarily carcinogenic for mice.

In 1980, I published in *Federation Proceedings*, a major journal, my concerns about the underlying rationale for this testing program, specifically the assumption that what's poison for the rat is also poison for the human. To investigate the species-to-species extrapolation assumption, I compared the results in mice with the results in rats. At that time, 192 chemicals had been tested for carcinogenicity. A total of 76 of these chemicals were carcinogenic, but only 37 (49 percent) were carcinogenic for both species. I concluded, "If this is the limitation of correspondence between two presumably closely related species, how then could one expect any greater correspondence between a selected laboratory animal species and the more distant human species?" In other words, if fewer than half the carcinogenic chemicals affected both rats and mice, it's likely that even fewer of them would have the same effect on humans.

Also, because the CBP focuses exclusively on the human-made chemicals, it ignores a significant source of environmental carcinogenicity: naturally occurring chemicals like AF. Such chemicals are not something we decide whether or not to add to our environment; they are already there. Since they cannot simply be legislated out of our food supply by ordering companies to stop using them, the CBP is forced to pretend that they do not exist.

What all this means, of course, is that we can't trust the CBP's findings, despite all the time and energy and money that the government has poured into testing all these suspected carcinogens. Instead of actionable knowledge, we're left with free-floating anxiety that "everything out there is dangerous and there's almost nothing we can do about it." Not exactly the sentiments of a well-informed and empowered population!

CARCINOGENIC MISDIRECTION

When a magician engages in misdirection, he attempts to distract his audience by focusing attention away from the main action of his trick. As he palms a card in his right hand, for example, he flourishes his left, or instructs a volunteer to shuffle the deck or open an envelope. As a result, the magician's palming technique need not be flawless since nobody is watching that hand anyway.

The CBP is essentially a giant exercise, however unintentional, in misdirection away from what the evidence shows to have a much greater impact on the development of cancer: eating too much of the wrong kinds of foods. It's based on the prevailing (but inadequate) theory that since chemical carcinogens are mutagenic, they are therefore primarily responsible for human cancer. In this model of cancer, nutrition is of little or no consequence. And with all available resources focused on doing reductionist research into the specific effects of specific chemicals on rats, without looking at the kind of wholistic evidence that would help determine whether or not those research studies were useful, there isn't a lot of manpower or money left over to investigate other causes and solutions to the cancer problem. As we've seen before, reductionist research tends to create its own rabbit hole, into which researchers can plunge ever deeper as they move further and further away from usefulness and applicability.

The CBP, which focuses on a disproved hypothesis and annually costs hundreds of millions of dollars, has been a huge distraction from the more likely causes of cancer. But no one involved in this program really seems to care, either about the program costs or, more important, about the misleading message being sold to a fearful and seemingly helpless public.

CBP CHEERLEADERS

During the 1980s and 1990s, I was one of the few voices shouting myself hoarse, "Don't focus on the chemical carcinogens. Look at nutrition!" Our lab was continuing to find evidence, in our own rodent experiments and in surveys of human populations like the China Study, that it was diet, not genes or carcinogens, that determined cancer development.

In the early 1980s, shortly after my presentations to the staff of the CBP's predecessor, the National Toxicology Program (NTP) in North Carolina's Research Triangle Park, the NTP organized a reasonably ambitious project at the carcinogen-testing laboratory in their Arkansas facility. One of the project goals was to investigate the role of nutrition in experimental cancer development, among other ideas. Dr. Ron Hart was put in charge, and he proceeded to focus his research program on the effect of calorie consumption on experimental cancer in a very large series of rodent studies. After some years, I invited Dr. Hart to present a seminar at Cornell to report some findings of that study. He brought along for me a large number of his publications. His findings were extensive and well done but, more important, they illustrated nutrition principles at work that were similar to those that we had found for protein. Both his research on calories and our work on protein and other nutrients clearly showed that it is the nutritional composition of the diet—not the chemical carcinogens in it—that primarily determines cancer occurrence.

During this same time, my lab was also turning out overwhelming evidence for the carcinogenic potential of nutrients like animal protein and fat. As I noted in that 1980 *Federation Proceedings* article, for example, based on CBP's own stated bioassay criteria, cow's milk protein should be considered a carcinogen: consuming it leads to cancer, and cancer halts or goes into remission once milk protein consumption is stopped. My comments at that time were based both on others' research studies on dietary protein and cancer from 1942 to 1979, and on our own laboratory's early research findings (we had not yet done the most convincing studies to establish this protein effect, especially the intervention experiments in which cancer was turned on with cow's milk protein and off when it was reduced or replaced).

In that article, I also pointed out the existence of a more reliable and less expensive way of testing chemicals for their cancer-producing potential: the Ames assay, developed by Professor Bruce Ames at the University of California, Berkeley. For a mere fraction of the dollars required for this Ames assay program (approximately 1 percent or less), we could evaluate chemicals for their mutagenicity and get more meaningful results.

In a nutshell, the Ames assay applies a suspected chemical carcinogen to an extract of rat liver, which is then incubated in a petri dish to see if mutations develop. A positive Ames assay indicates potential for cancer and other mutagen-initiated diseases. The recommendation for such chemicals would then be to avoid them and, if they were found capable of migrating into our food, water, and air, if possible, discontinue their use altogether.

Unsurprisingly, my views calling the CBP's methods into question did not make me a popular figure in the cancer research community at the time. The agencies that had organized and invested hundreds of millions of dollars in the program didn't agree with my views on its faults or nutrition's potential for cancer prevention and treatment. Mixing ideas about nutritional practices with the occurrence of cancer in the same discussion has been like throwing gasoline on a fire, sprinkled with a pinch of TNT. I believe there are three main reasons for this.

First, the research community is trapped within the paradigm that chemical carcinogens are the main causes of human cancer and, further, that these carcinogens are best identified in rodent bioassay experiments, despite all the evidence that these experiments are very poor estimators of what is carcinogenic for humans. As we've seen, once scientists start operating within a paradigm, it's very difficult for them to see, much less embrace, any evidence that calls that paradigm into question.

Second, unlike the attribution of cancer to genes and environmental toxins, linking cancer with poor nutrition smacks of "blaming the victim." If genes and carcinogens account for human cancer, then cancer occurrence is due to something outside our control—to fate. We're just lucky or unlucky; we bear no responsibility for either developing cancer or staying cancer-free. If nutrition imbalance is more important to causing cancer than chemical carcinogens—if our diets can turn cancer on and off—then cancer is something for which individuals possess some responsibility. Responsibility is not a bad thing; indeed, responsibility means empowerment. It means we have the power to control our health, through the simple act of choosing what we eat, rather than submit ourselves to random circumstance. But that power is not much comfort to those whose family and friends have already succumbed to disease.

Third, there are too many jobs, careers, and structures at stake. Three-fourths of the 75,000 experimental pathologists in the United States (an estimate given to me at my North Carolina seminar by the director of the toxicology testing program) are involved in evaluating the results of bioassay-type carcinogen testing programs. These people have no interest in hearing that their efforts are misguided, and the money they are paid produces little or no return in improved public health.

Those who vigorously defend the carcinogen bioassay program tend to believe that cancer starts with genes (and even progresses because of genes) and that chemical carcinogens are the most important agents of genetic change. In contrast, nutritional influence is often considered a second-class idea because, at best, it only modifies the development of cancer; it doesn't cause it. While that's technically true, it's like saying that grass seeds cause lawns, but watering, weeding, and providing sun only modifies lawns' development. Yes, you need the seeds to grow a lawn, just as you need genetic mutations to start growing precancerous lesions. But as anyone who has ever tilled a field can tell you, if you leave it alone for long enough the birds and the wind will happily seed it for you. Likewise, we live in a world where carcinogenic mutations abound, many of them from natural sources like the sun, viruses, and molds. Unless you want to live in a hazmat bubble (which probably contains mutagenic agents in the plastic), you can't avoid these carcinogens or the mutations they produce. The more effective method of prevention is to address what determines whether or not those mutations progress into cancer: nutrition.

THE CBP TODAY

The chief proponents of the CBP have continued that same drumbeat ever since those early days, against all the evidence to the contrary, and any serious dialogue on nutrition among these scientists is still missing. When CBP proponents do acknowledge that nutrition matters, they fall into the reductionist trap of identifying important individual nutrients. The emphasis on chemical carcinogens as the principal cause of cancer, especially their effects on genes, still predominates today.

Recently, one of this viewpoint's longtime proponents, along with two public activists, even recommended expanding the existing animal bioassay program from two to three years. They suggested the inclusion of in-utero (i.e., during pregnancy) exposure plus an additional year to observe the offspring in the hope that more chemical carcinogens might be discovered. In their 2008 paper, they claim as part of their justification that "chemical carcinogenesis bioassays in animals have long been recognized and accepted as valid predictors of potential cancer hazard to humans," mostly quoting the publications of their own inner circle.[4] Another author wants to refine and shorten the bioassay portion of this program by evaluating the so-called mode of action for each potential carcinogen.[5] Both of these proposed testing modifications would require massive amounts of new funding. And the focus still remains on chemical carcinogens as the chief causes of human cancer.

Although the CBP's methods are unreliable and wasteful, there's still a basic good in its aim (if restructured to use short-term assays at a tiny fraction of its current costs): to identify and ban certain harmful chemicals. Certainly my life would have been healthier and less painful had I not encountered dioxin along the way! But this cannot be the only, or even the primary, weapon we use in our efforts to prevent cancer, because if it is, we will continue to fail.

10

Reductionist
Medicine

*We can't solve problems by using the same kind of
thinking we used when we created them.*

—ALBERT EINSTEIN

In the last few chapters, I've shown how reductionism distorts the way
we do science, especially regarding the workings of our bodies. If the
only victims of this distortion were biology textbooks and organic chemistry final exams, it would be sad, but not a great tragedy. The problem
is, of course, that scientific theory and popular understanding of science
determine the way our society teaches, funds, and rewards the practice
of medicine. In this chapter, we'll see reductionism's fingerprints all over
the way we view and treat disease.

I began this book with the idea that something is fundamentally wrong
with the way we do medicine—that the so-called health-care system in
the United States doesn't really have much to do with health. Instead, it's
more properly called a disease-care system, because it just reacts to and
manages disease, producing the expensive and disappointing outcomes
we've come to tolerate and expect without knowing there's another, better

way. While many medical experts and politicians have floated proposals to improve health care and reduce costs, the vast majority of these proposals seek to tinker around the edges rather than address the root cause of the problem: its reductionist operating system.

THE DISEASE-CARE SYSTEM

In chapter four, I introduced the fable of the blind men and the elephant. Let's imagine that the blind men assumed responsibility for the elephant's health and well-being. What would this look like?

Obviously, none of the blind men would be tasked with monitoring the whole elephant—that would be impossible. Each would focus on his own area of "expertise": the leg, the tusk, the trunk, the tail, the ear, and the belly. If the elephant ate some moldy peanuts and began developing liver cancer, none of the blind men would notice, as none of the parts they were tasked with monitoring would be sufficiently affected yet. Only when the cancer reached a critical mass would its symptoms become noticeable: first as decreased appetite that the "trunk doctor" would notice, next as intestinal distress that the "tail doctor" would certainly smell, and ultimately as a fever that the "ear doctor" could sense and measure.

The blind men, limited by their experience of the elephant as a collection of individual, unrelated parts, have no ability to discern and deal with root causes that precede symptoms. By necessity, their treatments will react to problems that have already developed rather than preventing those problems in the first place. This is also the first major characteristic of our disease-care system: reactivity.

Because the blind men can discern symptoms but not causes, they treat those symptoms as if they were the entire problem. The trunk doctor might sugar-roast the moldy peanuts in an attempt to stimulate the elephant's appetite. The tail doctor, having no way to intervene in the elephant's gastrointestinal workings, might just fit the poor creature with a large carbon-filter diaper and explain that modern medicine doesn't really have a cure for that sort of thing. And the ear doctor might treat the ear fever with ice packs, and declare the elephant "cured" once the ear temperature returned to normal. This is also the case with our disease-care system: it focuses on treating symptoms as if they were root causes, and as a result, it tends to choose interventions that completely ignore the true root causes and thus make it highly likely that symptoms will reappear.

Since our reductionist elephant doctors ignore the entire system called "elephant," they cannot call upon natural means of healing that have evolved along with elephants, such as the leaves of certain trees that elephants know to eat to induce vomiting. Instead, they invent specific treatments that target the symptoms they observe, often causing new problems elsewhere. This, too, is emblematic of our reductionist disease-care system: a reliance on chemicals that don't exist in nature, that narrowly intervene in a small subset of our biochemistry while producing inevitable negative "side effects."

Let's move from metaphor to medicine, and explore how each of these reductionism-induced characteristics plays out in our disease-care system.

Reactivity

When you're talking about the kind of sudden, traumatic injury that sends you to the ER, reactivity makes sense. We don't go around giving people preventive casts on their legs or braces around their necks just in case they crash their motorcycle sometime in the future. But the entire system is as reactive as the ER, if you think about it. "Medicine" is practiced on people when they are uncomfortable, when they have just been diagnosed with an ailment or disease. As patients, we're trained and incentivized to avoid the doctor unless we have a presenting problem.

As I said, this makes sense in the case of traumatic injuries that occur suddenly and unexpectedly. You can't address something that hasn't yet happened. But medicine in the United States is almost entirely reactive. The medical profession treats all manner of diseases and disease progressions as if they are also sprung on us without notice. As if one day you're fine, and the next you've got cancer. Or one day your arteries are perfect, and the next you're in the operating room receiving a triple bypass.

We know this is crazy. By the time a biological process has progressed to the point of clinical symptoms, it's already been in the works for weeks, months, or, commonly, years. Yet the medical profession, through its reductionist guidelines and co-pays and ten-minute doctor visits, discourages patients from optimizing their health prior to full-blown disease.

"Wait until you're really sick," could be the motto of doctors and hospitals in the current system. "We can do nothing for you until your symptoms surpass the subclinical and reveal themselves in pain, loss of function, or a particularly worrisome test result. Until then, keep calm and keep eating the Standard American Diet."

Treating Symptoms, Not Underlying Causes

In the ER, it makes sense to first remove the steering wheel from the car crash victim's chest and set any broken ribs. Now's not the time to deal with the texting while driving, or drinking, or poor exit ramp design that was the root cause of the accident. That can wait until the victim's body has been stabilized. Similarly, when someone enters a hospital suffering from a heart attack, stroke, or diabetic coma, the first order of business is to ameliorate the most serious symptoms so the patient can survive the night.

But medicine stops at symptoms. With rare exceptions, we do not treat the causes of disease; we treat its effects. And we convince ourselves that those individual effects are themselves causes. Got hypertension? We better lower your blood pressure with an antihypertensive drug, because high blood pressure causes heart disease. We're not interested in why your blood pressure is high to begin with. Got cancer? Let's irradiate and chemo-poison the tumor. We don't care that the tumor may have been caused by a diet too rich in animal products. (As we saw in chapters eight and nine, the reductionist genetics movement wants us to believe there's nothing that *could* have been done—that cancer is inevitable because it's in our genes.) Had a heart attack? Let's put stents in your arteries so the blood can flow more freely in the future. The root cause of the blocked artery doesn't matter. The practice of medicine focuses almost exclusively on treating symptoms as the whole of the problem.

Can you see how crazy and counterproductive this is? By focusing on the symptoms, we steadfastly ignore the actual root causes, making it exceedingly likely that the symptoms will recur with a vengeance. If your lawn turns brown because you forgot to water it, you wouldn't paint it green and think you'd solved the problem, would you? But too often that's how the medical establishment thinks.

Prescribing Specific and Reductionist
Treatments That Make Things Worse

Clearly, a coat of green paint on your lawn won't solve the problem of not enough water to the grass's roots. But depending on the paint, that "solution" could also make things much worse. Standard paint contains formaldehyde, volatile organic compounds (VOCs), mercury, cadmium, lead, and benzene. These chemicals can kill the earthworms and bacteria that contribute to healthy soil. The VOCs can produce gas that harms the birds that eat bugs. So you see, treating the symptom of the brown lawn by addressing just that symptom—brownness—in isolation from its wholistic environment not only doesn't solve the problem, it makes it much worse.

As we've seen, Western medicine actually prefers treatments that are specific to particular ailments. The more targeted and less general the positive effects of a drug, the more highly regarded it is. Drugs are often chemically designed to act on specific events that lie in the pathway of disease development, perhaps involving a key enzyme, hormone, gene, or gene product. (Chemotherapy drugs are spectacular examples of this kind of super-narrow targeting; they are very specifically engineered to disrupt a very specific step on the pathway to disease formation,[1] as if all other contributing steps do not matter.) This practice of trying to be precise and specific is usually considered a hallmark of good science. But as you know if you've ever looked at the back page of a magazine ad for a new drug, this precision and specificity comes with lots of very unpleasant and often potentially life-threatening side effects. Just like the toxic green paint, the drugs that target specific nodes in the disease process tend to wreak havoc on other parts of the human body.

Relying on Unnatural Drugs

Most drugs originally came from plants. Humans (and animals) have known for millennia that certain plants have biological properties potentially useful in treating disease. Traditional healers the world over used the plants in wholistic ways to bring their patients' bodies back into balance. They saw these plants as having a "spirit" that embodied and channeled the healing effects.

From the modern medical perspective, this approach is fundamentally problematic. First, the idea that the entire plant has a spirit that needs to be honored in its wholeness—the idea that there is anything special about the plant as a whole—reeks of superstition and nonsense to the Western scientific mind. If the plant has healing properties, then somewhere in there is a chemical that can do all the work in isolation. Our job is to not just find it, but figure out how to recreate it, so that we can manufacture it in a sterile and scalable way.

Pharmaceutical researchers try to isolate and determine the chemical structures of the "active agents" responsible for healing properties of particular plants.[2] In the process of synthesizing these new, unnatural chemical structures, pharmaceutical companies try to maximize potency (i.e., efficacy) and minimize toxicity (i.e., side effects)—or so cheerleaders for the drug industry would have us believe.[3] In fact, the reverse is true. The more the natural chemical is structurally changed, the more problematic it becomes for the body. That's the source of the unintended and undesirable side effects common to all drugs. And this negative reaction to pharmaceuticals is often made worse by unnatural timing and dosage protocols, which sidestep the orderliness with which nature manages this extraordinary complexity.

Here's what happens. When the body senses that it's been poisoned (invaded by foreign chemicals), it raises the alarm and, among other responses devised through evolution, calls on its army of enzymes to convert the foreign chemicals to less harmful metabolites that can be excreted from the body. One of these enzymes is MFO. As I discussed in chapter seven, MFO performs a wide variety of biological activities, including the metabolism and disposal of drugs.

It's pretty ironic that specific drugs, formulated to target specific reactions within the body, all tend to evoke a response from the MFO enzyme system. But as we've seen, there's no such thing as a targeted strike when it comes to biochemistry. So the strategy of using these chemicals to treat disease is akin to the infamous Vietnam War strategy of "burning the village to save the village." Just as in actual war, it leaves in its wake a predictable killing field of collateral damage.

The story of side effects actually gets worse. To counteract the harm done by one chemical treatment, a second pharmaceutical may be administered, perhaps even a third or a fourth, each trying to mop up the mess left behind by the preceding drug. Also, as time elapses, drug doses often need to be increased, because the body gets progressively more efficient at detoxifying and voiding such chemicals before they can do their intended work. And we incorrectly take for granted that such a pill pile-up is normal!

A DISEASE BY ANY OTHER NAME

The reductionist nature of research, whereby scientists are encouraged and rewarded for looking very closely at very small areas of knowledge, contributes mightily to the blind-men-and-elephant problem that is our disease-care system. But the language our medical system uses, and the way we use it, reinforces those reductionist tendencies by making it difficult to think of the body as an integrated system in which all the elements interact with and influence one another.

Perhaps the most powerful example of this can be seen in the word *disease* itself. What do we mean when we use that word? Are the various diseases recognized by medicine actually individual entities? Or is the grouping of sets of symptoms into new diseases more arbitrary than that?

The history of disease classification goes back at least to 1662, when records on causes of death were first assembled and published in England.[4] A total of eighty-one disease types were recognized. Since then, this initial list has been revised many times; in its latest, tenth edition, it's generally called the International Statistical Classification of Diseases and Related Health Problems, or ICD-10. Its constant updating is maintained by the United Nations' World Health Organization. Many "new" diseases have been added, along with many subclassifications of disease and disease conditions. Today there are about 8,000 such entries—a bit more complex than the original eighty-one!

When we look at some of the historical disease classifications, we realize the limitations of our understanding and the arbitrariness of our disease taxonomy. Take, for example, one of the most common diagnoses of women in nineteenth-century Western Europe: hysteria. The word itself betrays the causal theory of the disease: a malfunctioning of the uterus (Greek name, *hystera*). The symptoms of hysteria included feeling faint, nervousness, sexual desire or lack of sexual desire(!), fluid retention, irritability, loss of appetite, and "a tendency to cause trouble," among many others. You have to wonder: Did men therefore not suffer this particular cluster of symptoms?

Thankfully, the diagnosis of female hysteria is a thing of the past. But why did it disappear? Obviously, the symptoms that characterized a diagnosis haven't gone away. Nobody got a Nobel Prize for curing hysteria. It's simply that Western doctors have stopped attributing these symptoms to a misbehaving uterus. The symptoms are real, but the "disease" is subject to cultural and gender bias. A disease is nothing more than a theoretical model applied to a cluster of symptoms.

Conversely, the medical establishment sometimes denies the existence of a disease—the relationship between a cluster of symptoms—that many people claim to have. Modern examples of this denial include chronic fatigue syndrome, chronic musculoskeletal pain, and fibromyalgia. When many doctors hear these disease names, they roll their eyes and translate them into a single diagnosis: hypochondria. The reason they don't consider them diseases is that their sets of symptoms cannot be correlated to particular, reductionist "underlying pathologies," like an infection or an immunological response. In other words, if a doctor can't reliably diagnose it through an objective test, it isn't actually a disease. See the circular logic at work here? The definition of a disease is whatever the medical establishment rather arbitrarily calls a disease.

The initial purpose for naming and monitoring disease occurrence was to detect patterns of changes in people's health that might forecast emerging epidemics. The naming system was also used to standardize medical records, so that health practitioners could more easily communicate with each other when patients changed doctors or when discussing hereditary conditions. Proper disease classification is crucial throughout the medical practice and research communities for the conduct of research as well, especially for epidemiological studies.

But the tendency to think of each disease as a separate, distinct entity has a dark side. It encourages tunnel vision, and promotes the idea that each disease has its own specific cause(s), its own unique explanatory mechanism, and its own targeted treatment (usually a specific drug).

The classification and treatment of disease isn't always so strictly reliant on this single-factor model. Medical professionals sometimes recognize that there may be more than one cause for a specific disease, or more than one drug to treat it. For example, many cancers are attributed to multiple possible factors: genes, environmental toxins, and viruses, working either separately or in combination. And most doctors can think of a few different antibiotics that are equally useful for bacterial infections, a few different analgesics for pain, or a few different antihypertensives for controlling blood pressure. This type of thinking definitely goes beyond the one cause/one disease worldview upon which much of medicine rests. But most practitioners view such instances as exceptions rather than the rule, and this line of thought still diverts attention away from the possibility that there are more effective natural ways of treating ailments. This is a shame, since really paying attention to the amount of overlap among causes, mechanisms, and outcomes could help more medical professionals break out of the narrow disease paradigm.

NUTRITION: WHAT WHOLISTIC MEDICINE LOOKS LIKE

Most people in the medical community of practitioners and researchers do not regard looking for global mechanisms of health and disease as proper science. Before admitting nutritional medicine to the "legitimate disciplines" club, they would want to know the precise details of how such a complex system works for each disease event. Short of that, they would insist on identifying the "active agents" of food, rather than simply accepting that the food itself is what's good for us. Of course, they are asking for something that is impossible, at least when it comes to nutrition—we don't know exactly how it works, because we cannot identify all the parts, what they do, and how they do it. We just know that it *does* work.

The medical community often cites the mantra that there is no such thing as "one size fits all," revealing their inability and abject refusal to fully embrace the idea of complexity and its implications. Nature does a far better job of arranging for proper biological functioning than we like to admit, and once we accept the ability of the body's infinitely complex system to attain and maintain health, then the one-size-fits-all philosophy begins to make sense. We can imagine "one size" being whole, plant-based foods, with an almost infinite number and variety of parts acting harmonically as one, as in symphony, and "fits all" as their ability to act on a broad variety of illnesses. While the one-size-fits-all approach cannot be applied within the paradigm of targeted drug therapy, it is immensely useful and powerful within the wholistic nutrition paradigm.

Another way to say this is that poor nutrition causes vastly more diseases than the disease-care system currently acknowledges; and that good nutrition, in contrast, is a cure for all those diseases and more. Poor nutrition is the root cause that all those blind elephant doctors can't see.

Nutritional solutions to disease should seem like just so much common sense at this point, but it's still worth taking a moment to look at how a medical system based on nutrition contrasts with the reductionist system we have today (see Figure 10-1).

Disease Management (reductionist)	Nutrition (wholistic)
Reactive	Preventive
Looks at symptoms	Looks at underlying causes
Prefers isolated treatments	Prefers systemic treatments
Uses unnatural chemicals	Uses natural foods

FIGURE 10-1.   Disease management versus nutrition

While the disease management system is reactive, nutritional medicine is proactive in preventing diseases before they develop. Disease management focuses on symptoms, while nutrition addresses the underlying causes of those symptoms. Disease management chooses isolated, reductionist treatments that attempt to target specific sites in our bodies, while nutrition simply gives the body the resources to select what it needs to maintain and regain health wholistically. And while disease management favors synthetic drugs that our bodies recognize as toxins, nutrition deploys the foods we have evolved to eat over hundreds of thousands of years, thereby avoiding side effects.

Medicine has become synonymous with ingesting foreign chemicals when our health deteriorates to the point that we have recognizable diseases. Medical practice means chemical practice—on our bodies. There is and always will be a place for the use of isolated chemical substances—even foreign chemicals—but only when all else fails. Reductionist disease management should, however, be a last-ditch accessory to health practice. It can't be the main game in town.

11

Reductionist
Supplementation

Science advances one funeral at a time.

—ANONYMOUS

Most of us know "alternative health"-minded people who are suspicious of the medical/pharmaceutical industries, and instead bet their lives on nutritional supplements: not only specific, identifiable vitamins and minerals, but also other "natural" ingredients like nutraceuticals, prebiotics, probiotics, omega-3 fats, and various whole food concentrates. The supplement industry has grown dramatically over the past thirty years or so; as of 2008, worldwide sales of dietary supplements were estimated at $187 billion.[1] Sixty-eight percent of American adults take dietary supplements, while 52 percent consider themselves "regular" users.[2] Forget apple pie—now nothing is as American as a multivitamin.

By now, I hope you recognize this as one more example of the reductionist paradigm at work, even when it's couched in natural and alternative terms. As we saw in chapter ten, one of the major problems with modern medicine is its reliance on isolated, unnatural chemical pharmaceuticals as the primary tool in the war against disease. But the medical profession isn't the only player in the health-care system that has embraced this element of reductionism. The natural health community has also fallen prey to the ideology that chemicals ripped from their natural context are as good as or better than whole foods. Instead of synthesizing the presumed "active ingredients" from medicinal herbs, as done for prescription drugs, supplement manufacturers seek to extract and bottle the active ingredients from foods known or believed to promote good health and healing. And just like prescription drugs, the active agents function imperfectly, incompletely, and unpredictably when divorced from the whole plant food from which they're derived or synthesized.

The reductionist sleight of hand goes something like this: Oranges are good for us. Oranges are full of vitamin C. Therefore, vitamin C is good for us—even when extracted from the orange, or synthesized in a lab and stuck in a pill, or "fortified" into a breakfast cookie. But there's no evidence that this is the case. As we'll see, not only do most supplements not improve our health, some that have been studied most intensely actually appear to harm us.

RUI HAI LIU AND THE REDUCTIONIST APPLE

Consider the humble apple. We all know the folk wisdom that "an apple a day keeps the doctor away." This insight is supported by all the evidence science has amassed that shows the apple is a food that contributes to health. But what is it about the apple that promotes health? Food composition tables tell us that the average apple contains a significant amount of the following nutrients: vitamin C, vitamin K, vitamin B_6, potassium, dietary fiber, and riboflavin. Also, it's got smaller amounts of vitamin A, vitamin E, niacin, magnesium, phosphorus, copper, manganese, and a whole host of other nutrients.[3] From this long list, can we figure out what really matters about an apple?

A friend and colleague of mine, Dr. Rui Hai Liu, got curious about this question, and he and his research team set about looking for the answer.

Professor Liu was among that early wave of Chinese students who came to the United States when our two countries began to open their doors (and their hearts and minds) in the early 1980s for scholarly exchange.

Because of my early work in China and the rapidly growing reputation of our joint project—the first research project jointly funded by the United States and China (and England)—Liu had sought me out to help him come to Cornell. He tells me that mine was the first American family and home that he visited. He did his PhD research program in Cornell's food science department, and I was a member of his graduate research advisory committee. Upon completion of his studies, an opportunity then arose for him to apply for an assistant professorship in the same department (he clearly demonstrated great potential). Again, he asked me to write a reference letter to support his application. Not long thereafter, he applied for and succeeded in getting some very competitive research funding from the NIH to enable him to develop a substantial research program. Since then, Liu's successes have been impressive. Now a tenured professor, he has amassed a very productive research career, establishing himself as an internationally prominent researcher and lecturer in his field.

The course of that career included his early findings about the health effects of the apple, an area of study that flowed naturally from his personal background. Professor Liu's father was a well-known herbalist in China, and, as a young boy, Liu helped his father make herbal preparations. He grew up in a family concerned with human health, within a culture that viewed health care wholistically. When Chinese doctors counsel patients, they traditionally consider the whole person: physically, mentally, socially, and environmentally. Their practice of "medicine" also considers the wholistic effects of whole plants, usually multiple plants, in their preparation of herbal remedies (plants comprise about 95 percent of remedies in traditional Chinese medicine). So Professor Liu was accustomed to looking at things not only in a reductionist way, as he was trained to in his Western biomedical schooling, but also in a more wholistic way, based on his familiarity with Chinese medical philosophy.

In studying the apple, Professor Liu and his research team began by choosing to focus on vitamin C and its antioxidant effect. They found that 100 grams of fresh apples (about four ounces, or half a cup) had an antioxidant, vitamin C–like activity equivalent to 1,500 milligrams of vitamin C (about three times the amount of a typical vitamin C supplement). When they chemically analyzed that 100 grams of whole apple, however, they found only 5.7 milligrams of vitamin C, far below the 1,500 milligrams that the level of antioxidant activity associated with vitamin

C indicated. The vitamin C–like activity from 100 grams of whole apple was an astounding 263 times as potent as the same amount of the isolated chemical! Said another way, the specific chemical we refer to as vitamin C accounts for much less than 1 percent of the vitamin C–like activity in the apple—a minuscule amount. The other 99-plus percent of this activity is due to other vitamin C–like chemicals in the apple, the possible ability of vitamin C to be much more effective in context of the whole apple than it is when consumed in an isolated form, or both.

Based on what I shared in chapter six, this just makes sense. The process of nutrition is profoundly wholistic, in that the way the body uses a particular nutrient depends on what other nutrients are ingested along with it. If we just take an isolated vitamin C pill, we miss out on the cast of "supporting characters" that may give vitamin C its potency. Even if we add many of those characters into the pill too, which some manufacturers have done with bioflavonoids, we are still assuming that whatever is in the apple and not in the pill is somehow unimportant.

The results of Professor Liu's study were published in the prestigious science journal *Nature*[4] and attracted considerable media attention. In that article, Liu's group concluded "that natural antioxidants from fresh fruit could be more effective than a dietary supplement [of vitamin C]." What a profound finding! The outcome of a fully reductionist study design (measuring the amount of vitamin C in an apple) demonstrated the utter fallacy of the reductionist toolkit.

Dr. Liu's subsequent research provided an even clearer picture of the mind-blowing complexity of a simple food like an apple. Once he discovered that an apple was far more powerful a vitamin C delivery system than it "should" have been, he wondered about the mechanisms that might explain that huge difference. His lab focused on searching for the kinds of chemicals that might account for the rest of the vitamin C–like activity in apples. Liu and his graduate student (now Dr.) Jeanelle Boyer eventually summarized their work—along with the findings of others—to show that there is a treasure trove of such vitamin C–like compounds in apples.[5] These include other antioxidants with names like quercetin, catechin, phlorizin, and chlorogenic acid found only in plants, each of which may exist in many forms within the apple. The list of these chemicals in apples and other fruits is long, and likely reflects just the tip of the iceberg. It's as if the inside of the apple is bigger than it looks from the outside.

Something else to keep in mind: This growing list of vitamin C–like compounds may have many important biological effects that may or may not depend on their antioxidant activities. Liu and his research group have used at least four laboratory tests to determine these various effects, including the ability of these compounds to inhibit the proliferation of cells (potentially stopping or even reversing cancer), decrease serum cholesterol (affecting cardiovascular disease and stroke), and generally block unwanted oxidation (implicated in cancer, aging, cardiovascular disease, and many other degenerative processes). Of course, there also are many other health functions that he could have tested as well.

It is now clear that there are hundreds if not thousands of chemicals in apples, each of which, in turn, may affect thousands of reactions and metabolic systems.[6] This enormous number and concentration of vitamin C–like chemicals in apples poses a serious challenge to the notion that a single chemical—vitamin C or anything else—is responsible for the major health-giving properties of apples. Even if we measure the amount of vitamin C two apples contain, we can't assume that one apple has twice the health value of a second just because it has twice the amount of vitamin C; the amount of vitamin C in a given apple may not tell us very much about that apple's antioxidant power. Add to this what we discussed in chapter six about the complexity of nutrition—that sometimes a combination of nutrients is more (or less) than the sum of its parts, and that the body plays a role in determining how many nutrients from the foods we consume are actually used—and it's hard to avoid the conclusion that knowing how much vitamin C (or even all vitamin C–like nutrients) there is in a given apple doesn't tell us anything of value.

This dilemma is not unique to vitamin C–like antioxidants, or any other fruit or vegetable for that matter. The same is true for any nutrient isolated from any whole food. Many chemically similar groups of health-giving chemicals present in food and circulating in the body are composed of dozens, if not hundreds or even thousands, of analogs that have the same kind of activities but very different potencies.

The problem here is not that we *can't* provide an accurate answer to how much of a nutrient there is in a given food, or even that we can't figure out how much we need for optimal functioning (though this is still currently beyond our grasp). The problem is that we are asking the wrong questions—questions based on a fundamental misunderstanding of the wholistic nature of nutrition. We're asking, "How much vitamin C are we getting?" when we should be asking, "What foods should we be eating to support our bodies' ability to maintain health?"

The reductionist mind cannot see the apple as promoting health and leave it at that. If apples are good for us, it can't be the whole apple. There must be some tiny part of the apple, some chemical inside the apple, that is responsible for its beneficial effects. And our job is to extract that thing from the apple and figure out exactly how much of it people need on a daily basis.

Under the reductionist mindset, healthy eating becomes a crapshoot of nutrient micromanagement—a list of individual nutrients that must be consumed in specific, regimented quantities. But in nature, you don't find beta-carotene on its own. You can't cut a slice of beta-carotene out of a carrot.

Unfortunately, that doesn't stop the supplement industry from trying.

THE SUPPLEMENT INDUSTRY

The two-part assumption inherent to this reductionist thinking about nutrition—that there is a single active ingredient in healthy foods, and that we can take it out of context while still maintaining its effect—is the foundation of the supplements industry. Founded on the techno-fantasy that we can get all our nutritional needs met by powders, pills, or cubes, this industry has been relentless in analyzing foods known to promote health so it can extract and synthesize their active agents. We've already seen how the medical community treats disease with individual chemicals synthesized or isolated from their natural origins. As should now be clear, so does the "natural medicine" community. And it's no more effective there than it is in mainstream medicine. More than that, supplements, as with their formally tested medical counterparts, can actually cause harm.

You may find it hard to swallow the truth of the ineffectiveness and potential harm of supplements. Arguably, the supplement industry has been even more effective in spreading their propaganda than the pharmaceutical industry. After all, supplements are "natural"; they are the same nutrients you find in food. And you can see ads for natural supplements in yoga magazines, at natural-living expos, and in your local health shop.

Your chiropractor may recommend or even sell some pills in his or her office. You may find yourself aligned socially, politically, and even spiritually with the supplement industry. But there's nothing natural about consuming these nutrients in isolation. And the main issue is not whether you like the marketing of natural pills, but what effects these vitamins and related supplements have on your long-term health.

There are many examples demonstrating the failure of individual nutrient supplements to do what they are expected to do. In fact, sometimes these supplements do exactly the opposite. While some individual studies may occasionally show a statistically significant health benefit for vitamin supplements in the short term (and a presumed benefit for the long term), when the findings of a large number of studies are collectively evaluated, there is little or no evidence that routine vitamin supplementation improves health. Researchers have looked long and hard, in vain and using lots of money, for verifiable reductions in cardiovascular disease,[7] cancer,[8] and total mortality[9] as a result of supplementation. Some of the best studies show that not only is reductionist supplementation not beneficial, it can actually be harmful. Let's take a look at three of the most studied supplements—vitamin E, beta-carotene, and omega-3 fats—to show what I mean.

Vitamin E

Vitamin E was first discovered in green leafy vegetables in 1922.[10] Since then, studies have shown that vitamin E is integral to a large number of biochemical functions, suggesting a wide range of health benefits. Indeed, the higher the levels of vitamin E in the blood, the lower the risk for a large number of diseases. Vitamin E is fat soluble (rather than water soluble), so it can work in fatty environments such as cell membranes, where it protects the membranes and their enzymes from oxidation damage.[11]

In recent years vitamin E has become a popular and routine supplement for the prevention of cardiovascular and other diseases,[12] on the theory that if vitamin E in food is so important to good health, then isolated vitamin E supplementation must be good as well. In the natural health community, vitamin E pills are widely thought of as the "wonder nutrient."

Even theoretically this doesn't add up. For one thing, vitamin E, like the other nutrients we've looked at in this book, seldom if ever acts independently; it can be substantially influenced by many other nutrients, including selenium, sulfur-containing amino acids, and polyunsaturated fatty acids. So removing vitamin E from its context within plant foods is like sending a general into battle without any troops. What's more, what we usually call vitamin E is actually not one vitamin, but a family of eight similar but slightly different varieties (called *analogs*).[13] While sharing many of the same functions, they vary significantly in potency[14] and the tissues they target.[15]

The market for vitamin E supplementation surged after a 1993 study found an association between higher vitamin E levels in the blood and lower incidence of major coronary disease.[16] What the study measured, however, was vitamin E that came from foods, not supplements. The authors made a small leap of faith when they concluded that high blood levels of vitamin E are what cause heart health (since the study was designed to detect an association, not a causal relationship), and a bigger one when they suggested that "vitamin E *supplements* may reduce the risk of coronary heart disease" (Emphasis mine). To their credit, the authors cautioned that more trials were needed before recommending widespread use of vitamin E supplements. But too many people have ignored the caution and interpreted this study to mean that vitamin E supplementation prevents heart disease.

The media hype about this study has fueled the huge market for vitamin E supplements over the past two decades. But all this interest has also brought about additional studies, which tell a very different story. Based on randomized controlled trials, vitamin E supplements do not decrease risk of cardiovascular diseases,[17] cancer,[18] diabetes,[19] cataracts,[20] or chronic obstructive lung disease.[21] These findings are broad based and quite convincing. Their size, their breadth (they look at multiple diseases), the number of studies, and the contrary researcher expectations support a compelling case: that vitamin E supplements do not work the way reductionists expect them to, based on the demonstrated benefits of vitamin E–containing foods. Although there may be a few special groups of people for whom vitamin E supplementation might offer marginal benefits, the vast majority of people receive no advantage from it.

And that's actually way too kind an assessment, according to recent research. One recent review of over six-dozen randomized trials involving nearly 300,000 subjects found that taking supplemental vitamin E (as well as vitamin A and beta-carotene, which we'll discuss below) was associated with greater overall mortality.[22] That's right; not only does supplemental vitamin E not make you healthier, it actually can contribute to your premature death.

Advocates of vitamin E supplementation have responded to these findings in a few rather expected ways. Some have blamed these studies' experimental design or the interpretation of their findings[23]—a fair, even desirable response among scientists, whose job it is to seek valid conclusions from imperfect data. But a responsible scientist can hardly ignore the growing consistency of findings among many studies questioning the supplemental use of this nutrient.

Other researchers have pointed out that the first four analogs of vitamin E (the tocopherols) were the ones used in these last trials. They've suggested that perhaps focusing on their brethren (the tocotrienols) might be a good idea because, in some systems, they are more active, supposedly to do good.[24] But this fails to mention that these analogs also may have more potential of doing bad.

Last, still other advocates of vitamin E supplementation have responded by searching for special groups for whom the benefits might outweigh the risks, including people with various genetic susceptibilities.[25] But this strategy still ignores the real possibility that a WFPB diet could do the same thing at lower cost and with fewer side effects like heart failure[26] and death.[27]

It's hard to argue with the mounting evidence: the beneficial effects of vitamin E are clearly lost when vitamin E is removed from its original plant-based environment and sold to us in bottles. But you wouldn't know it from the hype masquerading as legitimate research.

Omega-3

Like vitamin E, omega-3 fatty acids are essential to our bodies' functioning. As with all "essential" nutrients, we cannot manufacture these fatty acids, so we have to get them from our diet. There are three types of essential omega-3s: ALA, DHA, and EPA (although DHA is not usually considered essential under the right dietary conditions, as when one's diet includes adequate omega-3 in relationship to omega-6 and total fat). They are found in certain plants and also in some types of fish and edible algae.

Omega-3s appear to protect our bodies from inflammation; that is, they are anti-inflammatory, and thus being helpful in reducing rheumatoid arthritis and cardiovascular disease. Several small studies found that omega-3 fats improved clinical biomarkers of diabetes like glucose tolerance,[28] blood triglycerides,[29] and levels of high-density lipoprotein (HDLs, or the "good" part of one's total blood cholesterol),[30] which suggests that omega-3 fats may protect against diabetes.

Omega-3 fatty acids are one of the current darlings of the mainstream nutritional health world. To ensure we get enough of them, the media urges us to eat lots of fish, specifically fatty species like anchovies, herring, salmon, sardines, and tuna. (They don't often mention that one form of omega-3, ALA, which is found in certain nuts and seeds, can be converted in the body into the other forms, making fish consumption unnecessary.) And of course, we are also urged to take omega-3 supplements.

Supplement makers sell omega-3 to us mostly in the form of fish oil capsules. They focus on claims of "purity" for their products, contrasting them against the fatty fish we eat that contain dangerously high levels of mercury, PCBs, and other contaminants. The WebMD website goes so far as to warn pregnant women and children away from many species of wild and all species of farm-raised fish. So omega-3 supplementation would appear to be the smarter way to get what we need of this essential nutrient. In reality, however, this has proven not to be the case.

When the findings for a huge group of eighty-nine studies (this is a lot of studies!) were summarized, it was concluded that "omega-3 fats *do not* have a clear effect on total mortality, combined cardiovascular events or cancer"[31] (Emphasis mine). In a very large study of nearly 200,000 individuals over fifteen years,[32] increasing consumption of omega-3 fats (combined intakes mostly from fish but some from supplements) was actually associated with increased risk of Type 2 diabetes: the higher the omega-3 intake, the more likely the subject was to develop diabetes. In total, the study included almost 10,000 Type 2 diabetes cases, and as the omega-3 intake increased, the number of diabetes cases trended upward, so it's highly unlikely that this association is due to random chance.

Do higher intakes of omega-3 fats really increase Type 2 diabetes? What about those earlier, smaller studies that suggested omega-3s might prevent diabetes? How can we explain this discrepancy? When you look at these studies carefully, there is no discrepancy. The earlier, smaller studies were short term and looked only at biomarkers associated with diabetes. That's not the same as findings on the final occurrence of disease. Short-term findings are only isolated blips in a very complex sea of events. Yet supplement makers rely on these reductionist rushes to judgment, rather than waiting for meaningful long-term study results, to convince us that their products are effective.

Beta-carotene

A now-classic example showing this shortsighted rush to judgment based on short-term effects is the story of beta-carotene, the vitamin A precursor found in plants that our bodies convert into "real" vitamin A. Beta-carotene occurs naturally in green leafy plants and brightly colored red, orange, and yellow vegetables such as chili peppers, carrots, and pumpkins. In the 1970s, beta-carotene was discovered to be a powerful antioxidant[33] that could block the activities of free radicals thought to promote cancer growth. Also, beta-carotene-rich foods (i.e., vegetables and fruits) were associated with decreased lung cancer.[34] Together, these observations provided suggestive evidence that beta-carotene might protect against lung cancer, and perhaps other cancers as well.

About ten years later, however, a human study among smokers in Finland showed that beta-carotene supplements given for 6.5 years increased lung cancer deaths by 46 percent,[35] a very large and statistically significant effect. In addition, cardiovascular deaths were increased 26 percent for those taking the supplements.[36] This adverse effect was so prominent that the study had to be terminated early. That's right: beta-carotene supplementation increased death rates so dramatically that the trial was ended early to prevent further deaths.

Interestingly, in this same study, baseline beta-carotene consumption from food was associated with lower lung cancer risk. This difference was stark. Food beta-carotene was associated with less lung cancer, but supplement beta-carotene was associated with more lung cancer. This finding was confirmed in other big studies as well.[37]

Since that time, a consensus has emerged showing that beta-carotene supplementation does not decrease cancer or cardiovascular disease.[38]

SUPPLEMENTAL OBSTINACY

We now have a ton of studies showing all manner of mechanisms by which beta-carotene, vitamin E, and other antioxidant vitamins *ought* to prevent diseases like heart disease and cancer, but, when tested alone (e.g., in pills), they don't. Even though researchers are beginning to accept these specific findings, and are no longer recommending supplemental beta-carotene, vitamin E, or omega-3, they still tenaciously cling to the same old beliefs, claiming that, despite disappointments, we should continue to put our faith in preventing disease through isolated chemicals. What incredible stubbornness!

In the face of increasingly robust and consistent findings showing that isolated nutritional supplements are bad news, the supplement industry and its hired researchers are responding by digging their reductionist hole ever deeper. Some want to escalate the search for new antioxidant chemicals in plants, in the hopes that they have more pluses and fewer minuses than the current bunch.[39] Others suggest that a more customized selection of clinical biomarkers might help unearth new health benefits for the same antioxidants we're studying currently. That is, since the antioxidant effects that we're looking at now seem disconnected from meaningful health outcomes, we should instead look for different inter-mediate effects that do predict things we care about, like less disease and longer life. But the reason we use biomarkers as proxies for actual health—because it's cheaper and quicker to measure biochemistry than to follow study participants for years to see what happens to them—is exactly why biomarker studies are not appropriate for determining the true effects of a supplement on human health.

The reaction of researchers to the news about the failure of vitamin E, beta-carotene, and other isolated antioxidants to create health disheart-ens me. Many researchers are now aware of these failed studies.[40] They acknowledge the complex nature of antioxidant activity and the legiti-macy of several reports showing that vitamin supplements may in some circumstances cause toxicity. But rather than consider giving up on this dead-end approach to health, in some cases these researchers present still more technical details they hope will justify additional and more complex supplement research. After all these years and all these studies, they still fail to see the futility of continuing to go down this same very expensive and virtually useless path of searching for some new antioxidant analog that has the special ability to create health. Someday, perhaps, they'll find that needle in the haystack—the reductionist supplement that outperforms its natural counterpart. But I wouldn't count on it.

During the mid-1980s, when the nutrient supplement industry was initially emerging, I spent about three years giving substantial testimony, at the request of the National Academy of Sciences, to the U.S. Federal Trade Commission as to whether health claims favoring vitamin supplementation were justified by the then-existing evidence. I testified against the industry's proposed health claims both because reliable evidence did not exist and because, from the biological perspective I held then, it did not make sense. The perspective I held then is the same one I've presented here in this book a quarter-century later: nutrients rarely if ever act alone, or at least not properly so. After a few hundred billion (mostly) taxpayer dollars spent doing the research, we are now finally getting evidence that may prove helpful in moving this mountain.

Please understand: I'm not saying that there is no benefit for some people for some supplement preparations, especially when the chemical composition of the supplement begins to approximate the composition of whole plants, as in some dried herbal compounds. These products may be helpful under some conditions for certain people. But for me, the burden of proof is on those who make such assertions, and by "burden of proof," I mean objective research findings that pass the test of peer review. It is not appropriate to propose or even infer that these "natural supplements" are the best health option without also making clear that the routine consumption of whole, plant-based foods—from whence these products came—will produce far better health at a far cheaper price.

The danger of our increasing consumption of supplements is more than just the documented negative effects on our health. It's that our love affair with the magic bullet of supplementation lets us believe we're "off the hook" when it comes to eating right. Why eat your veggies when you can binge on hot dogs and ice cream and, if you get into trouble, make it all better with a pill?

Nutritional supplementation is proving to be the canary in the coal mine for the reductionist approach to health. While the pharmaceutical approach continues unabated, the supplement initiative, at least, appears to have reached a research dead end. Only by applying reductionist research methods—attributing too much significance to biomarkers and individual chemicals and refusing to look at real health outcomes—can the supplement industry defend its project of factory-formed fragments of former food as the road to good health.

12

Reductionist
Social Policy

Whatever we do to the earth, we do to ourselves.

—CHIEF SEATTLE

So far in Part II, we've been looking at reductionism in terms of nutrition and food policy, and how reductionism's effects impact individual health outcomes and quality of life through diet. But our reductionist approach to nutrition affects other areas of life, too. Social policy isn't my area of expertise, but as a member of several high-profile food- and health-policy expert panels, I've certainly considered the likely impact of dietary recommendations on social and cultural practices. Thus, I'd be remiss not to at least touch on the way reductionism affects the way we look at social problems, and how the nutrition information that reductionism discourages us from seeing—the benefits of the plant-based diet over one high in animal products—also affects the world we live in.

When you connect the dots of some of our biggest social, economic, and environmental problems, you can clearly see nutrition looming large as a causal factor and potential solution. It turns out that eating—how we literally absorb nature, or an artificial substitute, into our bodies—holds huge implications for how we treat the rest of nature and our fellow humans.

WHAT WE DO TO OURSELVES, WE DO TO THE EARTH

Every July 4th weekend, my adopted home town of Durham, North Carolina, hosts a wonderful crafts and music festival to raise money to preserve a local river. Bands come from all over the country to share their music in a beautiful state park. Vendors sell handmade jewelry, pottery, and clothing. Activists and environmentalists hold forth on solar energy, river cleanup projects, opposition to nuclear facilities, and various other causes. Every napkin, spoon, plate, and cup given out by food vendors is 100 percent biodegradable. In short, you couldn't hope to find a more environmentally conscious gathering.

Except for one thing: most of the food that festivalgoers shovel into their bodies. Deep-fried funnel cakes slathered in synthetic syrup and confectioners' sugar. Giant turkey drumsticks, hamburgers, chicken breasts, and corn dogs sourced from factory farms that pump hormones and antibiotics into their products. French fries submerged in fryers of genetically modified cooking oil. While we know that littering and polluting rivers and streams is bad, somehow we've accepted that polluting our own bodies is okay, as if what we eat has no impact on the rest of the environment.

I know many environmentalists whose commitment is manifest and commendable, but stops at their lips. It's understandable; many of our favorite "foods" (or, more properly, food-like items) are highly addictive. And our relationship with food is far more emotionally fraught than, say, our relationship with incandescent light bulbs or plastic shopping bags. But even these far-seeing and far-thinking activists are wearing reductionist blinders if they cannot see that their personal food choices matter at least as much as—and I would argue considerably more than—recycling and using energy-efficient light bulbs.

I began this chapter with a quote, attributed to Chief Seattle: "Whatever we do to the earth, we do to ourselves." You may have come across it, or some variation on it, before; it's often invoked by environmentalists to remind us that we can't clear-cut our forests, pollute our water, and spew toxins into our air without ultimately harming ourselves. But what's less obvious is that the reverse is equally true: what we eat has a huge impact on our environment. Specifically, our high consumption of animal-based foods contributes to environmental problems like soil loss, groundwater contamination, deforestation, fossil fuel use, and depletion of deep aquifers.

A Cornell University colleague of mine, Dr. David Pimentel, has documented many ways that our system of livestock production wastes precious resources and destroys the environment. He estimates that animal-based food requires about five to fifty times more land and water resources than the same number of calories of plant-based food (depending on various considerations, including animal species and whether the animal is pasture fed). In a world where human hunger is endemic, this inefficient use of resources is a tragedy.

Among Dr. Pimentel's findings:[1]

- Animal protein production requires eight times as much fossil fuel as plant protein.
- The livestock population of the United States consumes five times as much grain (which is not even their natural diet) as the country's entire human population.
- Every kilogram of beef requires 100,000 liters of water to produce. By comparison, a kilogram of wheat requires just 900 liters, and a kilogram of potatoes just 500 liters.
- A United Nations–sponsored workshop[2] of about 200 experts concluded that 80 percent of deforestation in the tropics is attributable to the creation of new farmland, the majority of which is used for livestock grazing and feed.

So we've got a host of interconnected problems that all stem from our addiction to an animal-protein-based diet. Simply put, our industrial system of animal production is unsustainable. We're using up our natural resources, such as fresh water and healthy soil, faster than we can replenish them. And the side effects of our animal-protein-driven food economy include environmental toxins and the poisoning of the very air we all depend on for life.

These are serious problems; each of them deserves a book of their own. And they're only the tip of the iceberg. If you want to learn more,

I highly recommend J. Morris Hicks's excellent work, *Healthy Eating, Healthy World*. For the purposes of this discussion, however, I want to focus on four problems that neither policy makers nor the media generally see as being connected to diet: two of the most significant environmental crises of our time, global warming and the depletion of America's deep underground water resources; and the cruelty and violence done to two of the most vulnerable groups on the planet, animals and impoverished humans. We'll see how reductionist thinking keeps us stuck, and how a wholistic approach can solve these multiple problems simultaneously.

OUR FOOD CHOICES AND GLOBAL WARMING

Let's start with the most prominent ecological crisis of our time: global warming. When you look seriously at the numbers, you find that switching from a meat-based to a plant-based diet would do more to curb and reverse global warming than any other initiative.

One of the intelligent criticisms of Al Gore's powerful and important documentary, *An Inconvenient Truth*, was that its prescriptions were woefully inadequate in light of the problem's magnitude. Tips like replacing incandescent light bulbs with compact fluorescents, lowering your thermostat by a couple of degrees, and keeping your car tires fully inflated may make you feel virtuous, but have little to no impact on the real problem. A tip sheet available from ClimateCrisis.net announces that reducing the amount of garbage you produce by 10 percent can save 1,200 pounds of carbon dioxide per year. When you do the math, you realize that the other 90 percent of your garbage still produces 10,800 pounds of CO_2 each year. Doing the same things a little less intensively is not going to turn global warming around, especially when the CO_2 we've already produced is going to be trapping heat in the atmosphere for hundreds of years to come. It's like we're all on a bus that's speeding toward the edge of a cliff, and the best idea we have is for everyone to stick their arms out the windows to increase wind resistance. Maybe someone should jump into the driver's seat and hit the brakes!

In 2006, the United Nations' Food and Agricultural Organization issued a report that highlighted the connection between animal foods and global warming.[3] Its contents are striking because this agency is chiefly responsible for developing livestock operations around the world. Being biased, if anything, toward observing the opposite effect, this report still concluded that eating animal-based foods creates 18 percent of global warming, more than the contributions of either industry or transportation.[4] This information, now six years old, is still not widely known.

On the relatively few occasions that food enters discussions on global warming, this 18 percent estimate is brought up. However, a more recent report concludes that this estimate of food's contribution to warming may be much higher. Robert Goodland, the longtime senior environmental advisor to the president of the World Bank, and Jeff Anhang, his colleague at the World Bank Group, have determined that livestock rearing contributes at least *51 percent* of total global warming.

The most famous greenhouse gas, the one that gets most of the attention from the media, activists, and policy makers, is CO_2. But CO_2 is not the only greenhouse gas, and is not in fact the one most sensitive to reduction efforts. Methane (CH_4) offers a more promising lever with which to push back global warming. Molecule for molecule, methane is about twenty-five times more potent in trapping heat than carbon dioxide. But more important, methane, with an atmospheric half-life of seven years, disappears from the atmosphere far faster than carbon dioxide, which has a half-life of more than a century. So almost as soon as we eliminate sources of methane, its contribution to the greenhouse effect begins to wane significantly. By contrast, even after we stop releasing CO_2, the gas that has already been released will contribute to global warming for decades.

When the amount of methane in the atmosphere is considered over a twenty-year period, its global warming potential is said to be *seventy-two times* that of CO_2.[5] And methane is largely associated with industrial livestock production. This means that reducing meat consumption, the main driver of the livestock industry, may be the most rapid way to affect global warming. It turns out that our present programs, focused on carbon dioxide reduction, are mostly a lot of hot air—in more ways than one.

If this new assessment of the methane contribution is correct, the implications are momentous. I am puzzled as to why more people in the environmental community aren't paying attention to this. Do they not want to challenge the livestock industry? Maybe we need bioengineers to figure out how to entrap and safely process cow farts. Failing this, maybe we should stop producing and eating the machines that do the farting.[6]

UNDERGROUND WATER
DEPLETION IN THE MIDWEST

As I write this in August 2012, most of the United States is in the grip of its worst drought in over a century. Scientists can debate the connection between this catastrophe and global warming, but there's no denying that rainwater is in short supply, crops are dying before germination, and vast amounts of groundwater will be needed if our country is to produce enough crops to feed its people. The trouble is, most of the available groundwater either already has been used up by the enormous demands of beef production (each kilogram of beef, remember, requires 100,000 liters of water to produce), or has been polluted by runoff from beef production (huge volumes of water run through feedlots to remove the vast quantities of manure).

The great Ogallala Aquifer, lying under eight Midwestern farming states (South Dakota, Nebraska, Wyoming, Colorado, Kansas, Oklahoma, New Mexico, and Texas), has been especially threatened by animal-based agriculture. Its water collected there ten to twenty million years ago,[7] and now contains an estimated volume equal to that of Lake Huron, the second largest of the Great Lakes. This water provides nearly all the water for residential, industrial, and agricultural use in this very large farming region, one of the richest agricultural production areas on the planet. "More than 90% of the water pumped from the Ogallala irrigates at least one fifth of all the U.S. cropland," according to a major report of the nonprofit Kerr Center for Sustainable Agriculture in Oklahoma.[8]

It's crucial that groundwater consumption doesn't exceed its replenishment by rain. But that's not what's happening with the Ogallala Aquifer. Water-intensive livestock farming is depleting it far faster than it can be refilled, to the point where this ancient resource has lost an estimated 9 percent of its water since the 1950s. In other words, we're using it up faster than rain can replenish it—a recipe for environmental disaster.[9]

Not only that, the Ogallala water is being polluted with chemicals used in growing feed for cattle production.[10] One of the more significant of these is nitrates, which are used in the commercial fertilizer used to produce animal feed and which can be quite toxic for pregnant women and children.[11] Saying no to factory-farmed meat from the Midwest can go a long way toward preserving the way of life of the thousands of farmers who provide plant-based food to millions of Americans, as well as improving the health of these millions wherever they consume this food.

ANIMAL CRUELTY, ANIMAL TESTING, AND THE MODERN LIVESTOCK FARM

Another consequence of consuming animal-based foods is animal cruelty: farming practices that, in making the production of animal-based foods more efficient, also increase those animals' suffering.

Concern for the rights of animals has drawn many people to eat plant-based foods, although as you saw in Part I, this is not what brought me to my present position. Although I certainly embrace the proposition that unnecessary acts of violence against animals should be avoided, it was the findings of experimental animal research—hateful to many in the animal rights community—that started me on the path that ultimately led me to my present position and, eventually, to my enlightenment on this issue. For myself, I am opposed to unnecessary violence of any kind: violence against people, violence against our environment, and violence against other sentient beings. Honoring life of all kinds is the holy grail that I seek.

However, I have much greater concern today regarding violence done to animals than before. In considerable measure, I've been spurred to this view because I have watched the emergence of the farming practice called confined animal feeding operation (CAFO), a fancy phrase for factory farming. The main difference between factory farming and the old-time farming of my youth is philosophical. My family and I thought of animals as sensory beings, capable both of comfort and suffering, while factory farmers, by virtue of their business model, see them as virtually lifeless units of production, much like the raw materials of any factory. Early in my career in the late 1960s, I remember well when the dean of the College of Agriculture at Virginia Tech excitedly told us about his consulting work, which led to the livestock operations that eventually became the CAFOs.

It was inevitable, as the economies of scale that CAFOs enabled became necessary for the bottom line of any farmer who wanted his operation to survive. The dean painted a technologically advanced picture of automated conveyor belts delivering precise amounts of nutritionally optimized feed to animals. Of automated machinery streamlining the milking of cows. Of contraptions for more efficiently collecting hens' eggs. All this, he claimed, meant more profit for the farmer.

Cows are mostly docile animals. They certainly feel and express emotions. In times gone by, they mostly spent much of their fifteen to twenty years in the pasture (in spring, summer, and fall) or in barns bedded with straw (in winter). In CAFOs, dairy cows live only three or four years, coinciding with their years of peak milk production. They are penned up in tight living (dying) quarters, never again to be pastured on green grass after they begin producing milk. I am constantly reminded of this practice on my jogging route in upstate New York, where I see cows that live in a giant CAFO poking their heads slightly out of their open-air building, as if they were craving the lush grass outside.

Young cows' tails are frequently chopped off (a practice known as docking), leaving only a stub a foot or so long, so that the person milking the cows avoids getting "switched" with a filthy, often manure-encrusted, tail—something I remember all too well. A stub for a tail doesn't do much to keep the flies off a cow's back—that's what tails are for—and if this irritation from flies affects a cow's milk production, she is drenched with a pesticide spray that can get into the milk we find in our supermarkets.

Most factory-farmed cows are injected with a growth hormone to increase their milk production that also increases their udder size, sometimes to painful dimensions—a physical condition that promotes inflammation called mastitis. Antibiotics are then required to reduce the resulting infections, increasing the amounts of antibiotics, pesticides, blood, and bacteria in the milk that we buy and consume. What a unique cocktail for human consumption!

It's a very different world these days on the farm—and it gets worse. Chickens unable to move in their cages because they're forced to stand in one place long enough for their feet to permanently wrap around the wire mesh on the cage bottom, fixing them in place. Unnatural, abnormal lighting cycles used to make hens lay more eggs and increase the producer's profit. Pigs that give birth to their young in so-called farrowing crates, in which the piglets must nurse from the other side of parallel bars arranged to keep them separate from their mothers.

Then there's the stench in which these animals are forced to spend their entire existence. Walk into a chicken house with thousands of birds and you can feel your eyes burn and tear up. And it's not just animals that can't avoid the smell; if you live near a factory farm, you know that humans are subjected to it, too. I know the smell of cow manure—I shoveled it enough! Today's cow manure has a pungent medicinal smell that is not what it was during my youth.

It's not just the animals that have suffered greatly in this transformation of American agriculture. Family farms, the kind I was raised on, are rapidly going out of business. As I travel through the countryside these days, I see so many once-beautiful barns now mere stick skeletons of old boards covered with weeds. The directive to "get big or get out" has bankrupted most non-factory operations. And government subsidies to the CAFOs obscure the fact that they are as unsustainable economically as they are environmentally.

If you think that it's natural for human beings to eat animals, consider just how unnatural are the lives and deaths of the animals that make up the American food supply in the twenty-first century.

HUMAN POVERTY

Animals and farmers are not the only victims of our animal-based diet. When small-scale agriculture is converted to industrial-scale animal production in the developing world, small land holders are forced off their subsistence plots, and have no way to afford the food being produced on their former land.

I have worked in several desperately poor areas of the world, where my eyes were opened to the connection between meat production and the economic enslavement of the poorest, most vulnerable people in those areas. I've been in the slums of Manila and Port-au-Prince and have seen firsthand desperately hungry children begging for food in a society where the elite eat steak produced on land stolen from the poor. I've seen long stretches of the best land in the Dominican Republic taken away from local farmers and handed to American and German firms, to raise livestock destined to become cheap hamburgers back home. I've heard stories of how this "best land" was "obtained" for cattle raising while small land owners were forced into the mountains, where food production is difficult if not impossible.

The simple math of industrial animal-protein production speaks volumes. In a world where millions of people die of starvation and starvation-related diseases every year, we still inexplicably insist on the gross inefficiency of cycling our plant production through animals before considering it "food." Feeding meat-producing animals rather than feeding humans directly means we lose upward of 90 percent of the calories otherwise available for our consumption. And, as "low-carb" advocates are fond of pointing out, animal-based foods have no carbohydrates, which should, in reality, comprise about 80 percent of a truly healthy diet. Factory-farmed animals on this planet consume more calories than all the humans, by a long shot. Through this lens, the issue of world hunger seems a lot less like a problem of production or distribution and more like a problem with our personal priorities.

Factory farming and large-scale livestock farming also erode the land they use, making it nearly impossible for impoverished nations to pull themselves out of poverty in the future. We see this most distressingly in Latin American countries, whose rainforests are daily logged and converted into fields to grow grain for cattle. After a few years, the soil fertility is spent, and rain and wind erodes what little topsoil remains. Industrial agriculture can eke out a few more grain harvests through heavy application of nitrogen-based fertilizers and herbicides, but after a couple of decades, all that remains is dead earth, a biological desert that will take millennia to recover. The multinational companies that wreak this havoc don't suffer, of course. They just move their operations to the next bit of fertile land—as long as they can still find some. Local farmers are left to pay the price.

If you are interested in solving the global problem of human poverty, you have many choices. You can "like" antipoverty status updates on Facebook. You can donate money to relief organizations that you trust. You can sign online petitions. You can volunteer to raise money. You can even join an advocacy or relief group and get involved on the ground. But one of the most important actions you can take is to say "no" to the system that expropriates subsistence-farming land and turns it into unsustainable feedlots that produce meat for us, cash for the wealthy, and misery, servitude, and starvation for the masses. You can stop consuming factory-farmed meat and dairy.

THE FOOD CONNECTION

We have a problem. No, we have many, many problems. Quixotically, we lament each problem, one by one, rarely seeing their connections to the food we choose to put in our bodies. We create specialists to help us solve each problem as if it stood alone. As a consequence, we fail to see interconnections, and we fail to see the whole. On several occasions, I've been invited to speak to environmental groups and have been asked to explain what I see as the obvious connections between environmental and health issues.

Choosing plant-based foods over animal-based foods reduces pain in so many ways. It alleviates our bodily pain.[12] It minimizes the pain animals experience by reducing CAFO farming. It also reduces human suffering associated with global poverty and hunger. Given all that, it's easy to see that investing in programs that promote, distribute, and encourage the growing of whole, plant-based foods in poor countries would be far more economical and effective than reductionist attempts to solve all these problems separately, as if they had nothing to do with one another.

The problems we face are far more connected than disconnected. Think of the way galaxies are made up of clusters of stars, held together by gravity; these social problems are clustered the same way, except the gravitational pull between them is the food we choose to eat.

The proportion of each of these problems that can be resolved by consuming whole, plant-based foods varies, of course. But for this discussion, those proportions don't matter as much as the fact that we can affect all of these problems in a positive way by doing the very same thing: eating better. There is no dietary or lifestyle strategy that is more comprehensive and effective in reducing and eliminating these problems than the routine consumption of whole, plant-based foods.

The single most important explanation for our failure to solve these problems, as with our failure to solve our health crisis, is our paradigm-driven inability and unwillingness to look for their larger context. The more I contemplate the meaning of paradigms and our failure to recognize them, the more I become aware of their subtle but powerful control over our thinking. The more I contemplate the role of reductionism within these paradigms, the more I become aware of the way reductionism makes it even more difficult to visualize paradigms and their boundaries. The reductionist mental prison is the main thing keeping us from doing grand things for ourselves, each other, and the rest of sentient life on earth. We need to learn how to look for the natural networks that connect many seemingly disconnected events and activities. Only through doing so can we finally find the answers that elude us—whether that's the answer to global warming, the solution to world hunger, or the effective and compassionate healing of our society's most fearful health problems.

PART III

Subtle Power
and Its
Wielders

As we saw in Part II, the reductionist paradigm functions as a mental prison, preventing the best and brightest minds in science, government, and industry from solving some of our biggest problems. More than that, reductionism actually causes and exacerbates many of those problems. In short, reductionist science is not producing health.

When we look closely at the prison of the reductionist paradigm, we notice that there's no lock on the cell door. We're free to stroll out of our mental prison and into a wholistic worldview any time we want. Throughout history, paradigms have arisen, exerted their influence, and then faded, to be replaced by other paradigms that more effectively captured reality and more successfully promoted the common welfare. We have the evidence that our current reductionist paradigm is incorrect (largely supplied, ironically, by reductionist science). So why aren't we walking out that door? The answer is that health information is controlled, and has been for a long time, by interests that are not in alignment with the common good—industries that care much more about their profit than our health. And those industries feel deeply threatened by the possibility of mass adoption of a plant-based diet.

In the next few chapters, we'll look at the groups and other forces exerting that control. We'll examine the obvious ones, such as the pharmaceutical, medical, and food industries, whose motives are transparently profit-seeking. But we'll also turn our attention to those under the sway of that subtle power, who dance to the piper's tune. We'll see that my own field of academic research is highly compromised, incentivized to chase reductionist research past any social use or relevance to health. We'll observe a scientifically illiterate media dutifully reporting the party line on the limited or nonexistent effect of nutrition on health. We'll witness a government in the thrall of industry-bought and pedigreed lobbyists. And finally, we'll examine the seamy underbelly of disease-focused fundraising institutions like the American Cancer Society (ACS) and professional organizations like the Academy of Nutrition and Dietetics (AND).

13

Understanding
the System

*The riskiest thing we can do is just maintain the
status quo.*

—BOB IGER

or the last few decades of my research career, I naïvely believed that
just sharing the facts about the benefits of the WFPB diet would be
enough to sway my colleagues, policy makers, journalists, and businesspeople. I had implicit faith in the evolutionary principle; I thought
that once people knew the truth (and more important, experienced it for
themselves), change would come naturally.

Looking back, my naïveté was immense. In that respect, I had no
more ability to discern the plain truth than my reductionist colleagues.
Despite example after example of human greed and fear of losing power,
I still thought sharing the facts would be enough. That someday the
weight of evidence would be so compelling, so overwhelming, that even
the AND and the ACS (two organizations whose names, in my mind,
mean essentially the same thing!) would bow to the truth and recognize

plant-based nutrition as the cornerstone of a healthy life, a healthy society, and a healthy planet. Scientists would come together with a unified
voice to advocate for a sane diet and social policies that would enable
all people to partake of it. Journalists would spread the very good news
and devote their talents to telling inspiring stories of change. Government officials would hastily abandon ill-conceived subsidies for deadly
foods and create nutritional guidelines and programs that could reduce
health-care costs by 70 to 90 percent in a few years. And industry leaders, as visionary entrepreneurs, would embrace plant-based nutrition as
the foundation of their cafeterias and health insurance plans in order to
maintain a competitive advantage in attracting, retaining, and profiting
from the labor of healthy and happy employees.

Despite the overwhelming evidence that supports a plant-based diet,
none of these things has happened. Plant-based nutrition is still marginalized and maligned as an approach to reducing disease rates, obesity, and
skyrocketing health-care costs. Journalists still tout gene therapy as the
road to redemption and ignore the benefits of eating more plants and less
meat and processed food. Lobbyists representing dairy, meat, sugar, and
other processed foodstuffs all but write government regulations and control the bulk of nutrition-related messaging. Our school lunch programs
highlight the government's lack of commitment to instilling healthy eating
habits in our population. And some companies have responded to the
crisis of health-care costs by cutting insurance coverage and outsourcing
jobs rather than addressing its root cause.

What I'm describing here isn't a vast, evil conspiracy designed to
keep the truth of the plant-based diet from you. Many of the players I've
criticized truly believe their own PR. Lots of cattle ranchers, dairy farmers, and high-fructose corn syrup manufacturers think they're providing high-quality calories to a hungry world. Many scientists are just as
confused as the general population about the big picture of nutrition and
human health. Many journalists report the results of each reductionist
study under the honest misconception that they're describing a comprehensive reality rather than a thin, misleading, out-of-context slice. And
many government officials, while privately acknowledging the immense
benefits of a plant-based diet, think that promoting such an idea would
be counterproductive to their political futures in the face of so much
deep-pocketed industry opposition.

The problem is not that humans are broken or evil. It's that the system is broken. I have spent my entire career in academia and professional research and, like most of my colleagues, I take pride in my institution's gentility, objectivity, and democratic tradition. Indeed, I believed that I experienced these virtues on many occasions. But that was before I realized I was living in a cocoon, unaware of the subtle way in which financial interests inform every part of the scientific process and beyond.

The thing about systems is that they're resilient. I've learned that the hard way, after spending years sharing the best scientific information with policy makers, businesspeople, and consumers and still not having much of an impact on the entire system. You can tweak all the details—you can correct the science all you want—but if the goal isn't changed, the system will continue to produce the same outcomes it always has. The logical goal of a health-care system would be to deliver health. That's the stated goal of ours, certainly. But that's not its actual goal. To discover that goal, as with any other system, we have to observe what it does, not what it claims to do.

If the goal of our health-care system were health, then it would operate in a way that promotes health. It might look clumsy, sloppy, and slow, but the connections built into that system would favor methods and technologies and interventions that move us all inexorably in the direction of good health throughout our lives. Obviously, that's not the case. The goal of our health system is not health; it's profit for a few industries at the expense of the public good.

That's right—profit is the goal at the center of our health-care system, and that skews everything.

A HYPOTHETICAL
HEALTH-CARE SYSTEM

When I say "health-care system" here, I mean more than just doctors, nurses, hospitals, drugs, and surgical apparatus. I mean everything in our society that affects our health, from our agricultural policies, to school lunch programs, to pollution laws, to public education about nutrition, to funding priorities for scientific research, to seat belt enforcement, and so on. This may sound unimaginably complex and hard to manage and restructure, and on a piecemeal basis it is. But let's imagine a hypothetical system in which the primary goal is better public health. In such a system, all these elements and policies would naturally tend to produce better health outcomes.

Since my training is in nutritional biochemistry, I often think of the world in terms of nutrient narratives. And the nutrient around which any healthy modern society is organized is information—in this case, information about health, a key product of science that individuals, governments, nonprofits, corporations, and the media consume. Figure 13-1 is a simplified diagram of how the nutrient information moves through the health-care system.

In an ideal society, the "information cycle" is driven by the goal of empowering people at all levels of society to enjoy healthy lives. That goal would drive the main input of the information cycle, questions that are significant to public health and worthy of research. Scientists would tackle these questions with great curiosity and enthusiasm, collaborating and competing to come up with the most creative, powerful, and valid study designs. Many different studies would be carried out, from the extremely reductionist to the extremely wholistic, which would generate more questions and some controversies. Eventually, a "weight of evidence" would accumulate, consisting of a model that would be tested by its ability to predict future health outcomes. It would not be "The Truth"—science never is—but it would be as close to it as a group of humans could get at that point.

This weight of evidence would then cycle into the rest of society. The media, both professional trade journals and public media organizations such as newspapers, would report it to the people, who would incorporate it into their individual lifestyle choices. Government would create public policy, based on the weight of evidence, designed to promote the general welfare. These two would be the chief sources of public health information. Industry's role would be to create health-related goods and services based on this evidence, since those things that work best tend to sell best. Businesses would compete to innovate and market new products and services that would better serve public health, based on the evidence. And professional and fundraising organizations would base their philanthropy and marketing on promoting and leveraging the weight of evidence to serve their communities. The result would be improved health outcomes,

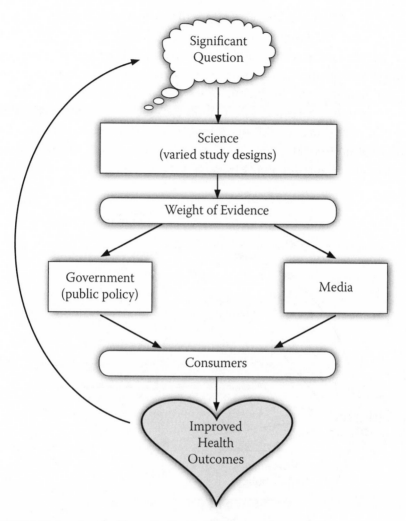

FIGURE 13-1. An ideal hypothetical health-care system

which would then lead to the next set of significant questions by showing where health research still needs to be done, in a continuous and never-ending quest for the best health possible.

It would be nice if our world actually resembled this diagram. But unfortunately, this idealized picture of a society whose goal is better health for its members is a very far cry from the way our system really functions.

OUR ACTUAL HEALTH-CARE SYSTEM

Let's take a look at reality—at the way the nutrient "information" actually moves through the health-care system, as in Figure 13-2. It's not in service of producing greater health outcomes, but instead in service of profit.

When the goal of the information cycle becomes profit rather than health, everything about it becomes distorted. Science, the producer of information from the raw materials of curiosity and funding, creates a monoculture of reductionist research that serves profit, not health. The

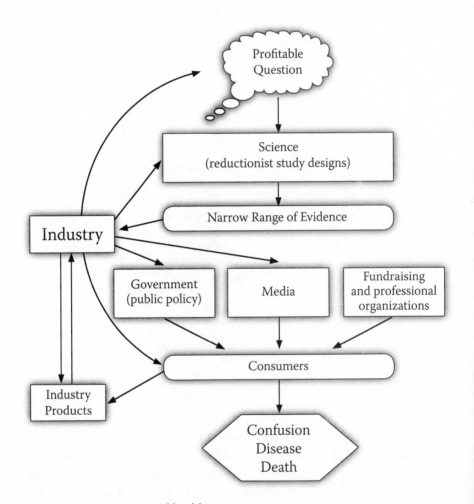

FIGURE 13-2.   Our actual health-care system

output of this research, a narrow range of evidence that precludes wholistic, simple, and powerful solutions, is then turned into myriad temporary and partial solutions that ultimately make things worse. Just as a diet of processed, nutritionally barren food cannot be metabolized for healthy functioning, a diet of processed, wisdom-barren information cannot be metabolized into wise, compassionate, or effective social policy.

Here's how the profit-distorted information cycle works. At the very top, the questions that are asked have more to do with the potential for profit than breakthroughs in human health. Why bother to think about something when you won't get the funding to pursue your research? Why build a career on questions that no one will pay for you to investigate? So already the system is excluding questions about how to get more people to eat healthy food, in favor of questions about how to make pills and potions that can be patented and sold at high margins.

These questions comprise what we currently call "science." All the labs and apparatus and test tubes and white coats are just a means to an end: answers to the questions science is called upon to answer. In contrast to a healthy information cycle, however, science in this case does not investigate the questions with the full range of study methodology available to it. Rather, it limits itself to highly reductionist experimental research designs, which are deemed the only appropriate means of gathering evidence. Not so coincidentally, those are the ones most suited to drug testing, and least suited to complex biology and behavior change. Of course, this systemic limitation produces a very narrow range of evidence, which is then reported and marketed as "the truth," as opposed to what it really is: a very narrow sliver of experience reflecting an even narrower set of questions posed by people with a hidden agenda. This evidence has two main audiences: the media (owned by industry and/ or funded by industry advertising) and those in government and private think tanks who determine the public health implications of the evidence and recommend policy to make use of it. But the way these two audiences receive and use this evidence is heavily mediated by industry.

Industry uses that narrow range of evidence—or at least what of that evidence the public seems to be responding to—to create new products (including goods and services) and to lobby the government to declare those products "the standard of care." Procedures and pills so labeled are all but forced upon doctors and hospitals, who fear lawsuits should they deviate from these treatments. Industry feeds press releases to a largely uncritical media emphasizing only the evidence that supports use of their products. And industry further distorts the evidence by spinning it to the public in the form of advertising, where the occasional benefits are hyped and the considerable side effects are shown in small print or quickly mumbled.

The evidence ends up filtered and distorted, and presented as broader and more meaningful than it is. Any information that contradicts expected narratives is downplayed or doubted. Intentionally or not, this makes it easier for industry to sell more things to us, be they drugs, procedures, nutraceuticals, supplements, expensive running shoe inserts, or diets in a bottle. The health advice we hear are all messages like, "You need dairy to get enough calcium so you don't get osteoporosis," and "If you have high cholesterol, you need to take statin drugs."

With this information, advocacy groups—professional interest groups and fundraising organizations—galvanize public support and collect and contribute money to the activities of science. Because of the limitations of the science they rely on, their donations go to those who seek magic-bullet cures for their diseases of interest. Advocacy groups also influence public policy through PR and lobbying; what politician wants to be branded a "friend of cancer" by not going along with the wishes of the American Cancer Society?

What all this means is that, in the current system, we don't have free choices; we have constrained choices. We're just deciding between equally ineffective magic bullet "cures" that don't work. We buy what is sold to us, enlist in the never-ending crusades against bad diseases, follow mainstream health advice (because to ignore it seems foolish and risky), and donate time, money, and energy to our favorite anti-disease society. All this in the name of achieving better health for ourselves and others, when all it produces is an endless cycle of ever greater confusion, disease, and untimely death while stuffing the wallets of those who control and manage this system. And when you look closely, you'll see that we the consumers, by unquestioningly buying the products created by a profit-obsessed industry, are funding the whole mess. That's why one of the most important things any of us can do is improve our own diet and health; we can "vote with our dollars" against this system by opting out. The less we buy, the less money industry can deploy to distort scientific research and government policy.

I need to emphasize that these negative outcomes are not the goal of the current system. They're simply an unavoidable side effect of the primary goal: ever-increasing profits for the several industries whose activities constitute and maintain the system. As I said, this isn't a story of nefarious individuals' intentions; to the contrary, most of the people contributing to the current mess truly believe they're doing good. They're waging the war on cancer. They're uncovering secrets of our genes. They're putting what are presumably much-needed nutrients in pills and foods. They're producing breakthroughs in surgical techniques. They're lowering the cost of calories for the poor. They're producing animal protein more efficiently. They're reporting new findings to a public hungry for advice about how to be thinner and healthier. And yet these wonderful intentions end up in the service of more profit and more disease.

I also want to be clear that I'm not arguing against capitalism, free markets, or profits. It's natural for all the elements in a system to do what they can to survive and thrive. In fact, that collective motivation is the basis for the stability and resilience of the entire system. Forests can last for eons (until people cut them down) not because all the organisms in the forest are unselfish and "nice" to each other, but because each is taking care of its own business in a way that contributes to the welfare of the other elements. But the goal of the system called "forest" is to achieve maximum biomass and biodiversity, so it rewards players who contribute to that end. Trees that drop their leaves are rewarded by the richness of decomposer life that turns those leaves into nutrients, which eventually make their way back into the trees. Birds that excrete nitrogen back into the soil are rewarded by a bumper crop of worms that live in the carpet of fallen leaves that grow from the birds' nitrogen. And so on. The problem in the case of our health-care system is not the selfish behavior of the individual elements; instead, it's which selfish behaviors are rewarded, and which are punished, by a system whose goal is profit rather than health. This problem is not inherent to the free market, but rather the result of a market manipulated by its most powerful participants, often through collusion with a government far removed from the people it is supposed to serve.

Systems naturally reinforce themselves; if they didn't, they wouldn't continue. Here, the operation of our health-care system generates powerful forces that reinforce the profit motive over the health motive. It generates equally powerful forces that keep the current system in place, allowing it to withstand all manner of scientific evidence that things could be done smarter, cheaper, and better. But systems do collapse when their resources can't sustain their goals on an ongoing basis. Such is the case when the high costs of our disease-care system, both economic and health related, threaten to bring down our entire society.

In a system that seeks the public welfare over profits for a few, companies and individuals could still make plenty of money, just as oaks and hickories can still get mighty big in the forest. They would just do it in a fashion that can be sustained indefinitely, because the other elements of the system would flourish, too.

THE REDUCTIONIST PROFIT CONNECTION

Before we explain how the pursuit of profit affects the health-care system, it's important to discuss the why. Why are reductionist science, medicine, and food so much more profitable than their wholistic counterparts? After all, isn't good health better for an economy than bad health? Healthy people make more productive workers and more avid consumers of the good things in life. And shouldn't we be measuring our economy by how well it contributes to everyone's well-being?

Reductionism goes hand in hand maximizing corporate profits because reductionism causes new problems as it solves existing ones. Each of those new problems, while costly for society as a whole, represents a further profit opportunity for some industry.

It's also easier to market reductionist solutions than wholistic ones. Picture a continuum of potential solutions to any problem, with "magic" solutions on one side and "realistic" solutions on the other (as shown in Figure 13-3).

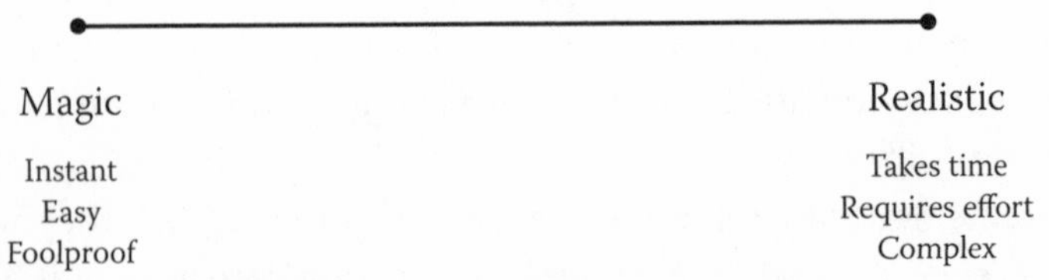

Magic	Realistic
Instant	Takes time
Easy	Requires effort
Foolproof	Complex

FIGURE 13-3. Magic versus realistic solutions to health issues

The magic solution, which is described as instant, easy, and foolproof, is much more appealing than a realistic solution that takes time, requires effort, and is complex to get right. You'll notice that most consumer advertising tends to favor the magic over the realistic. From weight loss solutions and financial services, to cleaning supplies and beauty products, the closer the product is to magic, the easier it is to sell and the more appealing it is to buy. This can produce a profit windfall for the person owning the intellectual property on which the magic solution is based, and indeed, these simple reductionist solutions can be patented, and thus owned, where others cannot.

Reductionist solutions, because they are formulated to address only a limited spectrum of a problem, are much more easily described as magical than as wholistic solutions. Worried about getting a heart attack? Well, all you need to do is take a couple of omega-3 capsules a day. It takes just a few seconds, and it's as easy as, well, popping a pill. Got diabetes? Hey, here's an insulin injector pen with a digital timer on the cap so you never have to think about doses and timing—or improving your diet. Overweight? Drink an appetite-suppressant shake, or just get your stomach stapled so you literally can't overeat or tolerate rich foods any more.

Magic solutions work by addressing symptoms rather than causes. Symptoms can be suppressed and managed quickly, while causes take greater effort, which often means more time to deal with. Temporarily addressing an isolated symptom is fairly simple. Causes are more complex, and require greater involvement by and responsibility from the person with the problem.

Now consider the wholistic solution to cardiovascular disease, diabetes, and extra weight: eat a WFPB diet. It works by eliminating the underlying cause, our bodies' attempts to deal with a diet high in processed foods and animal products. And while the *effect* of WFPB may be as quick as or quicker than a pill, a shot, or surgery, it requires continual upkeep; the reductionist interventions take far less effort to implement. Changing one's lifestyle can be challenging. It requires commitment and responsibility from the person making the change, and a willingness to be open to having new experiences and developing new habits and skills.

Our sound bite world, our hurry-up lifestyles, and our advertising-based economy all make the reductionist quick-fix a much easier sale than the long-haul, comprehensive, wholistic solution. That reductionist solutions create the need for additional products and services (drugs and other treatments to manage the side effects of the initial solution and to suppress other symptoms of the Standard American Diet, plus emergency surgeries when the initial solution fails) is an added benefit for industrial profiteers. And all that profit means the industries that make it have a lot of extra money to throw around to ensure they can make more of it in the future. In short, they have *power*.

SUBTLE POWER

When we think of people who abuse power, our minds go to Hollywood villains whose nefarious deeds keep entire populations cowed and craven: the banker Henry F. Potter in *It's a Wonderful Life*, Darth Vader in *Star Wars*, Nurse Ratched in *One Flew Over the Cuckoo's Nest*, among many others. These and other archetypal villains use violence, threats of violence, and cunning to create environments in which they benefit from power and grow it to near omnipotence. When someone uses these kinds of overt strategies, you notice. Money can be used this way, too, when you bribe a public official to look the other way as you break the law, or pay some thugs to frighten your opponents into silent submission. But there's another kind of power that's a lot less noticeable, which I call *subtle power*: power that operates so softly and effectively that its force and source are practically invisible.

By way of example, let's look at why millions of American school children drink milk, rather than water, with their school lunches, something that nets the dairy industry two huge benefits: huge financial return and early education of young people about the alleged health value of consuming milk. Obviously, the dairy industry does not post armed sentries in each school to force the administration to purchase the milk, the food service workers to serve it, and the students to drink it. They don't have to; the subtle influence they exert brings about even greater compliance than a heavy-handed use of power.

First, the dairy industry has spent a lot of money over the past sixty years lobbying the government to promote dairy as one of the cornerstones of good nutrition. When the current school administrators were children, they were indoctrinated in school that dairy was one of the "four basic food groups." The money the dairy industry spends to buy political influence extends to financial support for governmental agricultural policies that drastically subsidize milk production. For schools to offer the school lunch program with its subsidized foods, they must offer milk as an option. Federal authorities don't require children to actually *drink* the milk, but they don't need to. Local school authorities do the job. They've been well coached to believe that milk is needed for strong bones and teeth. The dairy lobby has also succeeded in compelling the federal government to buy billions of gallons of milk for use in other federal programs, including prisons, VA hospitals, and the military. Talk about your captive audiences!

In addition to the subtle muscle applied to our political apparatus, the dairy industry spends millions of dollars each year advertising the so-called health benefits of milk to consumers. The drumbeat has been going on for so long that we scarcely are aware that it's paid, commercially-motivated advertising, not a public service announcement. Most of us just accept that milk is good for us. And the highly successful "Got Milk?" campaign used popular role models to convince our young people that milk makes you thin, rich, healthy, and sexy.

Dairy interests contribute generous sums of money to many health-related nonprofits as well, thereby influencing their highly effective public pronouncements about the benefits of dairy. These nonprofits have to scramble for funding, so there's pressure not to upset large repeat donors. They also pay for academic activity that passes for "research," producing studies that start by assuming milk's benefits and then find increasingly creative and dishonest ways to "prove" those benefits. The mainstream media, to the extent that they are funded by "Got Milk?" and other dairy industry ads, conveniently ignores, underreports, and casts doubt upon the myriad studies that show that milk and other dairy products emphatically don't "do a body good." As newspapers and TV news struggle to stay afloat in the age of digital media, they also are susceptible to the dairy industry's subtle pressure to favor its side of the story.

So those school administrators have every reason to buy lots of milk. It's inexpensive (thanks to those government subsidies) and it's easy to procure with minimal paperwork (because the federal government has made milk the default beverage). Thanks to health education and advertising, students expect it, parents demand it, and it sells; milk brings in profits that pay salaries, whereas water from the water fountain is free. Just in case students haven't been brainwashed into viewing milk as a health food by thousands of images of celebrities with milk mustaches, the dairy industry "fortifies" school milk with sweeteners and appetizing chocolate and strawberry flavors to encourage children to drink up.

Similar subtle power operates everywhere: when people buy low-fat milk (because less fat is always healthier), reject the breakfast bagel in favor of two eggs and four slices of bacon (because carbs are bad for you), and choose their breakfast cereal based on its fortification with eleven vitamins and minerals (because it's the best way to get the nutrients you need). These choices feel self-generated, but in fact are heavily influenced by millions of dollars of spending by the dairy, egg, pig, and processed foods industries, respectively.

This confluence of power, by the way, is also responsible for the phenomenon of vegetarians constantly having to answer the question, "Where do you get your protein?"—as if protein were something that exists in animal products alone. It's also what gets us to agree to invasive medical procedures that earn the medical industry more money rather than improve our diets. Whenever you see large masses of people making what look like "free choices" against their best interests, you can bet that subtle power is at work in the background.

As you can see, money itself is a lever of subtle power. In a health-care system like ours, where profit is the ultimate goal, money is the most powerful force available, allowing those who have it to influence, almost invisibly, government policy, the media, popular culture, and the conversations that take place in the privacy of our own homes and minds.

Scientists are more likely to receive research funding and lucrative corporate contracts for research that can produce the next pill, supplement, superfood, or hospital treatment, so that research is more likely to get done. Media outlets are punished with the withdrawal of advertising for reporting unfavorably on advertisers' products, making them less likely to do so; journalists know their salaries depend on that revenue. Politicians who pass legislation and write statutes favorable to certain kinds of commerce are rewarded with campaign donations from industry groups who benefit from these laws and statutes. Nowhere in this process can you see violence or even green-stained fingerprints. No one called up those scientists, journalists, and politicians and threatened them; no one blackmailed them or offered them a bribe to do something they didn't want to. But behavior that supports the current paradigm is rewarded, and behavior that does not is disincentivized. These carrots and sticks are mostly silent, seldom pointed to, and never discussed.

This is how a system like ours—in which the goal of ever-increasing profits for the few is pursued at the expense of our health—can continue, even though that goal is not shared by the vast majority of people within it. Thanks to the rewards and punishments subtle power uses, people behave in ways they otherwise would not—ways that maintain the current system. The more industry profits increase, the more money is available to reward even more of the desired behavior. In other words, the money that is spent on subtle power achieves a return on investment that makes even more money available for the next round of subtle power. What we have is a vicious cycle that concentrates power more and more exclusively in the hands of those who already wield it.

If power corrupts and absolute power corrupts absolutely, then we should expect to see a lot of "legal" corruption in our health-care system. In the next chapter, we'll pull back the curtain on some of that corruption and see how it keeps us from moving toward true and lasting health.

14

Industry Exploitation
and Control

*I hope we shall crush in its birth the aristocracy of
our monied corporations which dare already to
challenge our government to a trial of strength, and
to bid defiance to the laws of their country.*

—THOMAS JEFFERSON

The wealthy and powerful industries that make up our health system have replaced its original goal—human health—with the pursuit of ever-increasing profits. Their money distorts research agendas, media reports on health issues, and government policies. And thanks to their skillful wielding of subtle power, they do so without leaving obvious evidence. My goal in this chapter is to make their fingerprints as visible as possible, especially when it comes to one of the main victims of industry control over how information is produced, distributed, and used: wholistic nutrition.

The medical, pharmaceutical, and supplement industries figured out long ago that a nation of healthy eaters would be disastrous to their profits.

They make much more money ignoring and discrediting the evidence for WFPB than by embracing it. So let's take a look at these three industries and how they maximize profits at the expense of human health.

THE MEDICAL INDUSTRY

The purpose of the medical establishment is to treat illness. Doctors go through many years of training to learn the best ways science knows to treat diseases. When we visit them as patients, we hope they will show us the best road to wellness. We trust them to know things we do not, and to hold only our best interests at heart. And so, when we are confronted with a life-threatening diagnosis, most of us take our doctor's recommendations for things like aggressive surgery, radiation, and chemotherapy, even if we sometimes wonder if another path is possible.

The medical establishment has all but cornered the market on legitimacy. And in my experience and to my knowledge, the vast majority of doctors are accomplished professionals who sincerely seek the best for their patients and pursue that goal as best they can, based on their medical training and ongoing education. But as we've seen, that training is limited by the reductionist way we do science. And like any group that "knows best," doctors can be blind to other options that might be more viable than their own skills and tools. Some of them, out of twin desires to cure and to remain blameless, use their power advantage to bully and silence skeptics who might want to explore wholistic methods of healing. As a result, even the bravest and most open-minded patients usually feel that drugs and surgery are their best bet.

Cancer and heart disease tend to reduce us to powerlessness in our relationship with the medical establishment. And too many doctors exploit the power difference to scare their patients into unblinking compliance while simultaneously and sincerely believing that they are serving their best interests. It's been said more than once that doctors are the clergy for a secular age, holding the keys to life and death in their hands and brooking no heresy. Like traditional clergy, they use symbolism and ritual to represent and reinforce their power (think of the waiting room, the receptionist behind the glass divider, the endless paperwork you fill out while you glance at the aging magazines). Far from maddening us, these and other rituals serve to comfort vulnerable patients who deeply desire to trust their doctors' opinions. At such moments the doctor–patient relationship is imbalanced, however unintentional this may be: one side desperate to save their life, the other perceived as capable of doing so. When the diagnosis is cancer, a doctor's unintended exploitation of this emotional vulnerability can lead to poignant, even tragic results. And not coincidentally, the treatment pathways they insist upon are those that deliver the greatest profits to the medical industry and its partner, the pharmaceutical industry.

When people find out that I have spent my career searching for ways to prevent and possibly cure cancer, they naturally ask my opinion about particular diagnoses: family members, friends, even themselves. Of course, I emphasize that I'm not a licensed physician and can't offer specific advice; their doctor has years of specialized education and training that I do not. But when faced with a diagnosis of cancer, many people persist. They ask, "What would you do if you or a family member were to receive a diagnosis of 'the Big C'?" At best, I can only share my interpretation of the scientific evidence, often advising them to get a second opinion while simultaneously trying to help them respect the advice of their personal physician. In 2005, my very best friend, after scratching a mole on her thigh and leaving a small scab, decided to have it checked and removed if necessary, because cancer was not infrequent in her family.

When test results were completed in a few days, her doctor phoned her to come for a visit. Being somewhat apprehensive, she asked me to join her. When the doctor entered the examining room, his demeanor was serious. The diagnosis? Stage III advanced melanoma, the most serious kind of skin cancer. He advised quick attention and referred her to a team of a surgeon and oncologist. Devastated, she experienced the usual emotions that every cancer patient knows so well: an all-encompassing fear and dizzying disorientation.

After getting two second opinions on the tissue specimens to confirm the diagnosis, she then scheduled her surgery. The cancerous tissue was removed from her thigh, along with a biopsied sample of the sentinel node of a nearby lymph gland to see if it had metastasized. The sentinel node is the part of a lymph gland to which cancer is most likely to spread first; if the sentinel node shows evidence of cancer, it is generally assumed that cancer has spread into the larger lymph gland "basin." Think of the sentinel node as the doorway to a room—in this case, the larger lymph gland basin. If melanoma cancer cells migrated to the sentinel gland, it is assumed they are also in the lymph gland basin, thus requiring its removal—a tactic akin to destroying a village in order to save it.

At about this same time, my friend met with her newly assigned oncologist to talk about her treatment options, depending on whether her new tests indicated lymph gland involvement. I did not accompany her on this visit, as she brought along her adult sons, but she told me after-word that the doctor told her of the treatment options patients generally consider, including chemo and radiation. She informed him that she did not want to undergo any of these treatments regardless what the biopsy results might indicate, and he seemed okay with this. She was to return in another few days after learning the biopsy results of the sentinel lymph gland. It was about this time that she learned that the results were positive: the sentinel node showed that the cancer had spread to the lymphatic system. Three pathologists confirmed the diagnosis.

Before we returned to the oncologist, I decided to inform myself more deeply about melanoma and its treatment. Among other things, this included a visit to a very open-minded and welcoming pathologist to see for myself the histologically diagnosed tissue (I had received training in histology and had done quite a lot of microscopic work in my laboratory research group).

I already had some familiarity with melanoma. About twelve years before, I had used a summary report of melanoma cases published in 1995[1] as recommended reading for my Cornell class on plant-based nutrition, because the summary showed a remarkable dietary effect on the rate of survival. This paper was significant not only because it was a relatively rare peer-reviewed report of a favorable effect of diet on a serious cancer, but also because the lead author had been a member of a distinguished science panel recommending how research results from alternative clinical databases should be interpreted and published. The report provided detailed evidence that a plant-based diet had considerable potential to inhibit the progression of melanoma, but it also mentioned a similar effect on other cancers. The patient cases in this study were provided with a diet of mostly whole, plant-based foods prescribed by the famous (or, if you prefer, infamous[2]) Gerson Institute in Tijuana, Mexico.

Survival was remarkably increased, even for cancers initially diagnosed as stage III and IV.

I also familiarized myself with the not very pretty consequences of lymph gland removal. The literature suggested that removing a major lymph gland in the groin often resulted in loss of use of the leg for about a year or so, with lots of side effects and discomfort, to say nothing of the serious compromise of the body's immune system. Indeed, the woman's doctor had told her that she should plan on being "out of commission" for a year.

I also learned that, to compensate for the lost immune system activity when lymph glands are removed, doctors often prescribe interferon, a powerful immunotherapy medication. I therefore sought and found a very recent review on interferon and related treatments for melanoma stage II and III patients.[3] It concluded that "at present there is no single therapy [including interferon] that prolongs overall survival in stage II and III melanoma." Research on this topic is exceptionally complex, involving different interferon types, drug dosages and protocols, and stages of melanoma, as well as lots of discussion of response details. Let's put it this way: it's definitely not bedtime reading. I don't see how someone without adequate background and experience—which includes most melanoma patients—could make sense of the research, let alone use it to advocate with an oncologist for a different treatment.

Probably one of the most interesting observations that came to our attention was found by my friend's oldest son, who is neither a doctor nor a medical researcher. He located a peer-reviewed publication by a group of researchers in London who summarized the case histories of 146 melanoma patients. In case you think any of the science in *this* book is a bit advanced, here's the title of that peer-reviewed article: "The Microanatomic Location of Metastatic Melanoma in Sentinel Lymph Nodes Predicts Nonsentinel Lymph Node Involvement."[4] Quite a mouthful!

Here's what the article reported: All 146 patients in the study, as with my friend, showed metastasis to the sentinel lymph node, a finding that is conventionally used to justify surgical removal of the neighboring lymph gland basin. Because all 146 patients in this study had melanoma cells in their sentinel nodes, their full lymph gland basins were surgically removed. But retrospective reexamination of their lymph gland specimens showed that only 20 percent actually had melanoma cells in the larger basin,[5] suggesting that 80 percent of these patients did not have to suffer removal of their lymph glands. For 38 individuals in that 80 percent, metastasis was limited to only a single region of the sentinel node, the subcapsular region.

These study results were startling. I called the study's lead researcher, Dr. Martin Cook, in London, and he emphatically affirmed the article's report. You can imagine how excited we were about this powerful and esoteric finding, as my friend's biopsy also showed that her metastasis also was limited to the subcapsular region. I gave copies of this publication to my friend's surgeon and pathologist, neither of whom knew of this information, while saving a copy for the upcoming visit with the oncologist.

With this information in hand and having examined the tissue specimens myself, I accompanied my friend on her return visit to the oncologist when he expected her to tell him which treatment option she preferred and when she could start treatment—even though she had previously said she did not want to undergo the recommended treatments. Her decision was, of course, hers to make, although I also believed that treatment was ill-advised in her case. Removing the lymph gland made no sense and would only lead to serious side effects. In clinical trials, interferon had been shown to be ineffective and laden with side effects. Furthermore, the presence of melanoma cells only in the subcapsular region of her sentinel node indicated a good prognosis, especially if she adhered to a WFPB diet.

My friend's oncologist did not know about my professional background in cancer research and, as far as I know, also did not know about my visit with the pathologist about Dr. Cook's study. He simply knew that I was there to support his patient, and I tried just to listen. As far as the oncologist was concerned, the facts were simple. It was "advanced" melanoma, as confirmed by the diagnosis, and it had already metastasized to the sentinel node of the lymph gland. Therefore, the remaining lymph gland needed to be removed and treatment with interferon or its equivalent needed to begin. All of this was urgently needed, in his opinion, and his personal demeanor left no doubt what he expected her to say.

Following this recitation of the "cold, hard facts," the doctor popped the question: "When will you be able to begin?"

My friend repeated what she had earlier said to him. "I am not going to do any of your suggested treatments."

Visibly shocked and annoyed, the oncologist now knew that his polite demeanor during the first visit was not working. He blurted out, "If you don't do this now, it's going to be too late when you come back!" He clearly expected "too late" to come sooner rather than later.

This kind of pressure from a medically informed superior given to an emotionally vulnerable and uninformed patient concerned for her survival is not a level playing field. It undoubtedly leads to acceptance of the physician's recommendation. Cancer patients intensely want to believe in their oncologist, whom they see as holding the key to their recovery.

Because of this reaction, I offered to share with him some of the literature that I had with me. Brusquely and rudely, he dismissed with a wave of his hand what he clearly considered to be nonsense. He had no interest in hearing anything but his own voice.

I can only imagine how many events like this occur in oncology offices across the country. Given the incidence of cancer in the United States, I'm guessing there are around 2,000 to 3,000 such events per day.[6] In most of these visits, the patient and their friends and family are neither capable of nor interested in questioning their doctors' opinions. I myself was taken aback by his certainty. I could not help but wonder: did I miss something? His behavior, laden with conviction and professional ignorance but also personal arrogance, was revealing—at least for me. He clearly had no interest in evidence suggesting anything other than "standard care" that favored traditional chemo treatments.

I have been told very similar experiences by dozens if not hundreds of cancer patients who are seeking information on nutrition and cancer, cases in which the research supports a nutritional approach, yet for which doctors insist on invasive, dangerous, and expensive treatments with poor success rates. However, I got much more involved in this case because the patient was my wife, Karen. And I know this melanoma case is a sample size of one and I did not professionally document it. It's anecdotal, period. But Karen opted to do nothing aside from continuing to eat only plant-based foods, has had no side effects, and eight years later is still in excellent health, now enjoying with me our fiftieth year of marriage. In fact, I feel that Karen's diet not only helped her after her cancer diagnosis, but in the years preceding it. The mole on her legs had been there for many years, and probably should have been checked out earlier. It is highly likely that this mole was cancerous prior to our family's conversion to a plant-based diet and that its progress was slowed or suspended, or perhaps even reversed, after this point. The results of the biopsy may even have showed the cancer retreating rather than spreading.

Looking back, this incident is representative of many similar stories that motivated me to write this book. Since I can't accompany every patient to high-stakes meetings with medical professionals, I wanted to do something to level the playing field—to give vulnerable women and men a voice, and to allow them to believe they have a choice when it comes to aggressive and expensive medical treatments for serious conditions.

On one level, the interaction between Karen and her doctor is simply a story of an arrogant professional pressuring a vulnerable patient to do what he believes to be in her best interest. He knows what standard care is. She doesn't. Period. However, when we take a step back and look at the fact that there are a few thousand of these interactions each day, we see the mark of a medical industry whose profits depend on doctors' unquestioning belief and persuasiveness—if not their arrogance. Let's take a minute and follow the money in this story. Where does it flow when the surgical/chemical approach is chosen over the nutritional approach, and who benefits?

First and most obvious, the more often chemotherapy and surgery and pharmaceuticals are prescribed to patients, the more money the entire industry takes in. Even if we were to assume that a chemical approach is equally as effective as a nutritional approach (though there is no proof of this), the medical industry benefits more from training and encouraging its members to choose the chemical solution. There's a lot of money to be made in cancer treatment. That's why drug and medical equipment companies dominate the advertising in medical journals. (That advertising explains why medical journals are loath to print results that call those industries' practices and effectiveness into question, but we'll look at trade journals more in chapter fifteen.)

Second, by passing referrals back and forth, the medical "old boys' club" keeps its members rich and busy. Karen saw three different doctors during her diagnosis, and each new doctor meant a new co-pay for her and high costs for her insurance agency. It's necessary to see so many doctors when going the chemical route, because each doctor is a specialist who focuses on a specific reductionist element of cancer. But the reason for their specialization has more to do with our misguided approach to disease than the best way of treating patients. It would only take one doctor to prescribe a WFPB diet and monitor the results—were this strategy ever used.

Also, the other doctors Karen was referred to were also very likely to back up her first doctor's point of view. They shared a paradigm, thanks to standardized educational training that does not include wholistic nutrition, and likely even shared a social circle. You can bet Karen's oncologists weren't playing golf with nutritionists who advocate WFPB diets!

I know that many people believe that the kind of behavior I've described here is symptomatic of the entire medical profession, but I would counter that. I have met many brilliant doctors who are sincerely devoted to their patients. It is not doctors who are responsible for this environment of coercion and hostility to suggestions of alternatives; it is the system in which they are trained and expected to practice. The structure of the medical industry makes it very difficult for decent and caring doctors to act contrary to the industry's selfish, profit-seeking, defensive attitude. Those who buck the system face not just ideological pressure, but ideological pressure backed up by the subtle power of money. In some cases, even their license to practice may be challenged.

THE PHARMACEUTICAL INDUSTRY

Our society embraces the sentimental notion promoted by Big Pharma that the pharmaceutical industry is a selfless group of scientists, motivated only by an intellectual hunger and desire to serve humankind, toiling away to discover the cure for cancer or diabetes or heart disease. That perception exists largely because Big Pharma is so skilled at pretending to be good while manipulating the public's emotions. There are plenty of sincerely good people in Big Pharma, but the economic imperatives of the system override their efforts to do good.

Big Pharma is an industry, and its constituent members are businesses. Most of them are publicly traded or, in the case of the newer gene-therapy companies, privately funded by investors looking to get massive returns as quickly as possible. Their only fiduciary responsibility to their share-holders is to turn a profit.

Okay, so, big deal. Every company is trying to turn a profit, right? If Big Pharma makes money by selling drugs that help people live longer and with less pain, why shouldn't they? We should celebrate their profit-ability, because this money returns to the system to fund the research and development (R&D) that creates new drugs and refines and improves old ones. That's just Business 101, simple enough even for a professor of nutritional biochemistry to understand. Unfortunately, Big Pharma is exempt from Business 101, because of the ingenious and insidious way they get their customers (us) to generously (and unwittingly) pay most of their research bill well before we pay for our prescriptions.

Do you pay taxes? If so, you're contributing to the research budget of the government's lead health research agency, the NIH, whose research priorities are heavily slanted to benefit Big Pharma. Have you ever made a donation to a private research funding agency, such as the American Heart Association, the ACS, or the American Diabetes Association? If so, you're directly funding research that frequently creates ineffective and often harmful drugs that are sold to the American people at a huge profit. And those profits go not to us, the real investors, but to the pharmaceutical companies that patent, manufacture, and market these products. We are paying twice for stuff that often does not work at best and at worst is killing us.

Big Pharma is not satisfied with this cozy arrangement, however. In a never-ending effort to increase their profits, they seek government protection from the free market even as they exploit it for all it's worth. Talk about having your cake and eating it too! Here's how it works (with a nod to Professor Donald Light of the University of Medicine and Dentistry of New Jersey and Professor Rebecca Warburton of the University of Victoria, Canada, whose recent work reveals some little-known and damning facts about Big Pharma's Big Claims about its Big Expenses).[7]

In an online review of their various published findings, Light and Warburton concluded the following: Big Pharma justifies its expenses and gargantuan profits by claiming very high R&D costs to bring a new drug to the market. The most commonly cited figure is a staggering $1.32 billion per drug. That's a lot of money when, according to independent review groups, 85 percent of new drugs are useless or no better than the drugs already available. But this $1.32 billion price tag turns out to be highly inflated by the drug companies. Light and Warburton say this is "to justify higher prices [in the marketplace and receive] more government protection from free-market competition and greater tax breaks." An inflated estimate of costs helps them cry poverty and dupe the government into passing anticompetitive legislation and relieving them of their tax burden. After all, a financially strapped pharmaceutical industry would be a national disaster and a tragedy—imagine if the cancer breakthrough that's just around the next corner never materialized because some drug company had to cut back on R&D.

After carefully evaluating and professionally publishing their findings, Light and Warburton say that "no one should trust any estimate" of drug development costs by Big Pharma. They found that these costs are far lower per typical drug, averaging only around $98 million for development (ranging from a low of $21 million to a high of $333 million) plus an uncertain amount for research. Research costs are almost impossible to estimate because it's impossible to know what scientific research should be counted as leading to which drug product. And most basic research is done at government expense with "84% of the world's funds for research [coming] from public or foundation sources," according to a National Academy of Sciences and other official reports.

When independent and reliable sources of cost estimates are considered, Big Pharma is scamming the system—by a Big Bunch. First, they came up with this $1.32 billion figure by using only the costs of 22 percent of the most expensive drugs (new chemical entities that are developed in-house) and implying that this was an average for all drugs. Second, the costs they claim on randomized clinical trials appear excessive, with twice as many subjects per trial as the averages reported by the FDA and costs per subject that are six times higher than NIH figures; overall, Big Pharma's trial costs are more than twelve times higher than independently reported averages. Third, their reported lengths of both trials and time it takes the FDA to review new drug applications for approval are significantly longer than those reported by the FDA.

The story gets worse! Big Pharma also inflates the interest rate they use to determine the cost of capital and ignores substantial tax savings related to R&D and their foreign tax havens. Those lost taxes, according to Light and Warburton, "might pay for nearly all pharmaceutical R&D costs."[8]

In all, the total costs industry pays for the development of a new drug (including the amount they receive from government grants) approach only $70 million—not the $1.32 billion they claim. And the extra $0.02 billion added to the $1.30 billion is silly. All that tells us is Big Pharma is using the marketing trick of false specificity to get the public to believe they have performed a mathematically accurate estimate.

Big Pharma has been telling this kind of Big Lie for decades. When President Lyndon Johnson spoke to a group of Big Pharma executives in 1969, he bluntly told them that they knew well that NIH was doing their research and, further, that the public was footing the bill.

They reinvest these profits strategically, buying air time to keep broadcasting the Big Lie. The United States is one of only two countries on earth (New Zealand is the other) where drug companies are allowed to advertise directly to the consumer instead of just to physicians.[9] Under the sway of advertisers, more and more of us are "asking our doctor about Viagra" and thousands of other brand-name drugs.

Big Pharma hasn't forgotten to "educate" our physicians as well. According to a 2008 report, Big Pharma spends, as of 2004, an average of $61,000 per year, per each and every physician in the country, to promote its products. It also organizes a massive number of promotional meetings for doctors, wining and dining them and giving away vacations and computers and other wonderful perks. In 2004, the last year for which I could find data, there were 371,000 such meetings in the United States, or more than 1,000 meetings each day of the year. That works out to an average of twenty physician-fests a day in every state of the Union.[10]

In a nutshell, Big Pharma gets Big Subsidies from the taxpayer to fund their research and they pay far less in taxes than they owe. They also vigorously seek—through inflated R&D costs—tax breaks from unsuspecting taxpayers, and they are permitted to advertise directly to the consumer without effective control of what they say. Unsurprisingly, this lax attitude leads to a recent estimate that "of the 192 advertisements for 82 unique products [that were surveyed], only 15 fully adhered to all 20 FDA Prescription Drug Advertising Guidelines. In addition, 57.8%... did not quantify serious risks and 48.2% lacked verifiable references."[11] Not only that, Big Pharma spends far more on this advertising than on R&D. In a 2008 report, they had, during the previous year, spent twice as much on promotion than on R&D.[12] Talk about misplaced priorities! Big Pharma's "selfless" agenda is simple: sell, sell, sell, sell, and in their spare time, lobby the government for tax breaks and more subsidies.

The annual revenue for Big Pharma, $289 billion in 2010,[13] exceeds the total national budgets of at least 80 percent of the countries in the world.[14] Arguably, this might be acceptable if the outcome—or even the goal—were increased health. But as we've seen, this is emphatically not the case.

As bad as all of this is, Big Pharma has more up its sleeve. A significant problem with the pharmaceutical business model is that healthy people tend not to take drugs. Vitamins and minerals and herbs, yes. Pharmaceutical drugs, no. Big Pharma's next step is therefore the development of preventive drugs that can be given out like candy to everyone at risk for common killers like heart disease, stroke, cancer, and diabetes—which, in our nutritionally ignorant country, is just about everyone.

One such troubling attempt at "prevention" is the proposal to develop a "polypill" to reduce the risk of cardiovascular disease (CVD).[15] This polypill might include a few seemingly effective drugs like "3 blood pressure lowering drugs from different classes each at half doses, aspirin, a statin and folic acid."[16] The stated rationale for this pill is the need "[to reduce] the burden of cardiovascular diseases [by] strategies that are applied to entire or large segments of the population."[17] What a boondoggle for the pharmaceutical companies!

The pill would hypothetically benefit and therefore be recommended for "all individuals with an established CVD and all those over 55 years without CVD"[18]—an impressive number of people. This estimate is based on considerable speculation and, it appears, was obtained by adding up the effect of multiple individual interventions for sustained periods of time. However, the combined effects of two or more agents are almost never additive. And the side effects of combined drug therapy are almost impossible to know beforehand. Making the matter even more troubling is the credence given to this idea by prestigious national and international health agencies.[19]

In their defense of the proposed polypill, the pharmaceutical lobby states that "primary prevention should include multiple strategies: health policy and environmental changes, individual behavioral changes, and use of proven and safe drugs."[20] They further claim that lifestyle interventions require behavioral modification—true—but then go on to say that such changes are too costly and "have only modest and unsustainable impact, and have failed to reduce CVD events when tested in large, long-term trials."[21] In other words, to echo a metaphor from chapter two, if an entire population suffers from headaches caused by hitting themselves over the head with hammers on a regular basis, it's too expensive and not effective enough to teach them to stop. Instead, we should implement health policy and environmental changes, such as public service announcements reminding everyone to wear their helmets, and recommend that everyone take painkillers with every meal.

The report[22] they refer to that supposedly damns lifestyle change as low impact and unsustainable was a meta-analysis of thirty-nine studies that only represented a collection of independently acting interventions. The studies reviewed in this report intervened first with drugs (for hypertension, lower cholesterol, and high blood sugar), and then with meaningless and independently acting (but not necessarily additive) interventions to reduce body weight, decrease fat intake, get more exercise, and stop smoking. In other words, giving people drugs and encouraging them to lose weight, eat less fat, and walk around the block once a day didn't miraculously make them healthy. That's what they call "lifestyle change"? Is anyone surprised that this approach doesn't work?

Big Pharma has used this collection of flawed studies as a straw man, claiming that "lifestyle change" doesn't improve health outcomes. But the combination of drug interventions (which fail to show adequate long-term benefits) with vague statements to reduce body weight (by any means, healthy or not?) and lower fat intake (another reductionist result that can be accomplished not by meaningful dietary improvement but rather by eating processed "low fat" foods) by no means can be considered a "lifestyle change." Lifestyle changes are wholistic, systemic, persistent, and comprehensive. A credible study of real lifestyle change to improve health would guide participants to transition to a WFPB diet, at a minimum. Yet most researchers in this field not only fail to acknowledge nutrition as a means to create and restore health, but also refuse even to become curious about its possibilities.

THE SUPPLEMENT AND
NUTRACEUTICAL INDUSTRY

Dietary supplements (which include not only single-nutrient supplements, but also a wide variety of food and herbal extracts) are a huge business—at recent calculation, it totaled $60 billion here in the United States—and one that has everything to lose under a wholistic paradigm. After all, supplements, as with pharmaceuticals, are the products of reductionist science, in which individual nutrients are seen as independent actors, each doing "a thing" in isolation from everything else in the body and the environment. As we saw in Part I, the limited efficacy of supplements reflects the limited science that created them: nutrients outside of their natural food context do little good and sometimes do considerable harm.

This hasn't stopped the supplement industry, though—and why should it, when there are so many studies to choose from and so much money to be made by choosing the ones, however faulty they may be, that support supplement use?

These days, the supplement industry has the process down to a "science." New scientific research on single nutrients generalizes in a very superficial way about their ability to promote human health. Companies put these newly discovered "nutrients" into pills, organize public relations campaigns, and write marketing plans to encourage a confused public to buy. But it wasn't always this way. The supplement industry rose from its modest origins to the multibillion-dollar behemoth it is today by exploiting relatively recent government policy toward deregulating the sale of certain health pills.

The nutrient supplement industry began in the 1930s, and for several decades had only modest growth. In the 1970s and early 1980s, however, it got a big boost, thanks to two events. First, in 1976, U.S. Senator William Proxmire and his colleagues succeeded in amending food and drug regulations to enable food companies to sell vitamins and minerals without a doctor's prescription.[23] Previously, a prescription was required for any preparation containing more than 150 percent of a recommended daily allowance. Second, in 1982, the NAS published that highly publicized report on diet, cancer, and nutrition, which we've already discussed,[24] that the industry spun to lend scientific justification to their products. That report—coauthored by thirteen scientists (including myself) and two years in the making—talked about individual nutrients as they existed within whole foods such as cruciferous vegetables. Though we mentioned certain vitamins and minerals, we had no intention of encouraging a nutrient supplement industry, and we made this clear in our executive summary. Ignoring our conclusions, the industry audaciously claimed that we had said the opposite, as if they knew better than we did what we had said!

This fledgling industry was now on a roll. The Proxmire amendment opened up the market, while the NAS report provided, in supplement makers' opinion, the scientific evidence to justify their products. What a combo! But an obstacle to growth remained: the industry couldn't yet make specific health claims that rose to FDA standards to help sell their products. Critics were right to be concerned about hyped-up claims, as evidence of such misbehavior had already surfaced with their gross misrepresentation of our NAS report. In fact, the NAS appealed to the Federal Trade Commission (FTC) to investigate the matter and asked me to represent the NAS in the subsequent court proceedings, which continued for about three years. My job was to examine the evidence the industry submitted to support their claims. I testified that most of their evidence was bogus and the FTC court agreed.

Neither the NAS nor the FTC had found any evidence to support these emerging health claims. Yet the industry still found ways to open doors for business, gradually gaining more and more liberty to make claims of improved health. Despite what, in my opinion, were (and are) minor restrictions on the health claims they could make, they essentially found ways—subtly but nevertheless powerfully—to advertise the health benefits of nutrient supplements and to grow their industry. I am not as familiar with the stream of regulatory and legal decisions paving the way for this growth that occurred over the next several years, because I was more involved with my research than with political shenanigans. But I do know that the industry has continued to grow—as did the lawyers' fees involved in ensuring the supplement industry had a friendly regulatory environment! Revenues climbed as more people succumbed to massive industry advertising and the belief that health could come from bottles of vitamin and mineral tablets.

The industry, now well established, received a further boost in 1994 with the passage of the Dietary Supplement Health and Education Act that amended the Federal Food, Drug, and Cosmetic Act. This amendment was designed to standardize specific supplement-labeling requirements, among other "housekeeping" chores, which gave supplements the appearance of scientific credibility and class. Most supplements and dietary ingredients could now be classified as food, a change the industry welcomed. By this point, the supplement industry had become as much a part of the American landscape as cars, churches, and apple pie. It had risen to become an elite class of food product, rather like dairy.

According to a 2008 report,[25] the variety of dietary supplement products has grown immensely over the last thirty years, all the way from the original alphabet vitamins (A, B complex, C, D, E) and minerals to prebiotics, probiotics, omega-3 fats, and various whole food concentrates. But almost all the health claims for these products rely on the same kind of short-sighted findings we debunked in Part II.

I've mentioned these statistics before, but they're worth laying out, all together, one more time. Sixty-eight percent of American adults take dietary supplements, while 52 percent consider themselves "regular" users.[26] As of 2007, the U.S. supplement market was $25 to $30 billion per year, with $7.4 billion spent on vitamins alone. More recent estimates have placed the U.S. market at $60 billion. Worldwide total dietary supplement sales in 2007 totaled $187 billion. Yet, with the immense growth of this "health" product market, the only thing getting any healthier is the supplement industry's bottom line.

BUSINESS AS USUAL

Many other books detail the ways in which corporate money has corrupted government and institutional policies, and not just when it comes to our health. I could write an entire book just on the examples I've seen personally, and I shared some of them in *The China Study*. As well, the three industries discussed here—the medical, pharmaceutical, and supplement industries—are not the only ones involved in our health system. The food industries, particularly the animal and junk food industries (which my son, Tom, and I examined in detail in *The China Study*), are also major players in the distortion of our health system, as we'll see in exploring these effects throughout the rest of Part III. But these three industries benefit most directly from the reductionist health paradigm, and have done the most to promote and maintain it.

What I want you to take away from the examples I've included here is just how much money there is to be made by suppressing wholistic nutrition in favor of reductionist health solutions, and just how far industry will go in pursuit of a larger share of that profit. In our current health care system, these examples aren't exceptions; they're business as usual. What looks like industry contributions to our well-being are often pure profit plays, dressed up as health initiatives. And it's to the many ways and places where industry encourages only those products, services, and beliefs that reliably generate corporate profits that we next turn—beginning with industry's influence on science itself.

15

Research and Profit

It is much easier to be critical than to be correct.

—BENJAMIN DISRAELI

At this point, you may be wondering: Why does the scientific establishment go along with these health-degrading schemes? Why do
scientists in health-related fields produce work that supports the
same strategies that have gotten us into this mess? The answer is that the
goal of Truth to which academic science has always aspired has been
replaced, in this distorted health system, by other goals: money, status,
influence, and personal security, among others. The basis of a healthy
information system is the quality of the information itself, and this industrial profit motive has distorted the very process by which the academic
research that produces this information is carried out.

Recall the way information moves through the health-care system in
an ideal society. The main input to that cycle is significant questions worthy of research. Scientists collectively address these questions through a
healthy diversity of study designs, ranging from the extremely reductionist
to the moderately wholistic and everything in between. This variety serves
a couple of purposes. First, when they all more or less agree, we can be
very confident in the results. Second, the reductionist studies provide new

questions, parameters, and constraints for the wholistic studies, and vice versa. And third, conflicting results gained from different types of studies show us the areas in which we may need to reframe our assumptions and pursue paradigm breakthroughs in order to get closer to the truth. As in any ecosystem, diversity contributes to the complexity, resilience, and health of the production of scientific information.

In our profit-driven system, the value added by this diversity of research is sacrificed. Instead of resulting from myriad perspectives, the weight of evidence is built from only the data deemed credible by the current paradigm—data that are the product of some form of reductionist study design. This narrow range of acceptable study methodology and research data is used to create more profit-generating "solutions" that in turn produce more problems that require research and treatment.

The question we need to ask is why. The answer, as you'll see, is that scientists are rewarded if they contribute out-of-context information that supports industry goals while contributing to our nation's poor health, and penalized if they don't.

THE IMPOVERISHMENT OF SCIENCE

At its best and most useful, science combines the arts of wholistic observation, reductionist observation, and experimentation in pursuit of human well-being. But today we almost completely disregard the art of observation of wholes, or systems, in favor of precise quantification and manipulation of minutiae. We mistakenly judge the quality of scientific investigation in the health disciplines by its precision and focus on tiny details—in other words, on how reductionist it is. "Real" scientists investigate parts, not wholes. But this diminishes the goals of true science. What most scientists are doing today really should be called technology, not science.

This distinction matters a lot. *Technology* refers to a means, a way of accomplishing some task. It's the last step in applied science, whereby the results of free and imaginative inquiry inform the creation of new products and services. When the "free and imaginative inquiry" phase is eliminated from the scientific roadmap, as it is in far too much medical research, we no longer have genuine science. Science is defined by the scientific method; it's an unbiased search for truth and a willingness to be proved wrong.

Technology is defined by market potential; only those questions that can be answered with dollar signs are deemed worthy of investigation.

Modern techno-biologists are expected to look deeply into DNA and cellular metabolism, but cannot express a professional interest in a topic such as human well-being. A pursuit that broad just isn't "scientific." Because we limit the permissible scope of scientific inquiry to reductionist details, we have lost sight of the true meaning of human progress. We equate advancement with the development of new technologies, of new products and services, rather than human well-being and happiness.

This isn't a new phenomenon. The subjugation of science to industrial profits has been going on for at least the past century, since capitalism devised the intellectual property protections that could fully reward those whose discoveries and inventions could be converted to products, sales, and capital. Once patent, trademark, and copyright instruments, among others, provided this protection, the engine of industrial capitalism could roar unhindered through society, using technological advancements to produce profits that were then plowed back into the system to fund more research and advancements. The system became self-replicating and self-perpetuating; initial market success provided the capital to fund subsequent market success.

The facts and information generated by science and used to create capital are the fuel that keeps the free-market engine running. The more useful the facts and information expected to be produced by a study—the better the fuel—the more likely the study is to get funded. If it won't end up with a barcode on it, it's probably not going to get funded.

As we've seen, a technological approach to nutrition—the kind that makes money for industry—includes drugs, supplements, and enriched and fortified foods. All of these are highly profitable and protected by intellectual property laws. There's plenty of funding for this type of science, and so plenty of it gets done. By contrast, research into the nutritional effects of whole plant foods doesn't really have market potential. You can't patent a recommendation to eat lots of fruits, vegetables, nuts, seeds, and whole grains. So there's no incentive for industry to invest in such research and no incentive for researchers to study and validate such claims.

Human health, happiness, and overall well-being cannot and will not be fully advanced by a corrupted free-market model manipulated by its most powerful participants. Instead of wholistic nutrition, the free-market engine gives us marketable fragments: supplements and nutraceuticals. When we get sick from lack of proper nutrition, the market engine obliges us with reductionist solutions: patented drugs and expensive surgeries. And through it all, the research community marches to the beat set by industry, masquerading as noble seekers of truth while churning out new ways to make money at the expense of our well-being.

FOLLOWING THE MONEY

Do you ever wonder who pays for medical research, the kind that investigates basic biological principles and lays the groundwork for later application? University professors—at least those who are tenured—are guaranteed a salary from their institutions,[1] but that doesn't cover the costs of dedicated lab equipment devoted to research, or the time of the graduate assistants and postdocs who do all the grunt work.

Just as politicians must spend much of their time raising funds for reelection, so must most research scientists devote many hours to applying for and maintaining grant funding. The main sources of research funding, aside from universities, are private industry and government. Since there are more researchers seeking funding than there is money to support their research, competition for dollars is fierce. Private companies and government agencies have to make decisions about what small percentage of research grants to approve.

What we call research ranges all the way from very basic, almost esoteric investigations, to very applied experiments that might more properly be called technology development (although the division between what is basic and what is applied is often vague and vigorously contested even within a single institution). While both types of research are useful, when it comes to funding, our system is biased toward the latter—even when the funding doesn't come from industry.

The majority of total health research, basic and applied, is funded by the pharmaceutical industry or by agencies beholden to it (such as the U.S. National Institutes of Health). Because the pharmaceutical industry expects a profitable return on that investment, its decisions on funding understandably tend toward applied science; the chief criterion they use for evaluating research proposals is usually how much money can be made. However, even government funding, via agencies such as the NIH or the National Science Foundation (which is the primary source for basic research), imposes reductionist criteria, either directly or indirectly, on just about all research into health and nutrition.

Unfortunately, over the last few decades I have observed a gradual encroachment by the corporate sector and its priorities into the domain of basic research at universities and related research agencies. The effects of this encroachment can be seen at nearly every level, from individual study design (what gets studied and how) and the way scientists interpret their findings, to the directions their careers take.

HOW FUNDING INFLUENCES STUDY DESIGN

If an applicant for basic research hopes to get funding, he or she is virtually required to ensure that the proposed hypothesis be "focused"—a code word for reductionist. To successfully compete for funding for this kind of research, applicants should want to study the detailed biological effects of a single nutrient rather than the food from which it came, or to search for the key biochemical mechanism that explains an effect rather than survey an array of possible mechanisms. In the pejorative jargon of the research community, wholistic research is described as "going on a fishing expedition" or "using the shotgun approach."

In basic research, each new reductionist finding usually leads to an obvious question: "What next?" The almost universal (and oftentimes legitimate) response from researchers is to recommend more research. (This certainly keeps our labs funded and running!) As a consequence, these researchers limit their ability to gain broader insight into the more fundamental phenomena that should be their mandate as basic research scientists. "What's next" is almost always another reductionist question that gets the results of the previous study closer to the marketplace. It doesn't matter whether or not we scientists give voice to our commercial interests in these research discussions; ultimately, research findings gain value and relevance when money can be made, and that affects how we think about our next steps. Whichever way these studies are designed and executed, they nonetheless represent steps on the pathway to commercial exploitation. Potential marketplace value has proven a powerful magnet toward which the research enterprise inexorably is pulled. In fact, as the years have passed, I have become more and more convinced that marketplace potential is the only goal of even the most basic, non-applied biomedical research.

I am not saying that individual researchers are even necessarily aware of these assumptions; they may be totally oblivious to this concern. Many researchers will be offended by these remarks and may deny that they are personally doing research for marketplace utility and possible financial return for themselves or their employer. But they are still working within a system whose primary motivation is a return on financial investment. Monetary return is the principal fuel that propels our biomedical system, and almost all professional biomedical researchers are part of and beholden to this system. The more a research investment is perceived as being able to yield a return, the more enthused and supportive the society at large becomes, from consumers and entrepreneurs to politicians and research-funding agencies.

HOW FUNDING COMPROMISES RESEARCH INTEGRITY

There's some evidence that funding pressure induces researchers to commit fraud to keep their funders happy. I'm not talking about egregious research sins like falsification or fabrication of data, but much subtler stuff. According to the colorfully titled "Scientists Behaving Badly" from the June 2005 issue of *Nature*, which reported on a survey of over 3,000 U.S.-based researchers who received NIH funding, 15 percent admitted to "changing the design, methodology or results of a study in response to pressure from a funding source."[2] When we break out the data by career stage, things get even more interesting. While only 9.5 percent of researchers in the early part of their careers reported engaging in this behavior, that number skyrocketed to 20.6 percent for those in mid-career. It seems that industry is quite good at training scientists to comply with their market motives. As well, this increase suggests that the longer established researchers are immersed in the system, the less they want to disturb that system. They've invested too much time, energy, personal identity, and professional status into their labs to put their funding at risk.

Two other admissions from the same survey help us see how these questionable practices conspire to damage the entire field of health research. First, 15.3 percent of health researchers admitted to "dropping observations or data points from analyses based on a gut feeling that they were inaccurate." Talk about seeing what you want to see and disregarding the rest! Even if an outlier bit of data managed to survive the reductionist study design, one-seventh of the researchers felt free to ignore it based on "gut feel," or, in other words, prejudice. Second, 12.5 percent of the researchers said they would overlook "others' use of flawed data or questionable interpretation of data" in informing their own research agenda and supporting their own conclusions. In other words, they would pretend that bad research that bolsters their own beliefs was actually good research, and quote it within their own papers to substantiate those beliefs. The sum total of all these admissions is a medical research engine that plays fast and loose with fundamental truths, picks and chooses data to support premeditated and prepaid conclusions, and is not very likely to contradict the sales and marketing agenda of the industries that sponsor its research.

I would argue for several reasons that the percentages in the previous paragraph are actually low. First, this behavior is so automatic that much of it is done unconsciously. Many researchers are literally unaware of the corrupting influence that their funders' expectations and pressures have on the integrity of their research. Second, "bad" behaviors are routinely underreported by survey respondents, even when assured anonymity as they were in this instance. And third, the survey response rate was just under 42 percent. It's probable that the 58 percent who declined to return the survey were even more susceptible to funding pressure than the respondents, as most voluntary surveys are completed and returned by those with the least to hide and who are least ashamed of their behavior.

The survey didn't look at the nature of the design or methodological changes to the altered studies, but my long experience as both a recipient of funding and a member of peer-review boards that evaluate grant proposals tells me that the research was almost certainly shifted in the direction of heightened reductionism—toward more specificity, more assumptions about causality, and fewer "messy" observational designs.

HOW FUNDING IMPACTS CAREER TRAJECTORIES

Nutritional scientists are rewarded for creating and perpetuating a system that focuses on single nutrients out of context, and they are effectively punished for examining real foods and real populations in the real world. This makes a difference not only in the case of individual studies, but when it comes to researchers' career choices. Take, for example, Chinese scientist Rui Hai Liu. Professor Liu, you may recall from chapter eleven, did early groundbreaking research demonstrating that the antioxidant activity of an apple is 263 times more powerful than the amount of vitamin C contained in the apple would suggest. Having learned this, Professor Liu was faced with a choice: what direction should his research take?

He could have chosen to demonstrate the same "the whole is greater than the sum of its parts" effect across a wide variety of plants and chemicals. His research, we now know from the research of others, could have discredited the misleading and often dangerous claims of the supplement and nutraceutical industries. He could have devoted his career to exploring the idea that eating plant-based foods is a superior option to the reductionist approach of consuming pills that contain only the "active ingredients" present in food.

But in academia, there is no funding for such a career trajectory. So, being the good researcher that he is (actually, he is outstanding), he chose the reductionist approach, his only option, because this is where the research money is. If he intended to advance in his profession and to secure tenure—if he wanted to afford the kind of equipment and assistance he needed to do any other research at all—this decision was a no-brainer.

Taking the reductionist path, Professor Liu was able to investigate many interesting ideas. He searched for other vitamin C–like compounds in apples that might account for the difference between the chemical and presumed biological activities of vitamin C. He confirmed their chemical structures, determined how they are absorbed and distributed after consumption, found out how they are metabolized, and learned how potent they are when doing these things. And in doing so, he has performed exceedingly well. Many would aspire to have his reputation and professional position. His are the kind of objectives that easily attract funding. He has had a relatively large group of graduate students whose research findings have been published in some excellent peer-reviewed journals.

The point is not that the reductionist approach is not interesting, or that it does not provide us with things that are valuable. I certainly loved the reductionist research I did; it was challenging and intellectually stimulating, and as long as I "focused" my proposed questions I always had plenty of public funding to be creative and to do the projects that seemed appealing. Graduate students use these studies to develop their critical thinking, experimental design, research, and writing skills—all highly useful to them, the scientific community, and society in general.

The problem is not that reductionist research is a career option. Rather, the problem is that it's the only career option. Professor Liu's career path is followed by thousands of newly minted young researchers every year, in areas ranging from very basic biology to the applied sciences. In one way or another, researchers are rewarded for following this conventional reductionist path. It's much easier to acquire funding this way. It's also a surer path to developing and enhancing one's scientific reputation.

Had Professor Liu fully honored his wholistic roots in Chinese medicine within the Western academy, it is my opinion that he would be scrounging for funds, bereft of a decent lab or motivated graduate students, and nowhere near a tenure track. Once scientists start doing well in reductionist research, shifting to a wholistic track is nearly impossible. If they do, they risk losing everything they've spent their lives working for: funding, facilities, prestige, and influence. And so, once established in a well-funded research career like this, a researcher becomes ever more subservient to his or her own research findings—and to the reigning paradigm of the discipline.

I do not mean to question my friend and colleague's choices, for I know and greatly value Professor Liu's dedication, perseverance, and sincerity in his work. Rather, my concern is for the environment that surrounds him. His example is an excellent illustration of the choices all researchers face—a choice that, given our system, is not actually a choice at all.

HOW FUNDING DRIVES
MYOPIC SPECIALIZATION

The reductionist agenda of research funders not only encourages reductionist study design, but also rewards narrower thinking about what is an important question. This has driven the development of more and more specialized areas of study.

Just as "human health" is too broad to be considered a real scientific discipline, so too has "biology" become a catch-all rather than a legitimate field of study. Instead of becoming a biologist, you become a biochemist, a geneticist, a microbiologist, a neurobiologist, a computational biologist, or a molecular biologist. There are no "naturalists" anymore. There are, however, animal physiologists, ecologists, evolutionary biologists, insect biologists, marine biologists, plant biologists, and biotic diversity biologists. And even these subdisciplines (which I copied from the list of concentrations on the Cornell University Biology Department website) sound quaintly general these days. Cornell's Department of Molecular Biology and Genetics (a completely different department than Biology, by the way) offers the following graduate programs: Biochemistry, Molecular, and Cell Biology; Biophysics; Genetics, Genomics, and Development; and Comparative, Population, and Evolutionary Genomics.

To some extent, this division into more and more subdisciplines was inevitable, as biomedicine learned more about our infinitely complex biology. There's so much to know that it's natural and useful to separate that knowledge into subdisciplines, including biochemistry, genetics, pathology, nutrition, toxicology, pharmacology, and so forth. Intellectual discussion of ideas is easier when like-minded people are able to converse in a more precise common language.

The problem is, these divisions reinforce the illusion that each group is studying something completely different from all the others. Each of these subdisciplines takes on its own identity and, in doing so, begins to form intellectual boundaries that filter out others who may be able to constructively contribute to discussions of broader health topics. To be taken seriously by pathologists, you must be a pathologist. No geneticist thinks he or she has anything to learn from a nutritionist. And so on. In effect, these enclaves (I think of them as tiny caves) become not just narrowly focused, but exclusionary and isolated.

As a result, becoming a highly competent researcher in a biomedical discipline or subdiscipline, while still having a good understanding of the broad umbrella of biomedical research of which that subdiscipline is a part, is discouraged. In an attempt to avoid being considered a "jack of all trades and master of none," biomedical researchers tend to focus exclusively on one trade. They may learn everything about how to hammer nails, but they often have no idea when a mortise and tenon joint, screwdriver, or a bottle of glue will do the job better.

Other writers have noted this problem many times before, and institutions have attempted to resolve it by developing cross-fertilizing and interdisciplinary programs to promote better communication among subdisciplines. But even within these interdisciplinary programs, group identities continue to exist. People still carry their labels with them. And here, as with research itself, expertise in individual disciplines is valued over a wholistic understanding of the relationships between them.

I accept and understand the ever-greater specialization of the biomedical research discipline. But it comes with a downside that is too often forgotten—and it is serious. Some of these specialized subdisciplines naturally produce more lucrative reductionist solutions than others, so they get a larger piece of available funding. And as they gain a larger share of research resources, they become ever more dominant within the broad community of researchers, thus giving them a platform to dominate public opinion as well. In short, without necessarily realizing it, they begin to control the conversation about the larger discipline of which they are a part. Instead of one perspective among many, theirs becomes the dominant one. And the reason for their dominance is not their perspective's greater value for solving the issue at hand, but rather its greater ability to generate a return on investment.

The public needs to know about this highly fragmented environment because this fragmentation is an important source of public confusion. The first subdiscipline makes known their views on a particular topic, while the second and third subdisciplines, with different perspectives, weigh in with their own views—and sometimes these perspectives conflict. The public, untrained in these matters, is left to guess who is right, when the answer may actually be none of them. Remember the blind men and the elephant? Each of these inward-looking subdisciplines is severely limited in their knowledge of the "full" story.

When someone has the qualifications of a biomedical scientist, that just means he or she has command of a fraction of a portion of a specialized subdiscipline. It does not necessarily mean that he or she is any more qualified than a layperson to comment publically on the umbrella covering the whole of biomedicine. Indeed, because such research specialists become so narrowly focused, they may be less qualified to speak about the larger context. It's a bit like a frog that has spent its entire life at the bottom of a silo telling us about the world outside.

Insofar as misguided scientific elitism is concerned, there is no better example in biomedical research than the individuals who call themselves geneticists—especially those within the subdiscipline of "molecular genetics." They now receive an unusually large share of the total funding for biomedical research and, as a consequence, have successfully positioned themselves as a dominant voice within both the professional and lay public communities. They have the money to create and relate their findings in ways that favor their own interests and perspectives. They may extend their boundaries to include other disciplines at times, but only on their own terms. For example, geneticists only acknowledge nutrition as a discipline completely unrelated to their domain—if they bother to recognize nutrition as a scientific discipline at all! Where the two do intersect, nutrition is defined as a subdiscipline of genetics, as in areas like "nutritional genomics" or "epigenetics." In this way, nutrition becomes secondary to genetics at best and completely irrelevant to health at worst. Geneticists control the conversation; this isn't an exchange of information between two equal partners, but geneticists using nutrition, because it's known to "play" well with the public, in a way that severely distorts and controls the vital importance of nutrition information to the public.

In addition, for-profit research funders benefit greatly from the fracturing and proliferation of the health sciences into more and more distinct disciplines. As in any free-market system, the more competitors there are for limited funds, the fiercer the competition—and the more the funding applicants are forced to exaggerate the importance of their research agendas and methodologies to please their deep-pocketed patrons.

HOW FUNDING DETERMINES
SOCIETY'S RESEARCH PRIORITIES

The sometimes subliminal "make a profit" agenda that attaches reduction-ist, market-focused strings to almost all funded research also has implica-tions for which disciplines get funding priority. Certain disciplines receive more funding than others. Genetics, as we've seen, is a much hotter topic than nutrition. The projected market potential of gene therapy to enhance the immune system drives much more funding than the possible market potential of broccoli. The money flows to genetics and drug testing not because these are the most promising or cost-effective ways to improve overall human health, but because they are the most profitable ways to address our need for human health—or, put another way, they are the best way to meet market demand.

Can you imagine the health gains in the U.S. population if the half-trillion dollars in annual Big Pharma revenue were allocated to educating the public about WFPB nutrition, and to making sure that fresh, organic, sustainably grown produce were available and affordable for all Americans? We can hardly imagine such an initiative; it seems utterly impossible within the current system. But why? Why, if the all-out promotion of WFPB would be such a positive thing, is it unthinkable that our society would coalesce around a nutritional Manhattan Project? Because we know that health research and programs reflect the priorities of for-profit industries, not science in the public interest. Such an initiative would pay dividends in health, not dollars (although in the long run, the results would pay off in dollars saved on health care, too!).

Here, too, the industry's emphasis on marketable reductionism influ-ences government funding, even though it is ostensibly not driven by the profit motive. Look, for example, at the NIH, a U.S. government agency that is also the most prestigious and wealthiest funder of health research in the world. The NIH comprises twenty-eight institutes and programs and centers, devoted to cancer, aging, eye health, alcohol abuse, and many other facets of human health and disease. But not one of them is solely devoted to nutrition! (Unless you facetiously count the Institute of Alcohol Abuse and Alcoholism, of course.) Of the meager research funding for nutrition at NIH (comprising only 2 to 3 percent of the heart- and cancer-specific institute budgets, and even less of other NIH institutes and programs), most of this money is being used to investigate the effects of isolated nutrients in randomized clinical trials, for optimal nutrition for patients who are taking specific pharmaceuticals, and/or for biochemical research on the function of individual nutrients. (Although a few of the NIH's projects occasionally considered the wholistic basis of health research and clinical practice in the past—without using the weird word *wholistic*, of course!—these studies were largely ignored in policy debates about food and health, and mostly remain in the realm of academic literature.) Sadly, the public has become convinced that these research priorities are the best way of achieving our health goals, when they are just the best way of achieving greater profit.

AN INSIDER LOOK AT
FUNDING AND RESEARCH

I know intimately how funding determines research priorities, both as a longtime applicant for research funding and as a peer reviewer for several research-funding agencies that determine which research grant applications receive funding and which do not. I know well both the frustration of having to force research questions into a form that research evaluation panels will find acceptable, and the pressure to find reductionist answers.

Over the years, my growing awareness of the limitations of reductionist research began to trouble me. I found it more and more difficult and disturbing to continue to teach the traditional (and reductionist) views of nutrition—the way I was taught—when my own views were changing. Even as I was chugging away in the reductionist paradigm, something within me knew there was something missing.

Then I began getting ominous warnings, such as the one I privately received from a former colleague, a member of an NIH research application review group (or "study section" in the jargon of NIHers) that was reviewing our latest (and in the end successful) grant application for renewed funding of our project in China. In the application, I had expressed enthusiasm for the biologically complex relationship of diet with cancer, and how our work in China might provide some unique opportunities to develop more complex disease causation models, perhaps reflecting the more wholistic nature of disease occurrence, instead of the linear mechanistic model. This apparently was a cause for deep concern on the peer-review panel. According to my colleague—who, by telling me this, ignored the code of silence generally imposed on reviewers—I had come perilously close in my proposal to a description of a wholistic research strategy, and he advised me that I should never again defend my research in reference to wholistic interpretation. I was being reminded that I was challenging a fundamental tenet of biomedical research and that, in doing so, I almost cost us the much-needed funding for the third and final three-year phase of this research project. I chose shortly thereafter to discontinue my very active experimental research program of thirty-plus years—a personally agonizing decision at the time because experimental research had long been my life's work, and I loved working with students. I could no longer bring myself to write research grant applications for funding to investigate only highly focused hypotheses on minute details out of context.[3]

But that choice—to opt out of the system, or even just to challenge it—is one that not every researcher has. Our program was, at that time, the largest, best-funded research group in a large nutritional science department long regarded as the best in the country, which gave me the freedom to explore questions that, in subtle ways, defied the prevailing paradigm. Others, especially those just starting out in their career and seeking tenure, are under much more pressure to adhere to the research community's industry-friendly expectations.

There is pressure on the other side of the table as well. From the late 1970s to the late 1980s, I was a member of a research grant review panel for the NIH's National Cancer Institute (among other cancer research agencies), and there were several occasions when an enthusiastic applicant proposed an investigation of a biological effect by considering a relatively broad array of causal factors—in other words, to look at a problem wholistically. Without fail, such "shotgun approaches" and "fishing expeditions" were summarily rejected without further review for funding priority. I generally went along with these rejections because, too often, the applicants did indeed lack any sense of focus or purpose. But not always. Our panel's knee-jerk rejections reflected something more, something that I find especially revealing, and troubling, in science: the belief that highly focused hypotheses—not fishing expeditions—were the only type that deserved to get funding.

Occasionally, I learn of more recent research that is being funded under a systems analysis model similar to our project in China. In earlier years, however, our work was the only such project that interpreted data in this way. What we learned in China, coupled with our laboratory work, has completely changed my understanding of nutrition; imagine what else we could learn if we funded a few more non-reductionist studies!

THE SOCIETAL COSTS OF PROFIT-SEEKING FUNDING

I know firsthand the personal passion and honest sincerity that the vast majority of biomedical researchers and practitioners bring to their work. But they are working in a system that, due to the pressure it puts on them to perform only reductionist research, makes it very difficult for that passion and sincerity to result in good, effective science.

As we discussed in Part II, reductionist research on its own is fundamentally inadequate. By definition, it lacks the understanding of the whole that is required to give meaning to its insights. Its solutions—as with a solution that works only for a spherical cow in a vacuum—do not hold up in the context of real life. But the profit motive doesn't just limit researchers' ability to do rigorous science through industry's funding priorities; it also leads to serious negative consequences, such as industry's push to translate questionable research findings into profit as quickly as possible.

Health products and services that arise from reductionist research are mostly delivered via syringes, pills, and potions, and their funders (or should I say "investors"?) rush these products and services to market very quickly, usually before the implications of the research on which they're based can be fully explored and integrated. Of course, companies test new products and services; in fact they run up big bills doing so, betting on their randomized control trials to show positive health benefits. Sometimes they do. However, calling those positive results truly promising requires assuming that narrowly focused, short-term results actually bring long-term health. That's a risky and generally unfounded assumption.

In short, the pressures of the market result in products that are based on unripe research insights and unpredictable in their long-term effects.

It shouldn't be much of a surprise that these products end up being of limited utility at best and actually harmful at worst.

Vitamin E, which we discussed in chapter eleven, is a good example. A prominent study suggested a correlation between vitamin E levels in the body and healthier hearts.[4] Industry began marketing vitamin E as a heart healthy supplement and rushed it to market. Then evidence started mounting that vitamin E supplementation actually increased overall mortality through, among other things, more prostate cancer and secondary heart disease[5]—evidence that industry has ignored for as long as possible. Researchers' responses to learning this new but damning information about vitamin E resulted in a consensus that the party must go on.[6] Everyone wants to find a way to save the market for vitamin E, or to find a replacement if vitamin E is beyond salvation. There is clearly great incentive to produce evidence that will justify the continued marketing of such products.

It is truly not the individuals within my community that I decry (although some could show more creativity and courage!), but rather our world of research, greatly influenced by market forces that define what is expected of us. Most of us know that money talks, as the old saying goes. But few of my fellow researchers and medical practitioner allies really know how corrupting money has been and continues to be. It is so pervasive that it is difficult to see from the inside. When we're in the belly of the beast, how can we know which beast our host is, or even that our host is a beast at all?

Too often, our research priorities are driven more by personal rewards than community good. But the public pays for this research and depends on its findings, and, in the current system, they are being penalized for it. Individuals within the research community may find personal success by adhering to the reductionist company line, but as a group, we are getting no closer to the goal of health.

16

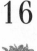

Media Matters

*Unthinking respect for authority is the greatest
enemy of truth.*

—ALBERT EINSTEIN

Scientific data underpin our decisions about health. They're used by the public to make lifestyle and buying choices; by doctors to diagnose and treat patients; by government officials to formulate policy; by industry to create and refine services, and to make health claims about those services; and by insurers to decide what diseases and treatments are covered. And that's only a portion of the ways the results of scientific research touch and affect our everyday lives.

The key link between research and these consumers is the media. Professional journals evaluate and publish research papers based on the editors' perceptions of the validity and importance of the findings. The mainstream media reports these results, making them accessible to lay readers and offering commentary and lifestyle advice based on the evidence. Without the media, scientific discoveries would languish, unacknowledged and unapplied, in the minds and lab notebooks of the scientists who made them. So the media plays an indispensable role in transporting information from the realm of its creation to that of its application.

Ideally, media is not just a conduit, unquestioningly conveying information from its creators to the social sphere. Media has traditionally served as a counterbalance to power, whether that power is governmental or scientific (the ability to peer deeply into nature and tell us its secrets is most certainly a form of power). This watchdog function of the media requires critical thought about data and their reliability. It requires that tough questions be asked. It requires journalistic independence. And it requires transparency of motive, so that the ultimate consumers of information can make informed decisions about how to evaluate the ways different media outlets interpret scientific evidence.

Unfortunately, this kind of independent, intelligent health journalism is rare. Neither professional journals like the *Journal of the American Medical Association* (*JAMA*) nor mainstream media outlets like the Corporation for Public Broadcasting can be relied upon for informed, courageous, and unbiased health coverage. I give those examples in particular because they are seen as the pinnacles of their type of media; the ones you'd least expect to fiddle with the truth. I don't mean to pick on them for being worse than other media; indeed, you don't have to look hard to find much less intelligent and honest health reporting in your newspaper and on the evening news. I just want you to understand that the problem isn't "a few bad apples," but rather the system in which the media is embedded, and the profit-seeking entities to which the media is beholden.

PROFESSIONAL RESEARCH JOURNALS

Research findings' first stop on the way to public consumption is one of the professional journals, which vary in influence and prestige. Articles in *Nature*, *JAMA*, and the *New England Journal of Medicine* (*NEJM*) often make the evening news if they seem interesting and relevant. Other prestigious journals are more obscure, known only to practitioners in the field the journal covers. Examples include *Cancer Research*, *The American Journal of Cardiology*, and hundreds of others that focus on specific disciplines and subdisciplines. Still other journals are known in the field as second tier, surviving on contributions that are considered "not up to snuff" by the top-tier publications.

The most important safeguard journals use against bad research is called peer review. This means that the editorial board sends manuscripts submitted to journals for publication to two, perhaps three, qualified reviewers (experienced scientists in that same field) to assess the quality of the research and the significance of the findings. The reviewers remain anonymous to the manuscript authors. This system is designed to filter out poorly done and unreliable research. When it is performed honorably, it is one of the most important guarantors of scientific integrity. Any supposedly authoritative article that has not passed through peer review should not, in my opinion, be invoked as proof of anything.

Peer review falters, however, when the reviewers bring their own biases to their decisions. When they decide in advance that certain research topics are out of bounds. That particular study designs (such as wholistic ones) are illegitimate. That certain conclusions just can't be right. In other words, when they cling dogmatically to their paradigm rather than seeking to expand or transcend it. Peer review can easily become an iron cage that stifles curiosity and creativity, discouraging many promising lines of research by all but assuring that they won't be published. This happens far too often. And it's no coincidence that a substantial reductionist bias permeates peer review, since that bias may serve the financial interests of the journals themselves—by attracting or keeping advertisers.

You may recall, from when we talked about reductionist versus wholistic study designs, that testing the effects of drugs was the subject most amenable to reductionist study design. It makes sense to study a reductionist phenomenon—for example, a single-function pill—via a reductionist lens. And, not surprisingly, medical journals make a lot of money when they please Big Pharma. Professional journals, like mainstream newspapers and magazines, are funded in large part by advertising. Marcia Angell, former editor of *NEJM*, reports that in 2001 the pharmaceutical industry spent $380 million on medical journal advertising. Without this income, the journals could not exist. So it's no surprise that the peer review process doesn't bite the hand that feeds those journals.

Big Pharma also funds medical journals in a more insidious way, through article reprints. When a study published in a prestigious journal supports the claims of a drug manufacturer, that's good news for sales, because one way the pharmaceutical company gets the word out to doctors who will prescribe the drug is through expensive, glossy reprints of the article that the drug rep delivers (generally accompanied by a box of donuts or fancier fare). The journals enjoy huge profit margins on these reprints, sometimes up to 80 percent, according to former *British Medical Journal* editor Richard Smith.[1] And a study published in 2010[2] correlated high reprint sales with industry-funded studies. In other words, the published studies that pharmaceutical companies paid for were much more likely to generate big reprint profits for journals. How much money are we talking about? It's not unusual for a single reprint order to cost millions of dollars.[3]

Setting aside the obvious question of whether the peer review boards of medical journals prefer studies that show positive drug effects, we can see that wholistic research is unlikely to become a reprint profit center. In whose financial interest is it to spread the word that eating processed food and factory-farmed beef, dairy, and poultry increases disease risk? Even "natural foods" retailer Whole Foods profits from processed foods; the *Wall Street Journal* reported in 2009 that CEO John Mackey admitted, "We sell a bunch of junk."[4]

Medical journals, in short, are given a financial incentive, if not outright pressured by their pharmaceutical benefactors, to publish reductionist studies that promote the efficacy of pharmaceuticals and other profitable interventions. Other models and viewpoints are seriously underrepresented in the medical literature, leading those who read that literature—doctors, researchers, policy makers, and the public—to believe mistakenly that the biased sliver of data that passes through the medical journal filter actually represents a larger truth.

I've seen publication bias of medical research journals many times in my own career. Although we were able to publish our findings on the effect of animal protein in highly qualified journals, further commentary on the broader significance of these findings has been another matter (one I intend to push even more vigorously after this book is completed).

Earlier, in chapter three, I mentioned the conversation I had with my colleague Peter Magee, the editor in chief of *Cancer Research*, the leading cancer research journal in our field. I told him of the new experiment my lab was planning, which would compare the remarkable protein effect on cancer growth with the well-accepted effect produced by a really potent chemical carcinogen, and which I suspected would show that a relatively modest change in nutrient consumption might be even more relevant for cancer development than exposure to the potent carcinogen. He was skeptical, but he agreed that, if we actually got such results, he would consider highlighting our findings on the cover of the journal.

Once we were ready to publish, however, my editor in chief colleague had retired. His replacement and the new editorial review board were inclined to dismiss nutritional effects on cancer. They wanted papers on ideas that were more "intellectually stimulating"—papers that looked at how cancer works in molecular terms, especially if these ideas concerned chemicals and genes and viruses. Despite our adhering strictly to reductionist experimental procedures, our investigation of nutrition's effects on cancer growth was almost akin to nonscience. Needless to say, *Cancer Research* did not publish our paper.

I received another cold shoulder from medical journals after collaborating with the director and founder of the True North Health Center, Dr. Alan Goldhamer. We coauthored a retrospective analysis of the dramatic effects of his fasting program on his clients with hypertension.[5] Every one of the 176 successive patients who were analyzed for the paper experienced a drop in blood pressure, most of which began within a few days of beginning the fast. The effect occurred relatively rapidly, was more substantial than that produced by any antihypertensive drug ever tested, and was free of side effects. It proved to be an unusually effective intervention. But journals like *JAMA* and *NEJM*, whose income depends on heavy advertising from antihypertensive medicines, declined publication in spite of reviewer recommendations to publish. They chose their wealth over your health.

The most egregious case of bias and muzzling I've witnessed on the part of a scientific journal revolved around a deeply flawed study[6] that purportedly proved that the dangerous Atkins Diet was more effective in helping overweight and obese women lose weight than three other diets, including Dr. Dean Ornish's low-fat diet. The study was published in *JAMA* in March 2007, despite the article grossly misrepresenting the study's results. One example: the authors claimed that their subjects on the Ornish diet were limited to 10 percent fat, as the diet recommends. But a careful review of the data table showed that over twelve months, participants supposedly on the Ornish plan actually consumed about 29 percent of their calories in fat. Yet the authors insisted that they had performed a fair comparison. In that deception they were aided by the *JAMA* Letters section editor, Dr. Robert Golub, who refused to publish a single critique calling attention to the study's very serious shortcomings, including commentaries submitted independently by Dr. Ornish himself, Dr. John McDougall, Dr. Caldwell Esselstyn, and myself. After *JAMA* ignored these submissions, I wrote to Dr. Golub, complaining about his journal's antiscientific actions, and urging him to publish at least one informed critique of this flawed study. His reply? A pithy:

> Dear Prof. Campbell,
>
> Your letter has been rejected, and we will not engage in further e-mail correspondence about it.

Dr. Golub should have been dismissed forthwith from his position with a reprimand. This is a lack of integrity of the highest order. But in the current system of medical publishing, it's just business as usual. After all, the Atkins Foundation is more than a diet; it's the propaganda arm of a billion-dollar business. They call the tune, in the form of funding grants totaling millions of dollars per year,[7] and the doctors and researchers who don't mind prostituting their professional credibility dance merrily across the pages of the most trusted medical publications in the world.

THE MAINSTREAM MEDIA

Most people don't read medical journals; instead, they get their health news from newspapers, television news, and news websites owned by large media corporations. Ideally, journalists who cover the health beat peruse the top medical journals, attend professional conferences, and interview scientists about new discoveries and ongoing research. They use their own scientific training and background (meager as it often is) to evaluate and interpret findings to a public that lacks scientific expertise—which includes most elected officials. One of the key contributions of health journalists is to set the context of new findings by showing how the new information fits into existing knowledge. Does it confirm, contradict, expand, or add nuance to the current paradigm?

In short, the public-facing media is supposed to be fair, thorough, and knowledgeable on the subjects they report. But they are too often none of the above. Most media bow to the subtle power exerted by the conglomerates that own them (in the case of the major networks and print media outlets), advertisers and/or underwriters, government regulators, and even elected officials (in the case of public broadcasting and other government-supported public media).

Both for-profit and the vast majority of nonprofit media simply echo the industry and government line. That line reinforces the reductionist paradigm and, as an extra bonus, produces some wonderfully gripping and sensationalist news to keep titillating the public: "A scientific breakthrough in the War on Cancer!" "New anti-obesity pill based on Amazonian superfood!" "Can chocolate cure depression?" You've seen many similar headlines and teasers, I'm sure.

If the mainstream health media were better—more scientifically literate, independent, and thoughtful—then the research establishment couldn't get away with the distortions of truth that come from shoddy study design and biased medical journals. The journalists, and the public they represent and educate, would demand more variety in study designs, clearer explanations of the limits of current knowledge, and more inquiry into questions that really matter. After all, we the people are the ultimate source of all the funding, whether through our federal taxes funneled through the NIH, or our health insurance premiums and co-pays going to pharmaceutical companies, or our charitable donations to disease societies and patient advocacy groups. If the media really were free and fair, they would represent our interests. Instead, they function, with little exception, as mouthpieces for industry, telling us the side of the story industry wants us to hear while pretending it's the whole truth. They spin the evidence positively and negatively to legitimize our broken health system and make it appear to be the only way things could be.

As we've seen, reductionist research may produce "truths" out of context that serve only to mislead and befuddle us. When the media report these minutiae as if they mean something important, it contributes to the public's sense of confusion. They share out-of-context details about fiber in oatmeal, lycopene in tomatoes, and vitamin A in carrots. One day they tell us that a glass of red wine a day will help us live longer, and the next day we discover that even one glass is toxic to the liver. Low-fat diets are great today; tomorrow, full fats are in. The result of all this reporting? Most consumers throw up their hands and alternate between false hope ("Hey, sardines prevent heart attacks!") and fatalism ("Looks like everything's gonna kill you. Might as well stop worrying about it."). This bipolar attitude toward nutrition serves the industrial profiteers who sell us these foods, as well as the ones who sell us the treatments for the diseases our poor food choices cause. All this confusion and noise also lets bad ideas sneak through and look good by comparison.

The reporting I've described here is unavoidably biased toward industry's interests. Bias does not necessarily mean lying. It can also mean exactly this: spinning minor details into major revelations.

Another form of bias involves omitting inconvenient data. The media can report only a small percentage of the biomedical findings that are produced every year. A legitimate media function is to act as a filter, choosing and sharing what's valid and most important while ignoring the rest. But some media outlets use this responsibility as an excuse for failing to report on some of the best and most important health information, because it doesn't fit into the reductionist paradigm or undermines the goals of an advertiser or sponsor.

Personal biases can also lead to the obfuscation of scientific truth—even by the nation's top journalists. Recently, *New York Times* science reporter Gina Kolata wrote about the discovery of genes that "cause" prostate cancer (just the latest in a long line of such stories, from Kolata and others). What really excited Kolata was the prospect that men could get tested for these genes for less than $300; now most men could find out whether, and possibly when, they would get prostate cancer. According to a surgery professor and prostate cancer specialist quoted in the Kolata article, this testing is part of "the boutique medicine of the future . . . we can know what diseases we will have to face in the rest of our lives." Kolata, perhaps the most influential health journalist working today, dutifully accepts and passes on this shameless plug for the genetic testing industry as scientific fact.

Kolata's reports don't simply inform the public on a day-to-day basis. They often become part of and guide our public conversations about health. And like many other journalists in love with the "next new thing," she has long emphasized the health promise of genetics research while subtly relegating nutrition research to irrelevance. In 2006, Kolata's front-page article "Maybe You're Not What You Eat" caused a national stir. It discussed the 49,000-subject Women's Health Initiative study, which had failed to show an expected decrease in breast cancer among women consuming a low-fat diet. Her conclusion: let's all stop worrying about food and instead get behind the future of high-tech medicine to save us from our faulty genes and misbehaving bodies.

This might be a defensible conclusion based on a study that actually showed no positive effect from a low-fat diet. The trouble is, the "low-fat" diet in question was a straw man, on two counts. First, the researchers' definition of "low fat" was 25-30 percent of calories from fat, a far higher figure than the studies they claimed to be refuting. And second, only 31 percent of the women in the study kept their fat intake below that already unimpressive level.

The problem with the journalism of Kolata and her ilk is not their inability to correctly report the technical details of research studies, but rather their prejudicial misunderstanding (or willful distortion) of some very fundamental science. Although well written and technically accurate, her story repeats the same superficial interpretations as her other writing about dietary findings. And taken as a whole, her body of work does not accurately reflect a balanced approach to scientific research done during her tenure, but rather a clear ideological position.

I cite these stories partly to suggest that media too often report on complex scientific issues in ways that reflect their own subjective preferences rather than the science, especially when it comes to issues of health. There is something very personal about these issues. We often discuss things like genetics and nutrition from a place of passion and ideology, ignoring facts to the contrary, and journalists are no exception.

Bias can't explain all the media's failures to give us good nutrition and health information. Another problem is the appalling lack of scientific expertise that many of the most influential reporters covering the fields of health and nutrition demonstrate. Because they are unable to assess critically the quality of health information that industry, government, and academia produce, they typically act as mouthpieces for these institutions rather than advocates for the public's right to know. Many articles consist of minimally rewritten corporate and government press releases, interspersed with expert interviews that corporate PR representatives conveniently hand them on silver platters. As a result, the reductionist half-truths that masquerade as scientific wisdom get passed on to us unquestioned and undigested. There's nothing wrong with nonscientists writing about science; I have no interest in limiting debate or silencing freedom of speech. But I do wish that journalists would acknowledge the limits of their expertise, rather than give the illusion of competence where none exists.

All in all, the story the media tells us about health and nutrition comes from a script written by the very people who profit from our pain and suffering. I've had far too many firsthand experiences of media manipulation, obfuscation, and suppression of the powerful connection between food and health to believe otherwise.

SPIN, OMISSION, AND INCOMPETENCE ON PBS

Around the same time I began working on this manuscript back in early 2007, there was an episode of the *PBS NewsHour* in which host Jim Lehrer reported an exciting news release from the ACS: cancer deaths in the United States decreased in 2004 for the second successive year.[8] Most notably, it was said to be a "big drop" from 2003. The way it was reported, it seemed that the tide in the War on Cancer, then thirty-six years old and counting, was finally about to turn. Later in the program, *NewsHour* correspondent Margaret Warner interviewed the chief medical officer of the ACS. Glowing with pride, he offered a few reasons for this big drop in cancer death rates, especially the decrease in cancers of the lung, breast, and prostate: better treatments, more screening, and less smoking. All in all, it was an upbeat report and interview that aired, coincidentally, just in time for the annual ACS fundraising campaign.

The next day, in my local Raleigh, North Carolina paper, the story dutifully made its appearance on the front page.[9] Shortly thereafter, President Bush was persuaded to go over to the nearby NIH laboratories and to declare that "the drop [in cancer rates] this year was the steepest ever recorded."[10] What's more, this "big" drop was all the more promising, the press regurgitated, because it followed what might be the beginning of a new trend that started the year before.

As someone who has spent most of his career seeking to eliminate cancer, I was fascinated by this wonderful announcement. Rather than depending on the TV and newspaper reports, I decided to dig a little and examine more closely the new figures in this report. Here they are: for every 200 cancer deaths in 2003, there was one less cancer death in 2004, a drop of about a half of 1 percent.[11] That's not the "big drop" that I expected based on the way it was reported. Although any such evidence favoring less cancer, however small, is welcome news, I doubt anyone who watched *NewsHour* that day, saw the subsequent media reports, or caught the president's speech would have estimated its magnitude at a measly half of 1 percent.

Furthermore, total cancer deaths from 2002 to 2003 had dropped by only 0.07 percent, a decrease of less than one death in every thousand. The numbers just don't merit the hype in the ACS announcement, which was diligently reported by media outlets aping one another without investigation or discernment, and which was publicly legitimized by the president. Watching this, I couldn't help but envy the cancer industry's control of the media and the bully pulpit of the presidency. What I could do with that kind of PR!

While most of the details of this cancer news item may be technically correct, its presentation is misleading. To say that a decrease in cancer deaths is "big" when it is less than 1 percent is simply wrong. To spend so much time talking about the reasons for this tiny decrease gives it, and its purported causes, far more significance than they deserve.

I know something about cancer. In addition to running my experimental cancer research program for about forty years, I was a member of several expert panels advising on policy concerning cancer causes, and I served on research grant review panels of the ACS, the NCI, the American Institute for Cancer Research, and the World Cancer Research Fund. In fact, I was responsible for organizing a couple of these panels. So when I say that the media is misrepresenting the truth, I speak from experience. Both my research background and my intimate involvement in the real story allow me a perspective that the average media consumer is denied.

The only message of this new ACS report likely to be remembered by the public is this: thanks to all our donations, the search for the cure for cancer is finally starting to pay off. Perhaps you think my concerns about this misleading report on cancer death rates are overstated. I disagree. In this age of information overload, we rely on sound bites like, "We are finally winning the War on Cancer," to tell us about the world and guide our actions. If winning this war means getting a minuscule change in cancer death rates after thirty-six years of spending tens of billions of dollars on cancer research (yes, billions, and largely by the U.S. government's NIH; its 2012 budget for cancer research is $5.9 billion[12]), it's going to be a very long war. This misguided overconfidence is our single biggest obstacle to truly overcoming cancer. Truly winning the war on cancer requires individual responsibility for our food choices; as long as we wait for the next pharmaceutical breakthrough or genetic engineering miracle to save us, we won't use the considerable power we already possess to end this scourge. In the meantime, the pharmaceutical/medical industry profits from our continued chase of cancer's cure, and the junk food and factory-farm conglomerates profit by suppressing knowledge about cancer's cause.

Had I been a reporter tasked with sharing the ACS press release with the public, here are just a few questions I would have asked: How big was the drop in cancer rates? Who chose the word *big*? Who funded the report? Which cancer rates declined, and which, if any, remained constant or even increased? (Not to mention: Why are overall cancer death rates in the United States so high compared to China and many other countries to begin with?)

Why didn't anyone on *NewsHour* ask these questions? Was it bias? Ignorance? I can't get inside the heads of the journalists who presented the story, so I can only guess that it was a combination of those sins, along with a relentless news cycle and ever-shrinking budgets that discourage slow and thoughtful consideration in favor of just running with a done-for-them press release.

ADVERTISING PRESSURE TO MISLEAD BY OMISSION

Shortly after publication of *The China Study*, I was interviewed on the phone by Ann Underwood, an informed and well-established senior editor of *Newsweek*. She told me at the top of the interview that her "senior editor" was *very* interested in the book. Our conversation lasted for almost two hours and she seemed personally interested in the implications of our message. Obviously, I was somewhat hopeful the interview I'd given would see print, although Ms. Underwood told (warned?) me that she first had to pass it by her editorial board for acceptance. From her especially articulate questions and her personal enthusiasm, I got the impression that I might expect a particularly good article. However, we heard nothing but silence over the next couple of months. I then received in the mail a copy of a *Newsweek* issue titled "Special Edition of the Future of Medicine"—an entire issue on health. *This is it*, I thought.

I opened the magazine to see what they had in store and counted more than twenty articles on various medical topics pointing to the future. Except for a rather superficial item on the relationship between diet and Type 2 diabetes, the articles ignored nutrition completely. They were all about new drugs and surgeries and genetics. Were I still in the experimental laboratory rather than wandering among the public, I could have easily become fascinated with the opportunities presented in this issue. Fundamental research into the workings of the cell is thrilling and mesmerizing. But this special *Newsweek* issue illustrated something far more important for the public. By omitting nutrition, the single most comprehensive contributor to health and well-being, *Newsweek* did its readers, at best, a massive disservice.

Disappointed, I browsed some of the boilerplate material in the front of the magazine to find this very thoughtful letter from *Newsweek* Chairman and Editor In Chief, Richard M. Smith:

> At *Newsweek*, we have a long and distinguished tradition of reporting on issues about science, medicine and health. Now, as biomedical research enters a new period of discovery we are proud to offer this special edition (a bonus issue for our subscribers) on the advances that are rapidly changing the face of medicine in the 21st century.
>
> We are pleased that Johnson & Johnson chose to be the exclusive advertiser for this special issue. As I trust *Newsweek* readers expect, the advertiser had no influence over the editorial content of this magazine.

Johnson & Johnson, one of the biggest medical device companies in the world, was the sole advertiser in the "Future of Medicine" issue of *Newsweek*, and I'm supposed to believe that *Newsweek*'s dependence on Johnson & Johnson's advertising dollars had absolutely no influence on its full-color ode to reductionist, for-profit, nutrition-ignoring health coverage? While I'm sure that a Johnson & Johnson senior executive wasn't sitting at *Newsweek*'s editorial meeting giving thumbs up and down to each article, the financially struggling news magazine could ill afford to displease such a powerful benefactor. (Yes, struggling: *Newsweek*'s revenues dropped 38 percent from 2007 to 2009, and in 2010 it was sold to audio pioneer Sidney Harman for $1, provided he assumed its $47 million debt.[13])

Shortly after the *Newsweek* inquiry, I got a call from Susan Dentzer, who was the health correspondent for the *PBS NewsHour*. The conversation lasted about an hour and was a good exchange. Ms. Dentzer certainly asked good questions and I thought she seemed quite interested, especially when she said she wanted to explore a possible interview for me with Jim Lehrer. She made no promise, but I nonetheless took some encouragement because I had been interviewed on that program before.

My hope eventually evaporated; an interview never came to pass. Why? I don't know for sure. But I did notice the increasing number of corporate sponsors now underwriting PBS who would not especially care for my views on nutrition. Someone on the *NewsHour* staff must have realized how unpopular my views would be with those big corporate sponsors. Why risk a funding backlash, when there are so many other stories out there that could be safely told?

In recent years, big corporations have gotten smarter about covering their tracks when funding supposedly impartial shows like *NewsHour*. One of the biggest current sponsors of the show is the John S. and James L. Knight Foundation, whose President and CEO, Alberto Ibargüen, serves on the board of PepsiCo.[14] Knight Foundation trustee Anna Spangler Nelson has been since 1988 a general partner of the Wakefield Group,[15] a North Carolina–based investment company that has a stake in many of the state's medical and biotech companies.[16] E. Roe Stamps IV, a Knight Foundation trustee since 2006, is cofounder and managing partner of the Summit Group, an investment company whose portfolio includes specialized molecular diagnostics laboratory ApoCell, Inc., which analyzes the effectiveness of oncology compounds for large pharmaceutical and biotech companies; specialized anatomic pathology laboratory company Aurora Diagnostics, LLC, whose website touts its "immediate access to cutting-edge laboratory procedures,"[17] including gene rearrangement; and several other medical technology and healthcare companies. Trustee Earl W. Powell endowed the Powell Gene Therapy Center at the University of Miami.[18]

My point here is not to criticize the Knight Foundation or its trustees; any of several other *NewsHour* underwriters, under scrutiny, would have produced similar results. As far as I'm concerned, the foundation does a lot of good work, and in fact generally supports "the little guy" against corporate interests. Furthermore, it makes sense for a charitable organization to fill its trusteeships with successful and wealthy people who can provide policy direction and aid in fundraising. But I do want to point out the inherent conflicts of interest that go undisclosed, unreported, and unaccounted for when a supposedly impartial news organization relies on a funding source whose trustees and executives are embedded in the very system that needs to be questioned and exposed.

I may be wrong to suspect such bias for a news program like *NewsHour* that is supported by public money, but a previous occasion with PBS about twenty years earlier turned me into a bit of cynic when it came to PBS's "journalistic independence." Back in 1992, a couple of years after the *New York Times, USA Today,* and the *Saturday Evening Post* had written lead articles on our project in China, PBS proposed the interesting idea to do a story comparing the diet and health habits of three rural communities: one in Italy, one in the United States, and one of our villages in rural China. At least, this is what I was told by a film group in Colorado who had been contracted by PBS (in Chicago) to put together footage. They visited Cornell, China, and the University of Oxford in England for the filming, and did a joint interview in China with me and Dr. Junshi Chen, my friend and Beijing counterpart.

Our conversation on camera in Beijing went well, I thought, especially when we talked about the health benefits of the low fat, mostly plant-based diet in rural China when compared with the typical high-fat, mostly animal-based American diet that the U.S. Dietary Guidelines Advisory Committee of the USDA (the group that produces the well-known Food Pyramid) generally favored. I offered then—and would do so with even more vigor now—that I was neither a fan of the typical U.S. diet nor of the Committee's politically sensitive government recommendations.

All went well, and the Colorado filmmakers kindly alerted us about two weeks prior to the upcoming TV show. They told us that we would like it, especially because the well-known news anchor Judy Woodruff would be providing the voiceover. Our friends and colleagues gathered around the tube at the designated hour, only to see nothing that had been promised. There was no comparison of the diets of the three rural communities, and the more significant discussions on policy had been purged. Dr. Chen and I were included in the credits at the end of the show, and that was about it. I called my contact in Colorado the next morning to ask what had happened. He said that when the final product was shown to PBS staff, they did not like my criticism of the dietary guidelines and the process by which the USDA constructs them. So those criticisms were simply omitted from the documentary, along with the supporting evidence Dr. Chen and I provided. What remained was a misleading, one-sided narrative that reassured Americans that our diet was fine and our government was protecting our health.

Is it possible that PBS, a celebrated media company known for its impartiality, is not so impartial after all? At the time the documentary aired in 1992, Archer Daniels Midlands (ADM), a company that, as of 2011, generates $70 billion in revenue from its worldwide operations, including sales of ingredients for livestock feed, was prominently featured as a major supporter of the PBS *NewsHour*. I could only wonder whether ADM's support was a consideration when the PBS senior management intercepted my comments in the documentary. Perhaps I'm wrong; I invite you to decide.[19] In any event, this early experience with PBS left a scar in my mind, which I could not help but recall when Susan Dentzer later interviewed me about *The China Study*.

I file both of these PBS experiences in a file labeled "Misrepresentation by Omission." When PBS edited out my comments on the U.S. dietary guidelines, it diminished its reporting. And, funnily enough, my comments at that time really were quite mild, compared to my present views!

SUBTLE POWER AND THE MEDIA

Nothing I've written here about the media is particularly dramatic. You couldn't make a gripping movie about *Newsweek* or PBS ignoring nutrition as part of its health coverage; I doubt Matt Damon is interested in telling my story on the big screen. Nobody lied, cheated, or conspired. As far as I know, there were no shady back room deals involving suitcases full of hush money. As far as I know, none of the journalists who slanted their stories were even aware of what they were doing, or what pressures they were responding to. These are decent, honest people just trying to fill airtime, entertain and inform an audience, avoid libelous statements, and keep their jobs by not offending those who ultimately underwrite their paychecks. That's the application of subtle power at its most effective and insidious: no fingerprints, no bruises, no blood, no foul. Just the seemingly innocent reporting of a scientific story as if it were the entire, obvious truth. But the cost of the missing part of the story, as we've seen, is nothing less than untold human suffering.

17

Government Misinformation

The only good is knowledge, the only evil is ignorance.

—SOCRATES

O ur federal government plays an important role in our health. It's responsible for funding health research, approving drugs and treatments, determining nutritional recommendations for federal institutions and school lunch programs, and establishing rules for nutritional labeling, among many other things. In the United States, we are supposed to enjoy a government of the people, by the people, and for the people. This should translate to a government whose policies seek to maximize public health by finding, funding, and promoting the most effective means of prevention and treatment of disease. Unfortunately, that's not the way things work.

I'm sad to say that in my experience around health policy and information, the people are getting the short end of the stick. We are being misled, with tragic consequences. The national debate on health-care reform wildly misses the mark, with Democrats and Republicans alike arguing about who's going to pay rather than about what would actually make people healthy. National nutrition policy panders to wealthy corporate interests rather than objective science. Governmental health agencies all but ignore nutrition as a factor in public and individual health. If someone asked you to create public health policy for which the goal was to mislead the maximum number of people in ways that would compromise their health while profiting the pharmaceutical, medical, and junk food industries, you couldn't do much better than what's currently in place. As my friend Howard Lyman, a former rancher and agriculture industry lobbyist, has said, "We have the best government that money can buy."

Are the people who create these policies so out of touch that they don't realize the effects are the opposite of their stated goals? Hardly. With unrestricted access to government officials at all levels, industry applies a mix of carrots and sticks to produce our government's pro-disease, pro-reductionist treatment policies that make them rich and the rest of us sick.

HOW INDUSTRY BOUGHT GOVERNMENT

Big Pharma, Big Insurance, and Big Medicine are among the biggest contributors to U.S. political candidates. According to the watchdog group OpenSecrets.org, health professionals (individual practitioners such as doctors, nurses, and nutritionists, plus large professional organizations such as the American Medical Association) ranked fourth in total giving to members of Congress in the 2011–2012 election cycle (almost $19 million), followed by the insurance industry at sixth (almost $15 million), and pharmaceuticals/health products at tenth (over $9 million).[1] And that means they have significant leverage when it comes to guiding health policy: they can coordinate millions of dollars in donations for candidates whose policies they support, and can deploy additional millions to defeat candidates who don't play ball. It was at an AMA convention that, in 2009, President Obama unveiled the public insurance option of his health-care reform plan.[2]

None of these industries have anything to gain by a more efficient and effective health-care system. To the contrary; if every American adopted a WFPB diet tomorrow, these industries would be in big trouble. You could argue that improving health care through nutrition and other lifestyle factors would even be "anti-growth," making it practically anti-American. After all, when someone avoids the operating room because they adopted a healthy diet, they aren't contributing to GDP. A diet of cheeseburgers, large fries, and Cokes is good for the economy when it's purchased, but it's even better when it leads to heart disease and a big hospital bill.

These industries can afford the best lobbyists, many of whom are hired for their connections as well as their persuasiveness. The "revolving door" between industries and the government agencies tasked with regulating them is spinning faster than ever.

Regulatory agencies routinely offer employment to industry lobbyists and so-called scientists who trade on their degrees to enhance their incomes. The departure of officials from government jobs for one in a related private-sector industry is common practice. In 2009, NIH director Dr. Elias Zerhouni resigned to take a position at Johns Hopkins University, according to a Johns Hopkins press release.[3] He lasted only four months in that position before joining French pharmaceutical company Sanofi as their new head of research and development[4]—a career move that was conveniently omitted from the NIH website, in contrast to those former directors whose subsequent careers involved a return to academia.

In 2010, Dr. Julie Gerberding, who headed the CDC from 2002 to 2009, found gainful employment at Merck Vaccines shortly after departing government service.[5] It's a relationship that benefits Merck greatly, allowing it to capitalize on Dr. Gerberding's contacts and influence in the federal government and the World Health Organization to help them sell more vaccines in the United States and around the world. But the career move also raises questions about impropriety. Certainly, at the very least, Dr. Gerberding's push to vaccinate all Americans against the flu each year of her tenure at the CDC (earning her the nickname "Chicken Little" for her annual predictions of a flu pandemic that never materialized) must have endeared her to her future employer.

We don't know; there isn't any evidence Dr. Gerberding intentionally promoted a vaccination policy that would enrich her future employer. But if you're a government official whose interest is in using vaccines as a primary strategy for controlling diseases like autism,[6] it must be hard to ignore the fact that your tenure is short and, if you play your cards right, a private sector job could be awaiting you at the end of it. Coupled with health policies that look like they could have been written by pharmaceutical marketing departments, this built-in incentive to please industry should make us a little less trusting that government agencies are seeking our good above all else.

On the industry side, lobbyists do more than shake hands and buy drinks after golf. They also write and edit legislation and regulations for grateful, understaffed legislators and agency heads. Their job, for which industry richly rewards them, is to strike out any language that might jeopardize profits. And the politicians play ball to protect their own careers. This fact, while not publicized, is common knowledge in Congress and on K Street, where industry groups have their lobbying offices. I've met with many high-ranking government decision makers over the years. While they often acknowledge privately that my views on nutrition and health should be public policy, I have learned that the political system will punish any elected official who advocates serious diet and health reform. Corporate interests don't just fund elections; they are willing and able to end political careers and derail progressive legislation as soon as they get a whiff of any move that might threaten their bottom line. And that means laws are enacted that further the interests of the wealthiest rather than the public good.

THE SO-CALLED HEALTH-CARE DEBATE

One of the hottest political debates of the past four years has been health-care reform. There's no question that our health-care system is seriously broken. But when you look at the evidence offered in public discourse, you begin to realize that virtually everyone is missing the point: the primary reason our very costly health-care system is broken is because it doesn't deliver health, and seems to have little interest in doing so. We're paying way too much money for way too little health. Every other problem is a symptom arising from that core truth.

In recent years, a virtual army of writers, scholars, politicians, and business leaders has offered opinions and proposed programs to solve the "health-care problem." Liberals point to the large numbers of uninsured people and insist the burden be shared by those who can afford to do so. Conservatives seek to protect the "free market" in health care, not realizing that this market is far from free. Sometimes the two sides find agreement, but such agreement is usually limited to how to streamline the delivery of health care.

For the most part, the debate over health care is focused on the supply side rather than the demand, with intense argument over who should pay the bill and not why the bill is so high.

We talk endlessly about shifting payment responsibilities among different groups—private sector or public sector, employer or employee—as if these programs are going to help control our country's back-breaking health costs: about two and a half *trillion* dollars in 2009.[7] Limiting these discussions and programs to matters of financing is too narrow. These political machinations, which are often fanned with much publicity and media coverage (or should I say hot air?), may please politicians and special interest groups from time to time, but they do little to address the main question of why we are so sick and why we are so unable to fix our sickness.

These discussions are not completely without consequence, however. They do serve to divert attention away from the really important question of how health might be improved—a question that leads directly to nutrition, not drugs and hospitals. Through this misdirection, they allow the system to continue to serve the profit motive at the expense of our health.

One of the best-known schemes intended for control of costs of health care is the HMO (health maintenance organization) legislation introduced in the 1990s. While health-care cost inflation slightly slowed for a couple of years with the introduction of HMOs, this trend proved short lived. Health-care costs have resumed their steady upward climb, with no new plateau in sight.

The initial savings generated by tough negotiations with doctors and efficiencies of scale did nothing to address the real problem: too many of us get sick, and the medical and pharmaceutical industries do a terrible job of making us well. Controlling costs is not the same thing as controlling disease. The HMOs talked about so-called preventive medicine, but in such a superficial way that the message had virtually no impact. Their dietary recommendations, by and large, boil down to "eat more veggies, drink fewer sodas, and choose leaner cuts of meat." That's like telling smokers to cut back from four packs a day to three—definitely a step in the right direction, but woefully inadequate. And because it was so superficial and inadequate, the "eat slightly better" message was universally ignored.

HMOs aren't the last word in cost-cutting. When money gets too tight, some private-sector employers eliminate health insurance programs, cut jobs, and close shops, or send their businesses and jobs outside of the country, where they are often legally able to ignore worker health and eliminate such coverage. The movement of much of the U.S. auto industry from Detroit to Mexico is a case in point. General Motors attributes at least $1,500 of the cost of every new car made in the United States to employee health-care premiums.[8] Ultimately, if we keep feeding the health-care monster everything we've got, it may bring down our entire economy.

HEALTH MISINFORMATION, COURTESY OF THE FEDERAL GOVERNMENT

We talked a little about the ways our government forwards the cause of reductionist nutrition in chapter five, focusing on the government's nutrient databases and RDIs. But their reductionist nature is only part of the story.[9]

RDI information printed on food packaging represents one of the most powerful, ubiquitous, and enduring ways the federal government tells people what to eat and what to avoid. As I noted in chapter five, RDIs are the ultimate in reductionist nutrition. Most packages list about a dozen nutrients, as if those were the only ones, or the only ones that count. The recommended amounts are also listed as percentages of daily value in grams. Last I checked, Americans weren't experts on metric weights or percentages. As we've seen, nutrition is nearly impossible to measure so precisely. And manufacturers are good at adjusting serving sizes to reduce the scary numbers of fat, sugar, and sodium—sometimes to zero, even though the product may contain a fair amount. In short, RDIs do a wonderful job of confusing the American public by appearing to be scientific while diverting attention from the simple truths about which foods support our health and which degrade it.

To make a bad system worse, for the vast majority of the population, most RDIs are much higher than they need to be. The establishment of the RDI for a nutrient generally begins with an assessment of the minimum amount of that nutrient needed to serve some particular function in the body for a sample group of individuals. This amount is sometimes referred to as the minimum daily requirement (MDR). For example, we might determine how much protein (measured as nitrogen) is needed to replenish the nitrogen lost by the sample group's bodies each day. But because the resulting number represents only a very small sample of the whole population, the MDR is then adjusted upwards to ensure that the majority of the people (say, 98 percent) will meet their needs. This considerably higher number becomes the RDI.

So even if we accept that the MDR is an accurate representation of what we need to achieve total health (a very risky assumption on its own), when we consume the RDI amount for a nutrient, nearly 98 percent of us are theoretically exceeding our minimum nutrient requirements. In addition, most people, including most health professionals, incorrectly assume that these *recommended* allowances are *minimum* requirements. This assumption encourages us to consume more of these nutrients than we need, which benefits companies who sell nutrient-based products such as supplements, fortified foods, and nutraceuticals.

There's more. These RDIs—as they are popularly interpreted—have in my experience long been biased on the high side for some nutrients to the point where they encourage the consumption of animal-based foods. Have you heard the myth that we need to consume lots of calcium to have strong bones and prevent osteoporosis? The calcium recommendation in the United States (1,200–1,300 mg/day) considerably exceeds the intake in countries that consume no dairy and less calcium (400–600 mg/day) but experience much lower rates of osteoporosis.[10] Convincing evidence favors a recommendation for lower calcium intake, but, suffice it to say, the dairy industry has long had a strangling influence on the committee making these recommendations, urging these "unbiased experts" (their words) to accept a high-calcium RDI.[11] The riboflavin (vitamin B_2) recommendation has long been set high as well, with the additional but false understanding that dairy is a rich source of this vitamin—a myth that started in the 1950s.[12] (In reality, dairy is not a rich source of riboflavin, at least as compared to certain plants.) In addition, the "daily value" for cholesterol is set at 300 mg/day. Cholesterol's inclusion in this list implies that it is needed as a nutrient. It is not! Our bodies, on their own, produce all the cholesterol we need. Dietary cholesterol comes only from animal-based foods, and a far healthier recommendation would be zero!

Then there is the epic story of protein, a nutrient that has long been the government's darling. The RDI for protein has for decades been 10–11 percent of calories, which is already more than enough (and not coincidentally, the average amount of protein consumed in a WFPB diet). Many people believe that a dietary average of 17–18 percent of calories from protein, also the current average level of protein consumption among Americans, is a good health practice. In 2002, the Food and Nutrition Board of the National Academy of Sciences (FNB) concluded, based on no credible evidence, that we can consume protein up to an astounding 35 percent of calories without health risk[13]—a number three times the longstanding RDI! At the time of the report, the director of the FNB was a major dairy industry consultant, and the majority (six out of eleven) of the members of a companion policy committee (the USDA "Food Pyramid" Committee) also had well-hidden dairy industry ties. Dairy groups even helped to fund the report itself. At this rate, before long, the government may start recommending a milk faucet in your kitchen next to the one for water.

The current system of developing and interpreting RDIs and guidelines according to industry interests is nothing less than shameful, not least because these industry-favoring standards and their supporting documents form the basis of so many government programs. These supposedly official items provide the scientific and political rationales for the way the national school lunch program, hospital meals, and Women, Infants, and Children programs are run.[14]

As a member of the expert panel that wrote the 1982 report on diet, nutrition, and cancer for the NAS, I recall that one of our central debates focused on what we should suggest as the appropriate goal for dietary fat to reduce cancer risk, based on existing evidence. Should we suggest reducing it to 30 percent of total calories (from the then 35–37 percent average), when the evidence clearly pointed to a much lower number? The debate was not about the evidence. Instead, we were worried about the political palatability of an honest dietary fat recommendation as low as 20 percent (still twice the level suggested by a WFPB diet). It was a statement that, thirty years ago, likely would have doomed our report to oblivion just on its own. Ultimately, we chose not to go lower than 30 percent, in deference to a prominent member of our panel from the USDA, who convinced us that doing so might result in a decrease in the consumption of protein and animal-based foods. That number, 30 percent, set the definition for a low-fat diet that remained part of the public narrative for many years thereafter. It gave the Atkins enthusiasts, among others, a false benchmark to use as a straw man in their argument that so-called low-fat diets don't work. Our committee's shading of the evidence in the policy statement in effect protected the animal foods industry and did nothing to promote human health.

While real nutrition is marginalized as a potential source of health, the federal government ignores and even covers up the truth about the deadly effects of the American medical system. As we saw in chapter one, the public CDC website conveniently omits the misfortunes of the medical system from the list of leading causes of death in the United States, despite the fact that "physician error, medication error and adverse events from drugs and surgery"[15] is the third leading cause of death, trailing just heart disease and cancer. These are deaths caused by the medical system, almost half of which result from the adverse effects of prescription drugs.

You might argue that the reason drug- and surgery-related deaths aren't included in the CDC list is because government has judged those death-by-health-care numbers to be incorrect; perhaps the researchers got it wrong. But this stark reality was summarized and reported in the prestigious *Journal of the American Medical Association*.[16] A federal entity, the Agency for Healthcare Research and Quality of the U.S. Department of Health and Human Services, was given responsibility in 1999 of monitoring medical errors nationwide in most U.S. hospitals. They have been diligent in getting all U.S. hospitals to systematically monitor such information, and have accumulated data for about five years as of this writing. The trend so far suggests not only that these statistics are correct, but also that the number of "medical errors" is increasing. Further, this may only be "the tip of the iceberg" with respect to the total number of avoidable deaths. An analysis of a subset of all hospitalized Medicare patients, for example, concluded that from 2000 to 2002, "over 575,000 preventable deaths occurred" nationwide.[17]

This more recent report confirms that these errors remain a "leading" cause of death; in fact, the report's authors agree that this number of deaths is so high that it should be considered an "epidemic." How is it possible that this cause of death might be an epidemic in one government report and not even be listed on a separate government website as a leading cause of death? Of course, such publicity would be bad for the disease business—and if the U.S. government cares about one thing here, it's the economic interests of the medical establishment, one of the leading donors to political candidates, parties, and political action committees.

THE CORPORATE AGENDA OF THE NIH

As we've discussed, the NIH devotes a microscopic amount of money to nutrition research, and most of that money supports reductionist studies on the effects of individual supplements, not whole foods. The NIH doesn't get a lot of public press, but its influence on the direction of medical research is huge. Its $28 billion annual budget funds somewhere between 68 and 82 percent of all biomedical funding in the United States, and a considerable amount around the world. Its two biggest institutes, based on funding, are the NCI and the National Heart, Lung, and Blood Institute, corresponding to the two leading causes of death. Of course, there's no Institute of Medical Error and Adverse Drug Effect Prevention, corresponding to the third leading cause! And, as I've mentioned, there's no Institute of Nutrition.

The NIH is thought to be an objective research organization, but of course there's no such thing as objectivity where funding priorities are concerned. Let's take a moment and look, in brief, at the way taxpayer money is allocated by the U.S. Congress. After receiving testimony and a proposed budget from NIH officials, Congress provides money to NIH in its general budget. NIH then apportions the budget among the directors of its institutes, each of whom divides the money into different program areas. Since institutes at various levels in the appropriation process essentially compete against one another for funding, they tend to be highly sensitive to the interests of powerful members of Congress. Regardless of how enlightened any individual institute director might be, she or he still must devote the lion's share of the money received to reductionist, profit-focused research, or else risk censure by Congressional representatives feeling their own financial pressure from industry lobbyists. There's not much money available for the type of systems analysis that could help us reprioritize our health spending in more efficient and compassionate ways. And almost nothing remains for studies of the social impact of health policies—trivial stuff, such as how real people's health is affected by RDIs and school lunch programs.

The NIH gives out money in the form of grants. The way they do this is by inviting qualified people to sit on grant application review panels and pass judgment on the many submitted proposals that are competing for the money. By "qualified," the NIH means something more specific and pernicious than "professionally qualified to evaluate study design and research potential." The people deemed qualified to pass judgment on research grant priorities are those who have been successful in getting NIH grant money in the past, a cycle that helps keep innovative wholistic research off the menu.

I have served on grant review panels both within NIH and nongovernmental cancer-research funding agencies. Several years ago, I was invited by two successive NCI directors to present my views on the link between cancer and nutrition in a Director's Seminar that included the director and about fifteen members of his staff. My second presentation followed my then-recent proposal for a new research-grant review panel called "Nutrition and Cancer" in hopes of giving some emphasis to this important topic. Although this new panel had been created, its name was changed to "Metabolic Pathology," thus negating its purpose. In my presentation, I expressed concern that this new name would obscure the goal of studying nutrition and its ability to prevent and reverse cancer—a phenomenon that I was demonstrating in my lab at that point, and that had been corroborated in humans in the China Study. I asked then-director Sam Broder why the word *nutrition* could not be in the title. After some heated discussion, he snapped, "If you keep talking this way, you can just go back to Cornell where you came from." Broder insisted that they were already funding nutrition research, but clearly our definitions of "nutrition research" were different. The NIH's nutrition research at that point comprised, as it does now, only about 2 to 3 percent of the total NCI budget, most of which was devoted to clinical trials of supplements. Two hours of discussion (all right, argument) got me nowhere.[18]

You can see the NIH's reductionist agenda clearly in what is and isn't included in its public pronouncements about the causes and future treatment options for currently "incurable" diseases. To cite an especially

pertinent example of an NIH-funded project laden with reductionist phi-
losophy, I turn again to the supposed link between AF and liver cancer.
The NIH website includes a page on this relationship, which I accessed
in March 2012, almost four decades after Len Stoloff (then chief of the
FDA branch studying mycotoxin) and I first published our doubts about
AF being a human carcinogen. This NIH page begins:

> For almost four decades, [National Institute of Environmental Health
> Sciences]-funded scientists have conducted research on the role
> in promoting liver cancer of aflatoxin, a naturally occurring toxin
> produced by mold. Their discovery of the genetic changes that result
> from aflatoxin exposure have led to a better understanding of the
> link between aflatoxin and cancer risk in humans. These discoveries
> are also being used in developing cancer prevention strategies....
>
> NIEHS-funded scientists at the Massachusetts Institute of Tech-
> nology were among the first to show that exposure to aflatoxin can
> lead to liver cancer. Their research also demonstrated that aflatoxin's
> cancer-causing potential is due to its ability to produce altered forms
> of DNA called adducts.[19]

See the reductionist assumption: AF causes cancer by altering DNA—
as if the process were that linear and uncomplicated and unmediated by
thousands of other reactions and interactions! But let's allow the NIH to
continue (while continuing to ignore the dominating nutritional effect on
the course of this disease):

> The Johns Hopkins University researchers are [...] the first to test
> the effectiveness of chlorophyllin, a derivative of chlorophyll that is
> used as an over-the-counter dietary supplement and food colorant,
> in reducing the risk of liver cancer in aflatoxin-exposed individuals.
> Studies conducted in Qidong, People's Republic of China, showed
> that consumption of chlorophyllin at each meal resulted in a 55%
> reduction in the urinary levels of aflatoxin-related DNA adducts.
> The researchers believe that chlorophyllin reduces aflatoxin levels by
> blocking the absorption of the compound into the gastrointestinal
> tract. The results suggest that taking chlorophyllin, or eating green
> vegetables that are rich in chlorophyllin, may be a practical and
> cost-effective way of reducing liver cancers in areas where aflatoxin
> exposures are high.[20]

Researchers have identified a biomarker—something they can measure that supposedly relates to cancer development. In this case, the biomarker is the level of AF-related DNA adducts in the urine. And they've identified a single nutrient—chlorophyllin—that can, in a straightforwardly reductionist fashion, block absorption of these compounds in the gastrointestinal tract.

Notice two fairly astounding things about this paragraph? First, green vegetables are mentioned, but in a throwaway tone. It's chlorophyllin that is "practical and cost-effective," not spinach and broccoli and kale. The NIH is coming down in favor of eating more green vegetables to prevent cancer in a way that won't actually undermine potential pill sales.

Second, this mechanism description relies on the completely unfounded assumption—not even acknowledged as such on the web page—that AF-related DNA adducts in urine correlate with cancer development. While it may be true, it's by no means a sure thing; you can't quantify cancer based on an adduct in urine any more than you can measure the amount of chocolate a child ate on Halloween by counting the candy wrappers in their bedroom trashcan.

The article concludes on a predictable note: the discovery of a gene that may explain why some people get liver cancer after AF exposure while others don't:

> In an effort to identify the genetic underpinnings of liver cancer, the Johns Hopkins University team has discovered mutations in a critical cancer gene, known as *p53*, in the serum of individuals who later were diagnosed with the disease. This discovery may eventually lead to new strategies for the detection, prevention, and treatment of liver disease in susceptible individuals.[21]

To recap: Our medical research establishment, funded by our government, responds to the scourge of liver cancer by recommending we take a pill to reduce gastrointestinal absorption of a carcinogen that has been shown to have nothing to do with the disease, and by promising much more expensive research into gene therapy that may one day save us from our own faulty bodies. No mention of nutrition at all, unless you count it as a vehicle for a nutrient more easily obtained as a dietary supplement!

I worked for a time with the researcher who led the team at Johns Hopkins mentioned in the article's conclusion. He is a chemist by training and, like most chemists, a reductionist in spirit. His journey into the question of what causes liver cancer began with a strong bias that the carcinogen AF is a major cause of human liver cancer (you'll recall I also once thought this could be true, early in my career). Thus he was focused on monitoring possible AF contamination in food, which necessitated routine analyses of food. He also was quite excited about a potentially lucrative company that he and his colleagues were launching to do just this. In addition, he and other Johns Hopkins colleagues were setting up an NIH-sponsored clinical trial in China to test the assessment mentioned on this NIH webpage, that chlorophyllin and related drugs might prevent liver cancer.

It was at this point in his career that he collaborated with my research group as part of our project exploring AF's connection to liver cancer. His laboratory had what I considered to be the best available method for analyzing urinary AF-to-DNA adducts as an estimator of AF exposure, and partnering with him enabled us to better assess its possible relationship with liver cancer mortality rates. Unfortunately for his interests (business and otherwise), there was no relationship—despite documenting AF exposure in three different ways and despite this being a more comprehensive survey on AF and human liver cancer than all other studies combined.[22] He refused to coauthor the paper of these findings. Also, his intervention project, in which chlorophyllin was administered to people in rural China, was abandoned after about eight years of NIH funding with no results, to my knowledge.

However, none of this appears on the NIH webpage, and this absence opens the door to and even encourages a variety of lucrative business practices, not least of which are chemical assays to analyze for insignificant amounts of AF (as offered by the company the Johns Hopkins researcher was starting).

This is reductionism—and your tax dollars—at work. Rather than preventing cancer, the NIH's approach actually serves as a psychological inoculation against true health: "There's no need to change your diet. You can if you want, but it's much easier and cheaper to take a pill. And don't worry, we've practically solved the problem by identifying the liver cancer gene. Just give us a few more years and we'll have a cure." Comforting words, with serious consequences.

This is the end result of all the political maneuvering and financial pressure we've looked at in this chapter, a version of reality shaped more by the profit agendas of Big Pharma, supplement makers, hospitals, surgeons, and suppliers of processed food and industrial meat and dairy than the truth. If these forces can so strongly influence the pronouncements of a powerful government agency supposedly looking out for our best interests, how can we trust our government's guidance on how to be healthy?

18

Blinded by the
Light Bringers

*When the search for truth is confused with political
advocacy, the pursuit of knowledge is reduced to the
quest for power.*

—ALSTON CHASE

When we make a list of "good guys" in the area of health, surely that list is topped by those selfless societies dedicated to defeating disease and spreading the gospel of good health practices. I'm referring, of course, to patient advocacy and fundraising groups such as the American Cancer Society (ACS) and the National Multiple Sclerosis Society (MS Society), which raise money and awareness in service of cures for very serious diseases, as well as professional organizations such as the American Society for Nutrition (ASN) and the Academy of Nutrition and Dietetics (AND, formerly the American Dietetic Association, until January 2012), which provide the education, networking, and leadership opportunities their professional members need to be as effective at their jobs as possible. But their donations and PR, their awards and fundrais-ers, just reinforce the system in which they are embedded—a system that lauds reductionist research and ignores nutrition.

The sad fact is that too many of these organizations are more likely to be found shilling for pharmaceutical companies and the food industry than advocating for patients or sharing scientific truths. And because these wolves clothe themselves in a sheepskin of selfless service, they are exceptionally good at pulling the wool over our eyes.

Patient advocacy groups like ACS and the MS Society ostensibly exist to eradicate specific diseases. The MS Society, according to its website, "helps people affected by MS by funding cutting-edge research, driving change through advocacy, facilitating professional education, and provid-ing programs and services that help people with MS and their families move their lives forward."[1] Replace "MS" with "cancer" or "diabetes" or "heart" or any number of diseases or parts of the body and you'll essentially have the mission statement of every such advocacy group. Professional medical societies have a similar goal; the main difference is their focus on a specific medical discipline, rather than on the particular disease or diseases that discipline treats. The AND, for example, "is committed to improving the nation's health and advancing the profession of dietetics through research, education and advocacy."[2] Both types of organization are as concerned with power and influence as they are with treatment and cure; the goal of most disease societies is to set themselves up as the "official" body that sets national policy on their disease, and professional societies typically seek the power to set standards and criteria for mem-bership in their profession.

These organizations see their gatekeeper roles as very important for protecting the public from fraud and incompetence, but this gatekeeping can just as easily stifle innovative approaches and fresh paradigms. Viewed cynically, these organizations begin to look like monopolies seeking to maintain their power at the expense of those who would challenge their worldview. At the heart of every disease society and professional organi-zation is an assumption about who is a legitimate practitioner and who is a "quack." These assumptions are generally unspoken until a challenger arises with a treatment protocol or research agenda that contradicts pre-vailing wisdom—and the prevailing wisdom in these organizations, as it is elsewhere in our health-care system, is the reductionist paradigm. As a result, despite the sincere efforts of many well-meaning people, these organizations actually get in the way of the treatment and cure of the very conditions they demonize in their PR and fundraising.

INDUSTRY DOLLARS AT WORK

In a healthy system, these organizations, especially the nonprofit ones, would be independent, beholden only to their members and the patients they serve. However, the main source of funding that supports these organizations is, as with the other groups we've looked at these last few chapters, the pharmaceutical and medical industries.

These organizations depend on industry in several ways. Most are funded largely by corporate donations, and they inevitably bend their policies and messages to benefit these funders. Many partner with deep-pocketed companies who cosponsor events and initiatives that the nonprofit could not have pulled off without such partnership. And here, as between industry and the government, there is a revolving door that provides an additional incentive for nonprofit executives and researchers to tune their actions to an industry-approved key. Those same industries might hire them as lobbyists or "thought leaders," also known as "key opinion leaders"—prominent physicians or medical researchers who have proven effective at influencing their peers—after their nonprofit stint ends.

Let's take a closer look at some of these nonprofits: two disease societies and two professional groups with which I'm quite familiar.

THE AMERICAN CANCER SOCIETY (ACS)

The ACS is dedicated to eradicating cancer worldwide. They fund research, sponsor patient education, galvanize the public into action, and remove the taboos against mentioning "the C word," all of which make the world a better place for cancer victims and their loved ones. The ACS's courageous campaign against the tobacco companies has significantly reduced smoking rates in the United States, and has succeeded in stigmatizing tobacco use. So who would be so Scrooge-like as to impugn their work?

Say a word against them and people respond as if you've confessed a fondness for cancer. But the ACS is one of the big obstacles to reducing cancer rates in this country. Called "the world's wealthiest non-profit" by Samuel Epstein, author of the 2011 book *National Cancer Institute and American Cancer Society: Criminal Indifference to Cancer Prevention and Conflicts of Interest*,[3] the ACS guides hundreds of millions of dollars per year into cancer screenings and medical research, and almost none into research or advocacy about diet. While Epstein's book focuses on environmental causes of cancer at the expense of nutritional ones, his exposé of ACS duplicity and conflicts of interest is required reading for anyone still under the ACS's spell.

If you were in charge of a wealthy and powerful organization dedicated to eradicating cancer, what would you want its positions on cancer research to look like? Mine would begin with a research program designed to understand the natural biological complexity of this disease, and then would try to take advantage of nature's tools to restore health. I'd encourage a wide diversity of research: reductionist and wholistic, mechanistic and dynamic, palliative and curative, reactive and preventive. (The more varied the research and interventions, the greater the chance of discovering something new—of stumbling upon a true breakthrough.) And I'd spend the vast majority of the funds I was given attempting to inform the public about what we do know regarding the role of nutrition in the prevention and treatment of cancer. By contrast, the ACS looks for simple solutions involving chemicals used to selectively kill cancer cells, a synthetic approach that ignores nature's means of restoring and maintaining health. In these aims, the ACS is indistinguishable from the PR departments of companies like AstraZeneca, the pharmaceutical company that has funded the ACS's breast cancer awareness drives, and, not coincidentally, manufactures and markets several breast cancer drugs; and Amgen, the biotech firm whose CEO, Gordon Binder, served as an ACS board member. In addition to AstraZeneca and Amgen, the following companies are on the ACS "Excalibur Donor" roster, signifying annual contributions of $100,000 or more: Big Pharma companies Bristol-Myers Squibb, GlaxoSmithKline, Merck, and Novartis; and biotech company Genentech.[4]

With one exception—the ACS's laudable and successful multi-decade crusade against smoking—the research and advocacy ACS funds is all about "preventive screening" (since when is a diagnosis of a late-stage existing condition considered prevention?) and molecular mechanisms of cancer development that might lend themselves to the latest toxic drug or genetic manipulation.

Mammography, the most common and lucrative form of breast cancer screening, is one of the pillars of ACS practice and philosophy. Epstein points out that five past presidents of ACS have been radiologists, and DuPont, a manufacturer of mammogram film, heavily funds the ACS Breast Health Awareness Program. The ACS's Breast Cancer Awareness Month culminates with National Mammography Day, an event underwritten by their corporate sponsors. ACS not only heavily promotes mammograms, it also ignores government guidelines on breast cancer screening when those guidelines threaten the pocketbooks of their sponsors. In 2009, the U.S. Preventive Services Task Force found that the risks of annual mammograms outweighed the potential benefits in women under 50 and so recommended routine biannual screening starting at that age.[5] The ACS, beholden to the radiation industry, still promotes annual mammograms for women starting at age 40.

The ACS doesn't just receive funds from pharmaceutical and health insurance companies; the junk food industry is also a generous and energetic contributor. ACS's Excalibur Donors list includes Wendy's, McDonald's, Unilever/Best Foods (maker of hundreds of food brands, including Rama margarine, Bertolli olive oil, Hellmann's mayonnaise, Knorr soup mixes, and Ben & Jerry's ice cream), and Coca-Cola. And, perhaps unsurprisingly, ACS does not take a hard stance on anything related to diet. ACS's diet recommendations (buried several directories deep on their website[6]) are vague and unthreatening to their funders' bottom lines. Examples of current diet recommendations include:

- Read food labels to become more aware of portion sizes and calories.
- Eat smaller portions when eating high-calorie foods.
- Limit your intake of sugar-sweetened beverages such as soft drinks, sports drinks, and fruit-flavored drinks.
- Limit your intake of refined carbohydrate foods, including pastries, candy, sugar-sweetened breakfast cereals, and other high-sugar foods.
- Choose fish, poultry, or beans instead of red meat (beef, pork, and lamb).
- If you eat red meat, choose lean cuts and eat smaller portions.

These recommendations hold no real financial risk for the meat and junk food industries. The ACS's recommendation to limit certain foods (not avoid them) is the equivalent of telling junkies to "limit your intake of cocaine." Not serious enough to make an impact on anyone reading them, and definitely not strong enough to make a meaningful difference in anyone's health. (How far this organization has strayed from its inception a century ago, when its founder, Frederick Hoffmann, advocated the study of nutrition as a key factor in cancer development! Hoffmann was removed from its board of directors three years later, then belittled at their first annual conference in Lake Mohonk, New York, in 1922.)

You may be wondering why I didn't include some tepid ACS recommendation about "limiting intake" of dairy products. That's because there is none. Despite all the evidence, the ACS doesn't mention avoiding or reducing consumption of milk or cheese, or dairy of any kind, in its recommendations. In fact, according to the January-February 2008 Digest of the National Dairy Council, the ACS recommends that both men and women reduce their risk of colorectal cancer by increasing their calcium consumption "primarily through food sources such as low-fat or non-fat dairy products."[7]

ACS doesn't content itself with promoting surgical, pharmaceutical, and radiological approaches to cancer treatment and prevention. The society actively funds vicious attacks on those who promote "alternative" cancer therapies, treatments, and prevention recommendations. Their Subcommittee on Alternative and Complementary Methods of Cancer Management (originally called, and still informally known among its staunchest administrators and supporters as, the Committee on Quackery[8]) denies funding to and in effect blacklists any practitioners who advocate natural, non-patentable, and nonmedical approaches to cancer treatment. (Just in case you're wondering if a WFPB diet qualifies as "quackery," two of ASC's "Signs of Treatment to Avoid" are: "Does the treatment claim to offer benefits, but no side effects?" and "Do the promoters attack the medical or scientific community?" Talk about being paranoid!)

I've experienced this ACS animosity personally, via a smear campaign against me and my research. In the early 1980s, diet and nutrition topics were off their radar screen almost entirely. Only begrudgingly did they give a passing nod to nutrition, when the NAS produced the 1982 report on diet, nutrition, and cancer that I coauthored. About that same time, a group of private fundraisers formed a new cancer research society, the American Institute for Cancer Research (AICR), for which I acted as the senior science advisor until 1986, and then again from 1990 to 1997. The AICR's sole mission was to emphasize the dietary causes of cancer. At first, I naïvely believed that a society dedicated to the eradication of cancer would welcome any research or policy avenue that showed promise in slowing or reversing the progression of the disease. I was wrong, though; the ACS turned out to be highly hostile to the AICR. I was surprised to find myself personally vilified in a memo about the AICR that the ACS president sent to their local offices around the country. The National Dairy Council promoted this memo to the press; it was even mentioned by advice columnist Ann Landers!

A few years later, after the AICR had become successfully established (and the ACS finally recognized it was here to stay!), the ACS invited me to be one of the six permanent members of their new panel of experts for evaluation of research grant proposals focused on the role of nutrition in cancer control. (By "permanent," I mean that I was allowed to hold the position as long as I wanted, based on their acceptance of my role in the initiation of the AICR.) I believed this represented a refreshing change of heart at the ACS, a new and sincere interest in the association of diet and nutrition with cancer. I served for a couple of years, then had to resign because of an overextended personal workload. Although I couldn't articulate it well at the time, I was becoming disenchanted with their focus on highly reductionist research.

A few short years later, with some new management and another change of heart, the ACS returned to their anti-nutrition roots by sponsoring the 2003 "Cattle Barons Ball" in Atlanta (their headquarters) as part of their annual fundraising drive. I questioned their behavior, given the known links between consumption of animal protein and cancer, and received a response from the then-president of ACS. She said that this ball was "not about beef," that the "event [had] no association or partnership with the beef industry or its interests nor does it articulate an endorsement of the beef industry by the Society." It was just a "fun" event.

I suppose some might accept this explanation based on a narrow technicality; they weren't suggesting those attending the event increase their consumption of beef. However, given the ACS's expertise in public relations—that's their business—it's hard for me to imagine they believed their own line. They've never held a "Marlboro Man Marathon" to raise money for cancer research.

The ACS may have avoided a formal partnership with the beef industry to avoid adverse publicity likely to arise from such a relationship, but it had a lot to lose if they were to advocate a plant-based diet, to the detriment of those cattle barons' bank accounts. The ACS very much supports the treatment of cancer with chemicals, and animal-product-free nutrition does not fit into such plans. Given its coziness with those cattle barons, it's not surprising that, to this day, serious research on the role of nutrition in cancer occurrence and treatment is an almost nonexistent priority for this all-American organization.

THE NATIONAL MULTIPLE SCLEROSIS SOCIETY (MS SOCIETY)

The MS Society provides another example of a disease organization whose impartiality and professed desire to improve human health is belied by the combination of its corporate funding and dogmatic anti-evidential stance.

Like the ACS, the MS Society depends on the food and pharmaceutical industries for the bulk of its donations. While direct donations from pharmaceutical companies total just 4 percent of the organization's 2011 annual revenue of $165 million[9] and other corporate donors provide another couple of million dollars each year, these companies are intimately involved with the events that drive the bulk of the MS Society's fundraising: the hundreds of walks, runs, and bicycle rides organized by good people who believe in their contribution to the cause. The big website sponsors of the Bike MS project are Pure Protein, a company that makes nutraceutical bars, shakes, and powders—"nutrition" that promises health but delivers a scary mix of processed ingredients, including sucralose, hydrolyzed collagen, sorbitol, maltitol powder, and palm kernel oil—and the pharmaceutical company Novartis, which manufactures and markets the MS drug Gilenya.

Poking at random through the MS Society website, I kept stumbling upon the society's financial dependence on companies that profit not from a cure but from the sale of processed foods that could contribute to onset of the disease. A local North Carolina MS chapter is sponsored by the Golden Corral restaurant chain. Sara Lee raised $111,000 in 2011 through their "Summer Bun Program." Sara Lee's parent company, Bimbo Bakeries USA (no, I am not making that name up), ran a summer 2012 promotion in supermarkets across the country to raise money for the MS Society through the sale of its other brands of junk food, including Stroehmann, Freihofer's, and Arnold breads and baked goods.

The MS Society clearly delineates the benefits of corporate sponsorship of its Women Against MS Luncheon as including "tangible marketing benefits," including "product sampling, brand exposure, and media exposure."[10] What isn't mentioned (but is understood loud and clear nevertheless) is that associating their corporate brand with the MS Society's name implies to consumers that the brand's products will aid in the "fight" against MS, or at the very least won't contribute to the problem of MS in the first place—something that, in the case of all these processed food sponsors, is not the case.

There is impressive evidence that high levels of milk consumption correlate with high rates of MS prevalence, and long-term studies show much lower death rates among MS patients who ate a plant-rich diet (5 percent, compared with 80 percent for those who consumed an unhealthy diet).[11] But the MS Society website has almost nothing to say about the role of nutrition in preventing and ameliorating the disease. The sum total of its general advice about nutrition:

> Maintenance of general good health is very important for persons with MS or any chronic disorder. A well-balanced and carefully planned diet will help to achieve this goal. MS specialists recommend that people with MS adhere to the same low-fat, high fiber diet that is recommended for the general population.[12]

In more detailed documents, the MS Society recommends lots of low-fat dairy (for calcium!) and lean meat (for protein!) as part of its MS diet, along with the usual lip service about eating fruits and vegetables. Not a peep about the demonstrated correlation between dairy consumption and MS. Not a word about the profound impact diet has been shown to have on MS survival rates. In short, the MS Society is all about whitewashing the causes of MS, coincidentally absolving its junk food sponsors of culpability while promoting its pharmaceutical sponsors' products and research initiatives as our best, only hopes of defeating this dread disease.

THE ACADEMY OF NUTRITION AND DIETETICS (AND)

Unlike the ACS and MS Society, the AND (until 2012, the American Dietetic Association) focuses not on a disease, but on a professional constituency. It exists to serve registered dietitians: those who advise hospitals, schools, clinics, daycare centers, government agencies, and the general public about what constitutes a healthy diet. The result is a substantial amount of influence over the way we think about nutrition in this country. Unfortunately for dietitians and the public they mostly misinform, the AND recommendations are tailored to the financial interests of its junk food industry sponsors.

While the AND gets much of its operating capital from member fees for services (including publications, accreditation, continuing education, and discounted attendance at annual meetings) and tax-deductible donations, they also solicit the for-profit private sector for donations. According to its 2011 annual report,[13] its generous "partners" include Aramark, The Coca-Cola Company, the Hershey Center for Health & Nutrition; and the National Dairy Council. "Premier" sponsors are Abbott Nutrition; Coro-Wise (a supplement-making arm of Cargill); General Mills; Kellogg; Mars, Incorporated; McNeil Nutritionals; PepsiCo; Soyjoy; Truvia (marketer of a sweetener manufactured by Cargill and Coca-Cola); and Unilever. The National Cattlemen's Beef Association and the National Dairy Council, along with many junk food manufacturers like Mars, PepsiCo, and Coca-Cola, were specially thanked in the report for donating at least $10,000 each to the AND.

I've lectured at the very large AND national meetings three times, at the request of a specialty group within the organization interested in vegetarian nutrition. The last time, in Chicago, prominently displayed on the outside of my registration bag were the names of the ADA partners, a veritable rogues' gallery of food and pharmaceutical interests. It was a nice mix of partners, with highly synergistic agendas:

one group (food industry sponsors) serves up soft drinks and milk products for school lunch programs across the country, while the other (pharmaceutical sponsors) peddles drugs for the ailments that these programs cause.

What I find especially repugnant about the AND is its stifling influence over nutrition education. The AND controls the content of the courses required for the registered dietitian degree in colleges and universities, as well as the criteria by which individual states license registered dietitians. The AND is also responsible for the training and licensing of other nutritionists across the country, through the Commission on Dietetic Registration (CDR). Only those nurses and dietitians who participate in AND's mandatory Professional Development Portfolio recertification system can maintain "registered" status, and the CDR determines who is allowed to provide this ongoing education, so crucial to those who wish to work in healthcare settings and be eligible for insurance reimbursement.

My friend and colleague, Dr. Pamela Popper, has experienced the AND's vicious anti-free-speech actions firsthand. She tells the story in harrowing detail in her excellent book *Solving America's Healthcare Crisis*. In 1993, she started a company that taught classes on plant-based nutrition in her home state of Ohio, thus incurring the ire of the Ohio Board of Dietetics. They investigated her, subpoenaed her to "name names" of other "non-dieticians" who were teaching nutrition so they could also be investigated, and actually threatened her with jail time. Beth Shaffer, the Board's compliance specialist, informed Popper that there are no First Amendment Rights in the State of Ohio when it comes to discussions about food and nutrition.[14]

Unlike most of the people bullied by the dietetic industry, Popper fought back. She spent tens of thousands of dollars of her own money, hired the top lawyers in the state, and ultimately succeeded in legalizing her business in Ohio. In an email, she shared with me a slide presentation given by the former Executive Director of the Ohio Board of Dietetics and current Chair of the AND Licensure Workgroup, Kay Mavko, urging and instructing local dietitians to "turn in" their competition to state licensing boards.[15] Just in case you think I'm being cynical or paranoid about the AND's real goals, I've reproduced a few of the slides in Figures 18-1 through 18-3.

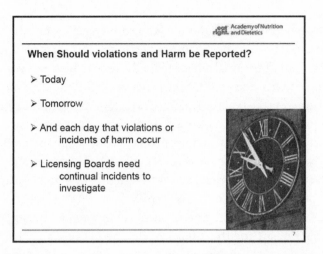

FIGURE 18-1.   Slide from an Academy of Nutrition and Dietetics presentation

Note that last bullet in Figure 18-1: "Licensing Boards need continual incidents to investigate." Without continual complaints, the Licensing Boards have nothing to do. Another slide warns of the danger of "sunset": that idle boards could be dissolved for lack of function. Dietitians must keep them busy! Again, the slide presentation says it far more eloquently than I can; see the slide in Figure 18-2.

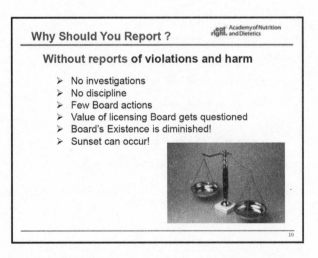

FIGURE 18-2.   Slide from an Academy of Nutrition and Dietetics presentation

But surely Kay Mavko and the AND are engaging in this witch hunt with good intentions. They're just trying to protect the public from what they see as bad nutritional advice from those who have not gone through the AND's rigorous accreditation process. Right? Again, Mavko's slide presentation sets the record straight. Take a look at the slide in Figure 18-3.

If registered dietitians are complacent, "other groups may gain a competitive advantage." You must protect "your scope of practice." Wow! You can see why this slide show isn't on the AND website, and why it was leaked to journalists by renegade AND members who were appalled at the idea of being turned into AND spies.[16]

The AND and its state board allies feel threatened by nutrition education that doesn't toe the official AND line because they fear for their jobs. That's understandable, as long as the public and regulators realize that the AND is, as Dr. Popper noted, "a trade group, not an authority on nutrition and health."[17]

Dr. Popper isn't, in AND's eyes, a legitimate source of nutrition information. So who is? The answer turns out to be the same industry and companies that pay the AND's bills. Some of the education providers approved by CDR include pharmaceutical giant Abbott Labs, food service providers Aramark, Sodexo, and Sysco, and front groups for the junk food industry, including the transparently named Coca-Cola

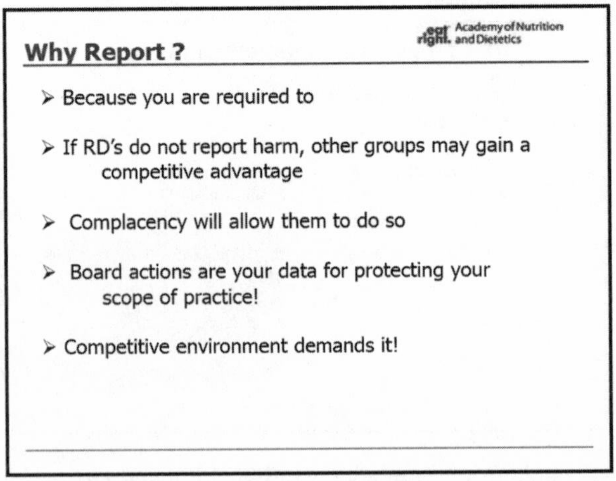

FIGURE 18-3.   Slide from an Academy of Nutrition and Dietetics presentation

Company Beverage Institute for Health & Wellness, ConAgra Food Science Institute, General Mills Bell Institute of Health and Nutrition, Kraft Foods Global, Inc., Nestle HealthCare Nutrition, PepsiCo Nutrition, and US Foods.[18]

Just in case some junk food manufacturers don't quite grasp the benefits of becoming an accredited provider of continuing professional education for AND members, the CDR website spells them out clearly under the heading "Marketing Opportunities":

- "[E]xposure to a market of over 65,000 credentialed dietetics professionals."
- "[P]romotion of individual CPE [continuing professional education] activities in the CDR CPE Database, which is available to practitioners via mail, fax, phone, and online."
- [L]isting "as an [sic] CPE Accredited Provider on CDR's website."
- "[A]pproval to use the CDR CPE Provider Accreditation logo while marketing CPE activities and materials."[19]

Talk about foxes teaching the hens about security fencing!

It is my experience that the education programs of all-powerful organizations very much defend the status quo, especially the so-called health value of dairy products for young people. They like to claim that they have a vegetarian subgroup in their organization, but it's treated more like a politically expedient stepchild than a true member of the AND family. As well, vegetarianism is still a far cry from the WFPB nutrition the research recommends; it cuts out meat, but still allows significant amounts of dairy products, eggs, and processed foods that prevent radiant health and freedom from disease.

The AND's work extends beyond educating (indoctrinating?) dietitians. In 2011, they also donated $62,000 to congressional candidates to promote their political agenda. What a great way for Coca-Cola, Pepsi, and others who donate to the AND to "launder" their political influence! AND, in effect, is turned into a highly credible PR agency for its corporate allies. Through its advocacy, public relations, and mandatory education partners, it serves as a front for the food and drug industries and their interests.

It saddens me to say these things because in my experience, the AND's individual nutritionist members are the most knowledgeable

professionals on nutrition I meet in my public lectures, skilled at presenting nutritional material to the public and unusually motivated in their
work. What I find repugnant is the organizational constraints placed on
these members, often without their awareness, about what is and is not
acceptable opinion.

AMERICAN SOCIETY FOR
NUTRITION (ASN)

I include the ASN (originally the American Institute of Nutrition) in
this discussion not because they're a particularly egregious offender, but
because I'm intimately familiar with the subtle and corrosive effect of
corporate money on this once-fine organization. To their credit, they
have developed a conflict of interest toolkit designed to root out obvious attempts at hanky-panky. Yet the influence of industrial profit is so
pervasive within the system that no overt attempts at self-regulation, no
matter how sincerely meant, can be truly effective.

I have been a member of this society for forty-five years and was very
active in it for many of them. They held their national research meetings
in conjunction with five (later six) sister biological societies, collectively
known as the Federation of American Societies for Experimental Biology.
At their peak, these annual five-day meetings attracted about 20,000 to
25,000 biological scientists. I greatly enjoyed the atmosphere and candid
exchanges with colleagues on our research findings. Some of my more
memorable recollections are of the awards given to my students, the
symposia that I organized or participated in, and the exchange of research
ideas in the formal presentations.

However, one thing always bothered me, and it only became worse
over the years: the so-called prestigious awards given annually to various
established researchers, usually along with award money provided by food
and drug companies. Each award was modest, ranging from $1,500 to
$5,000 apiece, but in total (approximately $40,000 to $50,000), the awards
represented a powerful monetary influence that steered the ASN away
from honest statements about nutrition. Industry knows that even small
rewards can buy loyalty from researchers who, given a range of topics to

study, simply find it easier and less uncomfortable to pursue research that does not implicate the products sold by their grantors.

When I became more involved in leadership positions of the society, I began to see the much-too-close involvement of these companies in its affairs. One of the more significant, at least for me, was the attempt by certain society members—prominent consultants to the American Egg Board, the General Mills Company, and other industries—to propose having me expelled from the society, the first time such an attempt had been made against one of its members in their forty-year history. Apparently, I had committed the ominous sins of (1) assisting as senior science advisor to the new cancer research organization, the AICR, to focus their efforts on nutrition with a bias toward plant-based foods; and (2) being a prominent member of the 1982 NAS committee on diet, nutrition, and cancer whose report brought focus to the cancer-prevention properties of plant-based foods. After an investigation, the society's eight-member executive committee voted 6–0 (with two abstentions) to absolve me of any wrongdoing. Still, this was an aggressive attempt by the industry-oriented members to silence me. As you can tell, it didn't work!

Professional societies protect their existence (and present and future funding) by aligning themselves with the traditional food and drug companies and their interests, avoiding as much as possible any mention of the possible health benefits of the WFPB diet. Having been part of several professional societies, I can assure you that they almost never accept findings that favor such a diet—and this includes the societies to which I have long belonged.

DAMAGING EFFECTS

Maybe you're wondering, what's the big deal? After all, these societies are free to publish, promote, and pay for any nonsense they like, and so are you and I. Training nutritionists and influencing research scientists isn't the same as dictating what we eat (how many of us have gone to a nutritionist?); these societies therefore seem easy to ignore. The problem is that because they are empowered by industry funding and granted quasi-governmental status to determine who is allowed to study and teach nutrition, and who can be marginalized or even disciplined for deviating from the party line, they are able to influence government policy, medical practice, and public perception far out of proportion to their financial weight, and in a number of different ways. I know something about this unprofessional behavior both from their investigation of my professional activities and from my tenure as liaison for the ASN and its sister societies to the budgetary process of the U.S. Congress.

First, they exploit the perception that they occupy some moral high ground in the battle against disease. To oppose them is to lend support to the enemy: the diseases that threaten us and our loved ones. Anyone who has had to explain to a neighbor suffering from breast cancer why they won't donate money for a pink ribbon, walkathon, race, bake sale, talent show, house party, reading group, or power lunch "for the cure" know the social ostracism that can result. As we've seen, most people suffering from a disease, as well as their loved ones, cling to hope in the medical establishment. After undergoing a surgery, drug regimen, radiation, or chemotherapy that improves function and staves off further degeneration, they may become active cheerleaders for current medical practice and evangelists for the "cure around the corner." Corporations like Astra-Zeneca and Merck can't command this passion and activism directly, but through nonprofits they convert well-meaning people's desperate energy into quarterly profits.

Advocacy and fundraising organizations in particular lay claim to a manufactured legitimacy that they have bestowed upon themselves, and few elected officials, journalists, or business people have the knowledge, incentive, or guts to question those credentials. When ACS puts out a press release, even the most respected journalists abandon impartiality as if they were local sports announcers openly rooting for the home team. *Three cheers for ACS and its success in the War on Cancer, NewsHour* and the rest of the mainstream press echo in tones of awed admiration.

Disease advocacy and professional organizations have also created the illusion of impartiality. All they care about, they tell us, is improving human health, either by wiping out their disease of interest or training their professional members in the best ways to deliver care. Because of this ostensible lack of commercial agenda, we trust their guidelines and research evaluations. When AstraZeneca tells us that tamoxifen is a safe and effective treatment for breast cancer, we know that, whether accurate or not, it is self-interested advertising. But when the ACS makes the same claim, we accept it as truth.

Perhaps the most serious effect of these nonprofits' collusion with industry is the "halo effect" that extends from these supposed saints to the corporations whose interests they promote. With industry's sales and marketing machines cloaked in mantles of charitable virtue, no wonder most Americans don't realize that the junk that passes for food is in fact the biggest contributor to our health crisis, and the junk that passes for medicine keeps us just well enough to continue to spend on both the food and the medicine.

THE ABDICATION OF PERSONAL RESPONSIBILITY

The upshot of this insidious industry influence over institutions that are supposedly helping us become healthier is a complete abdication on the part of most Americans of responsibility for their own health outcomes. It's not their fault; the nonprofits have indoctrinated us to believe that we don't have much influence over our own health—that all we can do is donate, march, run, and wear pink or yellow ribbons to help rid the world of these scourges. The fact that the vast majority of us can virtually eliminate our risk of premature death from cancer, heart disease, stroke, Type 2 diabetes, and dozens of other diseases is actively denied by the very societies who purportedly want to end these diseases. I'm sickened by the billions upon billions of dollars and the millions upon millions of volunteer hours that are redirected away from nutrition and toward reductionist, patentable, profit-generating distractions. And the most heinous misfortune of all is that the well-meaning people supporting these three societies honestly believe that they are doing socially conscious and constructive work to honor friends and family members who lost their lives to these diseases.

Here's an example that crossed my desk just as we were finalizing the manuscript: an October 3, 2012 blog post on the ACS website by Dr. J. Leonard Lichtenfeld, Deputy Chief Medical Officer for the ACS national office, with the title, "During Breast Cancer Awareness Month We Must Not Only Celebrate Our Success but Also Understand Our Limitations."[20]

The post, well-written and heartfelt, expresses sensitivity toward women whom the medical establishment could not help even while celebrating the contributions made by the latest screening techniques. Lichtenfeld writes:

> I understand the anger of women with advanced breast cancer who say, "What about me?" Among these women are those who did everything "right" when it came to early detection and treatment [....] These are women who pray for a breakthrough, who pray for a cure and wonder whether those who have not been diagnosed with breast cancer or who don't have advanced disease really understand.

These are moving, consoling, compassionate words. And yet they are utterly disempowering. Women with breast cancer, he advises, pray for a breakthrough. Pray for a cure. For your salvation lies in the hands of those who compound new drugs, who invent new radiation machines, who pioneer new surgical techniques, and who find new ways to manipulate genes. Even as he expresses humility and remorse on behalf of the medical establishment for having "oversold [their] magic," for having "overpromised and sometimes underdelivered," he's still selling reductionist treatment as these women's only hope. Not a word about prevention. About empowerment. About the fact that simple changes in diet may turn off cancer progression.

It's the same message everywhere in our health-care system, and this disempowerment—whether well-intentioned, as I suspect is the case for Dr. Lichtenfeld, or cynically in pursuit of profit—is the most obscene part of the whole story.

While the world is rife with unethical behavior, it would be a mistake to blame the problems I have discussed up to this point solely on individual morality. If we limit our sight to individual players, we'll never see the big picture. The issue is a systemic one, maintained by interconnected actors, all acting in their self-interest to further their goals. The trouble is not, or not always, the actors themselves, or their intrinsic motivations. Instead, it's the overarching goal of the entire system that's at fault: corporate profit above public health.

I've picked on the ACS, MS Society, AND, and ASN not because they're any worse than the hundreds of other disease advocacy societies and professional associations, but because they're the ones I'm most familiar with. They aren't "bad apples" in an otherwise good barrel; rather, the barrel itself, the system in which money talks and reductionism is the official language, is the source of the ethical rot. It rewards societies and associations that lend their moral might and PR prowess to expensive and ineffective reductionist approaches while ignoring or impugning the true preventive power of nutrition.

PART IV

Final
Thoughts

19

Making Ourselves Whole

*If a little bird were to take a grain of sand in its
beak from the seashore and somehow manage to
fly it to the furthest quasar in the universe, and if it
returned and repeated the process until all the sand
of the oceans both from the beaches and the bottoms
were gone, eternity would be just beginning.*

—ANONYMOUS, WRITTEN ON THE WALL OF THE
MATÉ FACTOR CAFE, ITHACA COMMONS, NY

If this book does nothing else, I hope that it convinces you that we need
to change the way we think about health. We must recognize nutrition
as a cornerstone of our health-care system, not a footnote. We must also
recognize the limitations of our reductionist paradigm and learn to accept
the validity of evidence beyond what that paradigm allows us to perceive.
If we are truly to understand the meaning of nutrition, its effect on the
body, and its potential to transform our collective health, we must stop
seeing reductionism as the only method by which to achieve progress and

start seeing it as a tool, the results of which can only be properly evaluated within a wholistic framework. And we must be willing to embrace wholism beyond the realm of nutrition. The body is a complex system; bodies gathered together in societies are even more complex; and human life, interwoven with all of nature on this planet, is complex beyond our imagining. We cannot afford to ignore this complexity any longer.

I realize that what I'm proposing here is a tectonic shift in the way we think about nutrition, medicine, and health. The process may not be easy. But it is possible. I know, because this shift is one I experienced myself over the course of my career.

My doctoral dissertation, written over fifty years ago, was on the greater biological value of animal-based protein. I believed then, as firmly as any meat-loving cattle baron, that there was no better, more beneficial food than the protein we received from meat and milk. But as you have seen here and in *The China Study*, my position today is very different. I am now convinced that there is no healthier way to eat than a whole food, plant-based diet, without added fat, salt, or refined carbohydrates.

For me, the source of that shift was evidence—the empirical, peer-reviewed evidence produced over many years by my own research group. It was bolstered in later years by the evidence produced by my colleagues in clinical medicine, who have been independently and convincingly documenting the WFPB diet's ability to reverse serious diseases in ways unmatched by pills and procedures.

But this shift in thinking required more than just evidence. It also required a shift in my understanding of the body, and therefore in the way I understood evidence related to the body's functions. And this shift is one that I hope this book will help you achieve, as well.

Early on in my career, even before I began the work on AF and MFO we've talked about at some length here, I had a conversation with a nutrition professor of mine at Cornell about a set of research studies that looked at the role played by four nutrients in two diseases, encephalomalacia (softening of brain tissue) in chicks and muscular dystrophy (progressive muscle weakness) in calves. It turned out that the activity of any one of these four nutrients could substantially change the activities of the other three, leading to changes in the body's response to the diseases.

When I asked my professor how common interactions like these were for other nutrients, he replied that although they were quite common, they did not get much attention in experimental research; they were too difficult to study and almost impossible to interpret adequately. Although nutrients act in complex ways in nature, we still had to think about their activities in a simple, linear way to produce acceptable scientific evidence. In other words, even though we could see the applicability of the wholistic framework, we still had to pursue our research as if reductionism were the whole truth.

That we ignored this complexity was something that troubled me greatly, and in a way it drove the direction I chose in my research into AF and MFO. I might not have begun this research had I not been willing to question what appeared to be an unquestionable, reductionist fact: AF causes liver cancer. If I had not been so interested in the idea of complexity, I might not have looked for factors other than AF that could affect the development of liver cancer. I might not have discovered that, in fact, AF was not even the most important factor affecting liver cancer development. And I would not have gained the much deeper understanding and appreciation of our biological complexity that I now possess and seek to share with you.

This understanding of biological complexity was crucial to changing the way I viewed the findings of reductionist studies. It made me realize how important it was to view such findings not as truths that are complete in and of themselves, but as pieces of a larger, more meaningful puzzle.

Any individual finding—say, that MFO's catalysis of AF leads to liver cancer, or that beta-carotene protects against lung cancer—does not tell the whole story. Therefore, choosing a course of action based on that individual finding, without looking at the larger wholistic framework— avoiding AF to avoid liver cancer, or taking beta-carotene supplements to prevent lung cancer—has the potential to be either significantly less effective than other ways of addressing the same problem, or even outright dangerous.

The findings in our reductionist experiments with MFO and animal protein are important, but not for their specific results (e.g., animal protein is a critical causal factor in liver cancer) so much as for the biological principles they suggest. These principles have helped me understand how cancer works and how nutrition, taken as a whole system, affects the development of cancer and possibly other diseases as well. The fundamental biological properties these MFO experiments revealed suggested a need to investigate the impact of animal protein in real people, in the real world, in all its complexity.

It was with this mindset that we designed the project in rural China that came to be known as the China Study. We wanted to investigate not single chemical mechanisms, as I had been doing for so many years in the research lab, but patterns of causes and effects that might help explain complex diet-disease relationships. We were looking for the larger context that might confirm or challenge findings like mine with MFO. We found it, and the shift in my view of nutrition and health was complete.

Looking back, it's easy to wonder why this shift was so difficult and took me so long. But I had to struggle against the same beliefs and assumptions that now plague my efforts to convince my colleagues, as well as the public, of what I have learned.

The first is our reverence for animal protein. Our society believes so passionately in the health value of milk and meat that it is hard for us to conceive that we might be wrong—that these foods might, in fact, be very *un*healthy. It is too far outside of what we have been taught for decades for us to believe it easily, no matter how true it may be.

Second is the reductionism paradigm that leads us to focus on parts of things separate from, and to the exclusion of, the whole. The body is a wholistic, interconnected system, but we are accustomed to thinking of it instead as a collection of individual parts and systems, in which solitary chemicals do solitary, unrelated things. Through the lens of reductionism, we see nutrition as a matter of individual nutrients rather than a comprehensive diet, and as an isolated field of study rather than the most influential determinant of our health as a whole. And although thinking this way about our bodies and our health has not yielded effective answers, we persist in believing that, if we stay on the same path, we will eventually find those answers—instead of admitting that there is something wrong with our approach. Trapped within this paradigm, it is difficult to grasp the idea of something that reductionism cannot measure in its entirety.

Third is the profit-oriented system that discourages us from behaving in non-reductionist ways. There's much greater profit in reductionism, with its quick and easy fixes, each targeted to one of thousands of different potential problems, than in wholism. And so long as industry is a driving force in determining what research questions get asked, what studies get funded, and what results are published and publicized and turned into official policy, breaking out of the reductionist paradigm will be an uphill battle.

Biology is incomprehensibly complex. The way our bodies create and maintain health is the result of millions of years of evolution—not just of individual cells, not just of organs, not just of functional systems, or even of the entire body, but of the body as a part of the food web and all of nature. Yet, either due to ignorance or motivated by avarice, some of us mere mortals want to tinker with the separate elements, taking the whole apart and using the pieces to create our own false reality. Disease, disability, and untimely death are the inevitable results.

So how do we put a stop to this?

I have tried for years to enact change from the top down, and it simply doesn't work. Even when individual leaders believe in what my colleagues and I have found, their hands are often tied by responsibilities to those who help put them in office (including the corporations who fund their election campaigns). And even if that does not derail their good intentions, they are still at the mercy of the political system. There are many ways to steer good but inconvenient ideas through a bureaucratic maze that results in watered-down, virtually worthless programs and guidelines bearing little resemblance to the original ideas.

But government decision makers are also beholden to their electorates—and that gives us, as individuals, power. This idea, like a seed, will sprout only from the bottom up; only after it grows roots can it produce fruit.

I've given much thought to the next steps that individuals who are sufficiently convinced by what I've shared, both here and in *The China Study*, and who want to help create change, might take. The most important step is to change the way you eat. The diet is simple: eat whole, plant-based foods, with little or no added oil, salt, or refined carbohydrates like sugar or white flour. (Though it may take some research, there are cookbooks out there that will fit your needs—more of them now than ever before.) There is nothing more convincing than experiencing the change for oneself. That crucial shift in the way we think about our health will happen, one person at a time. Eventually, policy will begin to change. Industry, deprived of the income produced by ill health and our ignorance, will follow.

It's time for us to begin a real revolution—one that begins by challenging our individual beliefs and changing our diets, and ends with the transformation of our society as a whole.

Acknowledgments

There are so many people whose support has been incredibly meaningful to me in the writing of this book.

First and foremost, I could not have done this without the support of my wife, Karen. She read drafts, tolerated my being on the computer when we could have been enjoying things she might have preferred, and was a very serious listener and critic of my ideas. After fifty years of marriage, she knows my work well, and after hearing at least 400 of my lectures during the past decade, she has also gotten to know what the average reader and listener might like to hear. She keeps my feet on the ground.

Howard Jacobson (PhD in the health sciences) added literacy to my manuscript as my "with" author. Howard is a brilliant writer. (I especially liked his metaphors.) He, together with Leah Wilson, our editor at my publisher, BenBella, made this book more readable, rearranging some of my chapters and connecting them into a sensible story. I can hardly be more complimentary about their professionalism and their dedication to this project. I am privileged to have acquired the best editorial team possible, and their deep investment in the book's message is especially gratifying. I want to acknowledge as well the considerable interest in my work shown by Glenn Yeffeth, publisher of this book and its forerunner, *The China Study.*

There are many others who contributed to my career in experimental research and policy-making: undergraduate honors students, graduate students, technicians, visiting scholars, and support staff in the laboratory and in the office. In addition, I greatly benefited from hundreds of colleagues who coauthored research papers, served on expert committees with me in the development of food and health policy, and critiqued our research findings for publication. Also among those who deserve my sincere thanks are the staff members of my foundation, headed by Micaela Cook and her predecessor, the late Meghan Murphy. I am most appreciative of their generous, sincere support. I could not have written this book without their contributions. Thanks are due also to my eldest son, Nelson, a true scholar of things social, entrepreneurial, and linguistic, for his careful reading of the final manuscript and putting me right on issues that could have gotten me in trouble.

Most importantly, I am grateful to the American taxpayer, who provided generous amounts of funding for my research (obtained competitively and mostly from the U.S. National Cancer Institute of NIH), thus providing for me an unusual opportunity to conduct experimental research free of any direct industry bias.

Finally, I am very grateful also to Cornell University, which recruited me to a full, tenured professorship at age forty. Director of the Division of Nutritional Sciences Mal Nesheim, Dean of the School of Nutrition Dick Barnes, Dean of Agriculture Keith Kennedy, and President Dale Corson each interviewed me and together granted me a position that provided an almost unparalleled opportunity to reach for the skies. Mere words cannot adequately express my gratitude for their expressions of support; the exemplary personal philosophies of these gentlemen gives meaning to the idea of academic freedom, a concept that needs all the support it can get in these challenging times.

About the Authors

For over fifty years, **T. Colin Campbell, PhD**, has been at the forefront of nutrition research, authoring more than 300 professional research papers. His legacy, *The China Study*, coauthored with his son, Thomas Campbell, II, MD, has been a continuous international bestseller since its publication in 2005. He holds the position of Jacob Gould Schurman Professor Emeritus of Nutritional Biochemistry at Cornell University, has coauthored several expert food- and health-policy reports, and has lectured extensively worldwide on resolving the health-care crisis through the little-known but remarkable effects of nutrition. He has founded a unique and highly successful set of online courses on plant-based nutrition as a partnership between the T. Colin Campbell Foundation (tcolincampbell.org) and Cornell University's online subsidiary, eCornell. Dr. T. Colin Campbell will be blogging at www.wholevana.com and participating with his sons in an effort to launch a grassroots health revolution. Together, they are launching a program intended to bring the empowering message of plant-based nutrition to individuals, worksites, and communities everywhere.

Howard Jacobson, PhD, is an online marketing consultant, health educator, and ecological gardener from Durham, North Carolina. He earned a Masters of Public Health and a Doctor of Health Studies from Temple University, and a BA in History from Princeton. Howard runs an online marketing agency, and is the author of *Google AdWords For Dummies*. He speaks, coaches, and consults on individual health and planetary sustainability, and can be reached at howard@permanator.com.

Notes

Part I

1. Nanci Hellmich, "U.S. Obesity Rate Leveling Off, at about One-Third of Adults," *USA Today*, January 13, 2010, http://www.usatoday.com/news/health/weightloss /2010-01-13-obesity-rates_N.htm.
2. U.S. Centers for Disease Control and Prevention, "Crude and Age-Adjusted Percentage of Civilian, Noninstitutionalized Population with Diagnosed Diabetes, United States, 1980–2010," last modified April 26, 2012, http://www.cdc.gov/diabetes/statistics /prev/national/figage.htm.
3. United States Environmental Protection Agency, "Cardiovascular Disease Prevalence and Mortality," last modified June 2011, http://cfpub.epa.gov/eroe/index .cfm?fuseaction=detail.viewPDF&ch=49&lShowInd=0&subtop=381&lv=list .listByChapter&r=235292.
4. International Diabetes Federation, "Morbidity and Mortality," August 3, 2009, http:// www.idf.org/diabetesatlas/diabetes-mortality.
5. B. Starfield, "Is US Health Really the Best in the World?," *Journal of the American Medical Association* 284, no. 4 (2000): 483–85.
6. *Ibid.*
7. Centers for Disease Control and Prevention, "10 Leading Causes of Death by Age Group, United States—2010," accessed December 2, 2012, http://www.cdc.gov/injury /wisqars/pdf/10LCID_All_Deaths_By_Age_Group_2010-a.pdf.

CHAPTER 2

1. R. A. Vogel, M. C. Corretti, and G. D. Plotnick, "Effect of a Single High-Fat Meal on Endothelial Function in Healthy Subjects," *American Journal of Cardiology* 79, no. 3 (February 1, 1997): 350–54.
2. Miranda Hitti, "FDA Approves New Angina Drug: Ranexa Is for Patients Who Haven't Responded to Other Chest Pain Drugs," WebMD, February 7, 2006, http:// www.webmd.com/heart-disease/news/20060207/fda-approves-new-angina-drug.
3. Kristin Johannsen, Ginseng Dreams: *The Secret World of America's Most Valuable Plant* (Lexington, KY: The University Press of Kentucky, 2006); Kim Young-Sik, "The Ginseng 'Trade War,'" accessed February 12, 2013, http://www.asianresearch.org /articles/1438.html.

4. L. M. Morrison, "Arteriosclerosis: Recent Advances in the Dietary and Medicinal Treatment," *Journal of the American Medical Association* 145, no. 16 (1951): 1232–1236; L. M. Morrison, "Diet in Coronary Atherosclerosis," *Journal of the American Medical Association* 173, no. 8 (1960): 884–888.

5. N. Pritikin and P. M. McGrady, *The Pritikin Program for Diet and Exercise* (New York: Bantam Books, 1984): 438.

6. Caldwell B. Esselstyn Jr., *Prevent and Reverse Heart Disease: The Revolutionary, Scientifically Proven, Nutrition-Based Cure* (New York: Avery Trade, 2008); C. B. Esselstyn Jr., S. G. Ellis, S. V. Medendorp, and T. D. Crowe, "A Strategy to Arrest and Reverse Coronary Artery Disease: A 5-Year Longitudinal Study of a Single Physician's Practice," *Journal of Family Practice* 41, no. 6 (1995): 560–68.

7. Dean Ornish, *Eat More, Weigh Less* (New York: HarperCollins, 1993); D. Ornish, S. E. Brown, L. W. Scherwitz, J. H. Billings, W. T. Armstrong, T. A. Ports, S. M. McLanahan, R. L. Kirkeeide, R. J. Brand, and K. L. Gould, "Can Lifestyle Changes Reverse Coronary Heart Disease?", *Lancet* 336, no. 8708 (1990): 129–33.

8. Esselstyn et al., "A Strategy to Arrest and Reverse."

9. C. B. Esselstyn, Jr., "Updating a 12-year Experience with Arrest and Reversal Therapy for Coronary Heart Disease (An Overdue Requiem for Palliative Cardiology)," *American Journal of Cardiology* 84 (August 1, 1999): 339–341.

10. Miranda Hitti, "FDA Approves New Angina Drug: Ranexa Is for Patients Who Haven't Responded to Other Chest Pain Drugs," WebMD, February 7, 2006, http://www.webmd.com/heart-disease/news/20060207/fda-approves-new-angina-drug.

11. You can find the exact number of data points that *are* required in the appendix of any sufficiently sophisticated statistics textbook. The main point here is that Esselstyn's study, with its remarkably profound results, could be accomplished with small numbers, while most drug trials cannot.

CHAPTER 3

1. T. V. Madhavan and C. Gopalan, "The Effect of Dietary Protein on Carcinogenesis of Aflatoxin," *Archives of Pathology* 85, no. 2 (February 1968): 133–37.

2. Gerardus Johannes Mulder, "On the Composition of Some Animal Substances," *Journal für praktische Chemie* 16 (1839): 129–52 (the paper where he named protein, according to H. N. Munro in *Mammalian protein metabolism*, Vol. I, eds. H. N. Munro and J. B. Allison, Academic Press (1964): 1–29); Gerardus Johannes Mulder, *The Chemistry of Vegetable & Animal Physiology*, trans. P.F.G. Fromberg (Edinburgh, Scotland: W. Blackwood & Sons, 1849).

3. D. A. Schulsinger, M. M. Root, and T. C. Campbell, "Effect of Dietary Protein Quality on Development of Aflatoxin B1-Induced Hepatic Preneoplastic Lesions," *Journal of the National Cancer Institute* 81 (1989): 1241–1245.

4. L. D. Youngman, "Recall, Memory, Persistence, and the Sequential Modulation of Preneoplastic Lesion Development by Dietary Protein," Cornell University: Masters Thesis (1987 , T. C. Campbell, mentor).

5. G. E. Dunaif and T. C. Campbell, "Relative Contribution of Dietary Protein Level and Aflatoxin B1 Dose in Generation of Presumptive Preneoplastic Foci in Rat Liver," *Journal of the National Cancer Institute* 78 (1987): 365–69; L. D. Youngman and

T. C. Campbell, "Inhibition of Aflatoxin B_1-Induced Gamma-Glutamyl Transpeptidase Positive (GGT$^+$) Hepatic Preneoplastic Foci and Tumors by Low Protein Diets: Evidence That Altered GGT$^+$ Foci Indicate Neoplastic Potential," *Carcinogenesis* 13, no. 9 (1992): 1607–13.

6. J. Chen, T. C. Campbell, J. Li, and R. Peto, *Diet, Life-Style and Mortality in China. A study of the characteristics of 65 Chinese counties* (Oxford, United Kingdom; Ithaca, NY; and Beijing, People's Republic of China: Oxford University Press, Cornell University Press, and People's Medical Publishing House, 1990).

7. M. F. Muldoon, S. B. Manuck, and K. A. Matthews, "Lowering Cholesterol Concentrations and Mortality: A Quantitative Review of Primary Prevention Trials," *BMJ* 301, no. 6747 (1990): 309–14.

8. G. N. Stemmermann, A. M. Nomura, L. K. Heilbrun, E. S. Pollack, and A. Kagan, "Serum Cholesterol and Colon Cancer Incidence in Hawaiian Japanese Men," *Journal of the National Cancer Institute* 67, no. 6 (1981): 1179–82.

9. Madhavan and Gopalan, "The Effect of Dietary Protein on Carcinogenesis."

10. T. V. Madhavan and C. Gopalan, "Effect of Dietary Protein on Aflatoxin Liver Injury in Weanling Rats," *Archives of Pathology* 80 (August 1965): 123–26.

Part II

CHAPTER 4

1. David Foster Wallace, "David Foster Wallace, In His Own Words," *More Intelligent Life*, September 19, 2008, http://moreintelligentlife.com/story /david-foster-wallace-in-his-own-words.

CHAPTER 5

1. I still remember my final oral examination for my master's degree at Cornell in 1956, in which I was supposed to name each of the then-known amino acids and their chemical structures. I wasn't able to, and they nearly failed me. I still don't know them all by heart, even though I taught this stuff for years!

2. R. S. Preston, J. R. Hayes, and T. C. Campbell, "The Effect of Protein Deficiency on the In Vivo Binding of Aflatoxin B1 to Rat Liver Macromolecules," *Life Sciences* 19, no. 8 (October 15, 1976): 1191–98.

3. K. D. Mainigi and T. C. Campbell, "Subcellular Distribution and Covalent Binding of Aflatoxins as Functions of Dietary Manipulation," *Journal of Toxicology and Environmental Health* 6 (1980): 659–671.

4. "MonaVie: Discover the Beat of a Healthy Heart," Monavie.com, accessed December 2, 2012, http://www.monavie.com/products/health-juices/monavie-pulse.

5. Office of Dietary Supplements, "Dietary Supplement Fact Sheet: Multivitamin /mineral Supplements," accessed December 2, 2012, http://ods.od.nih.gov/factsheets /MVMS-HealthProfessional.

6. K. S. Kubena and D. N. McMurray, "Nutrition and the Immune System: A Review of Nutrient-Nutrient Interactions," *Journal of the American Dietetic Association* 96 (1996): 1156–1164.

7. T. C. Campbell and J. R. Hayes, "Role of Nutrition in the Drug Metabolizing System," *Pharmacological Reviews* 26 (1974): 171–197.
8. N. W. Tietz, *Textbook of Clinical Chemistry* (Philadelphia: W.B. Saunders Co, 1986).

CHAPTER 6

1. The placebo effect, whereby patients get better because they believe they will, is one of most powerful documented interventions ever studied. Some researchers believe that fully 30 percent of the effect of any intervention is attributable to the self-fulfilling prophecy of patients improving because they think they've taken a powerful drug.

CHAPTER 7

1. T. C. Campbell and J. R. Hayes, "Role of Nutrition in the Drug Metabolizing Enzyme System," *Pharmacological Reviews* 26, no. 3 (September 1974): 171–97; T. C. Campbell and J. R. Hayes, "The Role of Aflatoxin in Its Toxic Lesion," *Toxicology and Applied Pharmacology* 35, no. 2 (February 1976): 199–222.
2. In this chapter, I've used AF as a generic description for all of the aflatoxin group, but my work largely dealt with AFB1, the most common and the most carcinogenic of the group.
3. K. Sargeant, A. Sheridan, J. O'Kelly, and R. B. A. Carnaghan, "Toxicity Associated with Certain Samples of Groundnuts," *Nature* 192 (1961): 1096–97.
4. M. C. Lancaster, F. P. Jenkins, and J. M. Philp, "Toxicity Associated with Certain Samples Of Groundnuts," *Nature* 192 (1961): 1095–96; W. H. Butler and J. M. Barnes, "Toxic Effects of Groundnut Meal Containing Aflatoxin to Rats and Guinea Pigs," *British Journal of Cancer* 17, no. 4 (1964): 699–710; G. N. Wogan and P. M. Newberne, "Dose-Response Characteristics of Aflatoxin B1 Carcinogenesis in the Rat," *Cancer Research* 27, no. 12 (December 1967): 2370–76.
5. Lancaster et al., "Toxicity"; Butler and Barnes, "Toxic Effects."
6. T. C. Campbell, J. P. Caedo Jr., J. Bulatao-Jayme, L. Salamat, and R. W. Engel, "Aflatoxin M1 in Human Urine," *Nature* 227 (1970): 403–4.
7. T. C. Campbell and L. A. Salamat, "Aflatoxin Ingestion and Excretion by Humans," in *Mycotoxins in Human Health*, ed. I. F. Purchase (London: Macmillan, 1971): 263–69.
8. T. C. Campbell, "Present Day Knowledge on Aflatoxin," *Philippine Journal of Nutrition* 20 (1967): 193–201.
9. *Ibid.* The practical message if you're looking to avoid AF, by the way, is that when you're shelling peanuts for your own consumption, you should throw away the shriveled, discolored kernels.
10. Urine samples are generally a more reliable estimate of AF consumption than asking people what they've eaten. People forget, under- and overestimate quantities, and sometimes "improve" their families' diets to impress the questioner, a problem all too common in many dietary surveys.
11. Campbell et al., "Aflatoxin M1 in Human Urine"; T. C. Campbell, R. O. Sinnhuber, D. J. Lee, J. H. Wales, and L. A. Salamat, "Brief Communication: Hepatocarcinogenic Material in Urine Specimens from Humans Consuming Aflatoxin," *Journal of the National Cancer Institute* 52 (1974): 1647–49.

12. Campbell et al., "Brief Communication."
13. *Ibid.* This test system was run by Dr. Russell Sinnhuber at Oregon State University.
14. Wogan and Newberne, "Dose-Response Characteristics"; R. S. Portman, K. M. Plowman, and T. C. Campbell, "On Mechanisms Affecting Species Susceptibility to Aflatoxin," *Biochimica et Biophysica Acta* 208, no. 3 (June 1970): 487–95.
15. Portman et al., "On Mechanisms Affecting Species."
16. R. Allcroft and R. B. A. Carnaghan, "Groundnut Toxicity: And Examination for Toxin in Human Food Products from Animals Fed Toxic Groundnut Meal," *Veterinary Record* 75 (1963): 259–63.
17. A. H. Conney, "Pharmacological Implications of Microsomal Enzyme Induction," *Pharmacological Reviews* 19 (1967): 317–66.
18. M. Maso, "Decrease in Mixed Function Oxidase Activity in Rat Liver Over Time," Cornell University: Undergraduate Honors Thesis (1979, T. C. Campbell, mentor).
19. Madhavan and Gopalan, "Effect of Dietary Protein on Carcinogenesis."
20. W. L. Elliot, "Bioenergetics: Pathways of Human Energy Metabolism," HealthBuilding .com, http://www.healthbuilding.com/metabolism.htm. A full color version of this image is available for purchase in poster size at HealthBuilding.com.
21. R. L. Lewis, *The Unity of the Sciences Volume One: Do Proteins Teleport in an RNA World?* (New York: International Conference on the Unity of the Sciences, 2005).
22. Madhavan and Gopalan, "The Effect of Dietary Protein on Carcinogenesis."
23. Madhavan and Gopalan, "Effect of Dietary Protein on Aflatoxin"; Madhavan and Gopalan, "Effect of Dietary Protein on Carcinogenesis."
24. J. R. Hayes, M. U. K. Mgbodile, and T. C. Campbell, "Effect of Protein Deficiency on the Inducibility of the Hepatic Microsomal Drug-metabolizing Enzyme System. I. Effect on Substrate Interaction with Cytochrome P-450," *Biochemical Pharmacology* 22 (1973): 1005–14; M. U. K. Mgbodile, J. R. Hayes, and T. C. Campbell, "Effect of Protein Deficiency on the Inducibility of the Hepatic Microsomal Drug-metabolizing Enzyme System. II. Effect on Enzyme Kinetics and Electron Transport System," *Biochemical Pharmacology* 22 (1973): 1125–32; J. R. Hayes and T.C. Campbell, "Effect of Protein Deficiency on the Inducibility of the Hepatic Microsomal Drug-metabolizing Enzyme System. III. Effect of 3-Methylcholanthrene Induction on Activity and Binding Kinetics," *Biochemical Pharmacology* 23 (1974): 1721–32.
25. Madhavan and Gopalan, "The Effect of Dietary Protein on Carcinogenesis."
26. R. C. Garner, E. C. Miller, J. A. Miller, J. V. Garner, and R. S. Hanson, "Formation of a Factor Lethal for *S. Typhimurium* TA1530 and TA1531 on Incubation of Aflatoxin B_1 with Rat Liver Microsomes," *Biochemical and Biophysical Research Communications* 45 (1971): 774–80.
27. W. P. Doherty and T. C. Campbell, "Aflatoxin Inhibition of Rat Liver Mitochondria," *Chemical and Biological Interactions* 7 (1973): 63–77.
28. J. R. Hayes, M. U. K. Mgbodile, A. H. Merrill Jr., L. S. Nerurkar, and T. C. Campbell, "The Effect of Dietary Protein Depletion and Repletion on Rat Hepatic Mixed Function Oxidase Activities," *Journal of Nutrition* 108 (1978): 1788–97; L. S. Nerurkar, J. R. Hayes, and T. C. Campbell, "The Reconstitution of Hepatic Microsomal Mixed Function Oxidase Activity with Fractions Derived from Weanling Rats Fed Different Levels of Protein," *Journal of Nutrition* 108 (1978): 678–86.
29. J. R. Hayes et al., "Effect of Dietary Protein"; L. S. Nerurkar et al., "Mixed Function Oxidase Activity"; Preston et al., "Effect of Protein Deficiency I."

30. A. A. Adekunle, J. R. Hayes, and T. C. Campbell, "Interrelationships of Dietary Protein Level, Aflatoxin B_1 Metabolism, and Hepatic Microsomal Epoxide Hydrase Activity," *Life Sciences* 21 (1977): 1785–92.

31. K. D. Mainigi and T. C. Campbell, "Effects of Low Dietary Protein and Dietary Aflatoxin on Hepatic Glutathione Levels in F-344 Rats," *Toxicology and Applied Pharmacology* 59 (1981): 196–203.

CHAPTER 8

1. The importance of medical hygiene was known to midwives for centuries, but only made its way into the medical establishment after Louis Pasteur, Robert Koch, Edward Jenner, and others demonstrated the existence of microbes and the mechanisms of contagion. That's another pitfall of reductionism: Until scientists have the means to isolate and measure things, they insist those things don't and can't exist, and anyone who says otherwise is ignorant and superstitious.

2. John Markoff, "Cost of Gene Sequencing Falls, Raising Hopes for Medical Advances," *New York Times*, March 7, 2012, http://www.nytimes.com/2012/03/08/technology /cost-of-gene-sequencing-falls-raising-hopes-for-medical-advances.html.

3. *Ibid.*

4. Having four letters that can form only two base pair types (A-T or G-C) may not sound like it can generate very many word possibilities, but a string just two base pairs long can be arranged in sixteen different sequences, while a string comprising four base pairs can be arranged in sixty-four such sequences. In addition, each base pair can theoretically be used in sequence an unlimited number of times. Imagine, for example, eight to ten successive units of one letter, say, followed by one or a few units of a second, maybe a couple more of the first, one of a third, and several units of a fourth. The possible combinations are close to infinite.

    If you are not yet sufficiently awed, then consider this: There are about three billion total bases—that's billion, not million—strung along the length of a single molecule of DNA. If those bases were placed only one millimeter apart along this chain, its total length would stretch 1,824 miles—more than 6,600 times the height of the Empire State Building! Their order may look random, but it is not. Imagine just a few dozen of those three billion bases as pearls strung along a normal length of necklace. Now, imagine picking up the necklace and letting the pearls fall off the end of the strand into a pile, mixing them up, then trying to put them back exactly in the same order. If it seems impossible at a few dozen, imagine doing so for three billion.

5. We cheated a bit, actually; 95 percent of our genetic material, which scientists don't yet understand, has been labeled "junk DNA" and swept under the carpet. Only very recently have geneticists begun to take seriously the possibility that this junk DNA is actually important information that humans just haven't been able to decode.

6. U.S. Department of Energy Office of Science, "Gene Therapy," Human Genome Project Information, last modified August 24, 2011, http://www.ornl.gov/sci/techresources /Human_Genome/medicine/genetherapy.shtml.

7. *Ibid.*; J. Lazarou, B. H. Pomeranz, and P. N. Corey, "Incidence of Adverse Drug Reactions in Hospitalized Patients: A Meta-analysis of Prospective Studies," *Journal of the American Medical Association* 279, no. 15 (1998): 1200–5, cited on U.S. Department of Energy Office of Science, "Pharmacogenomics," Human Genome Project Information, last modified September 19, 2011, http://www.ornl.gov/sci/techresources /Human_Genome/medicine/pharma.shtml.

8. Lazarou, Pomeranz, and Corey, "Incidence of Adverse Drug Reactions."

9. *Ibid.*

10. *Ibid.*

11. *Ibid.*; U.S. Department of Energy Office of Science, "Pharmacogenomics," Human Genome Project Information, last modified September 19, 2011, http://www.ornl .gov/sci/techresources/Human_Genome/medicine/pharma.shtml.

12. Committee on Diet, Nutrition, and Cancer, *Diet, Nutrition, and Cancer* (Washington, DC: National Academies Press, 1982).

13. R. Doll and R. Peto, "The Causes of Cancer: Quantitative Estimates of Avoidable Risks of Cancer in the United States Today," *Journal of the National Cancer Institute* 66, no. 6 (1981): 1192–1265.

14. *Ibid.*

CHAPTER 9

1. K. K. Carroll, L. M. Braden, J. A. Bell, and R. Kalamegham, "Fat and Cancer," supplement, *Cancer* 58, no. 8 (1986): 1818–25; B. S. Drasar and D. Irving, "Environmental Factors and Cancer of the Colon and Breast," *British Journal of Cancer* 27, no. 2 (1973): 167–72; J. Higginson, "Etiological Factors in Gastrointestinal Cancer in Man," *Journal of the National Cancer Institute* 37, no. 4 (October 1966): 527–45; J. Higginson, "Present Trends in Cancer Epidemiology," *Canadian Cancer Conference* (Honey Harbour, Ontario: Proceedings of the Eighth Canadian Cancer Conference, 1969): 40–75; J. Higginson and C. S. Muir, "Epidemiology in Cancer," *Cancer Medicine*, edited by J. F. Holland and E. Frei (Philadelphia: Lea and Febiger, 1973): 241–306; J. Higginson and C. S. Muir, "Environmental Carcinogenesis: Misconceptions and Limitations to Cancer Control," *Journal of the National Cancer Institute* 63, no. 6 (December 1979): 1291–98; E. L. Wynder and T. Shigematsu, "Environmental Factors of Cancer of the Colon and Rectum," *Cancer* 20, no. 9 (September 1967): 1520–61.

2. Michael Tortorello, "Is It Safe to Play Yet?" *New York Times*, March 14, 2012, http://www.nytimes.com/2012/03/15/garden/going-to-extreme-lengths-to-purge-household-toxins.html.

3. C. Campbell and L. Friedman, "Chemical Assay and Isolation of Chick Edema Factor in Biological Materials," *Journal of the American Association for Agricultural Chemistry* 49 (1966): 824–28. My exposure occurred long before I adopted a WFPB diet in the 1980s.

4. J. Huff, M. F. Jacobson, and D. L. Davis, "The Limits of Two-Year Bioassay Exposure Regimens for Identifying Chemical Carcinogens," *Environmental Health Perspectives* 116 (2008): 1439–1442.

5. S. M. Cohen, "Risk Assessment in the Genomic Era," *Toxicologic Pathology* 32 (2004): 3–8.

CHAPTER 10

1. Y. Singh, M. Palombo, and P. J Sinko, "Recent Trends in Targeted Anticancer Prodrug and Conjugate Design," *Current Medicinal Chemistry* 15, no. 18 (2008): 1802–26; Y. H. Lu, X. Q. Gao, M. Wu, D. Zhang-Negrerie, and Q. Gao, "Strategies on the Development of Small Molecule Anticancer Drugs for Targeted Therapy," *Mini Reviews in Medicinal Chemistry* 11 (2011): 611–24; R. Munagala, F. Aqil, and R. C. Gupta, "Promising Molecular Targeted Therapies in Breast Cancer," *Indian Journal of Pharmacology* 43, no. 3 (2011): 236–45; H. Panitch and A. Applebee, "Treatment of Walking Impairment in Multiple Sclerosis: An Unmet Need for a Disease-Specific Disability," *Expert Opinion on Pharmacotherapy* 12, no. 10 (March 2011): 1511–21; J. Rautio, H. Kumpulainen, T. Heimbach, R. Oliyai, D. Oh, T. Järvinen, and J. Savolainen, "Prodrugs: Design and Clinical Applications," *Nature Reviews: Drug Discovery* 7, no. 3 (2008): 255–70; P. Ettmayer, G. L. Amidon, B. Clement, and B. Testa, "Lessons Learned from Marketed and Investigational Prodrugs," *Journal of Medicinal Chemistry* 47 no. 10 (May 2004): 2393–2404.
2. This does give drug companies an interest in preserving tropical rain forests as a resource for potentially useful drug candidates, but this may be the only positive side effect.
3. Singh et al., "Recent Trends."
4. Gale Encyclopedia of Public Health, "International Statistical Classification of Diseases and Related Health Problems," Answers.com, accessed November 11, 2012, http://www.answers.com/topic/icd.

CHAPTER 11

1. C. Thurston, "Dietary Supplements: The Latest Trends & Issues," *Nutraceuticals World*, April 1, 2008, http://www.nutraceuticalsworld.com/issues/2008-04/view_features/dietary-supplements-the-latest-trends-amp-issues/.
2. *Ibid.*
3. "Apples, Raw, with Skin," *Self*NutritionData, accessed November 11, 2012, http://nutritiondata.self.com/facts/fruits-and-fruit-juices/1809/2.
4. M. V. Eberhardt, C. Y. Lee, and R. H. Liu, "Antioxidant Activity of Fresh Apples," *Nature* 405, no. 6789 (June 22, 2000): 903–4.
5. J. Boyer and R. H. Liu, "Review: Apple Phytochemicals and Their Health Effects," *Nutrition Journal* 3, no. 5 (2004), http://www.nutritionj.com/content/3/1/5.
6. *Ibid.*; K. Wolfe, X. Z. Wu, and R. H. Liu, "Antioxidant Activity of Apple Peels," *Journal of Agricultural and Food Chemistry* 51, no. 3 (January 29, 2003): 609–14.
7. C. D. Morris and S. Carson, "Routine Vitamin Supplementation to Prevent Cardiovascular Disease: A Summary of the Evidence for the U.S. Preventive Services Task Force," *Annals of Internal Medicine* 139, no. 1 (2003): 56–70.
8. U.S. Preventive Services Task Force. "Routine Vitamin Supplementation to Prevent Cancer and Cardiovascular Disease: Recommendations and Rationale," *Annals of Internal Medicine* 139, no. 1 (2003): 51–55.

9. *Ibid.*

10. H. M. Evans and K. S. Bishop, "On the Existence of a Hitherto Unrecognized Dietary Factor Essential for Reproduction," *Science* 56, no. 1458 (1922): 650–51.

11. D. Farbstein, A. Kozak-Blickstein, and A. P. Levy, "Antioxidant Vitamins and Their Use in Preventing Cardiovascular Disease," *Molecules* 15, no. 11 (2010): 8098–8110; B. B. Aggarwal, C. Sundarum, S. Prasad, and R. Kannappan, "Tocotrienols, the Vitamin E of the 21st Century: Its Potential against Cancer and Other Chronic Diseases," *Biochemical Pharmacology* 80, no. 11 (2010): 1613–31.

12. C. H. Hennekens, J. M. Gaziano, J. E. Manson, and J. E. Buring, "Antioxidant Vitamin-Cardiovascular Disease Hypothesis Is Still Promising, But Still Unproven: The Need for Randomized Trials," *American Journal of Clinical Nutrition* 62 (1995): 1377S-1380S.

13. B. C. Pearce, R. A. Parker, M. E. Deason, A. A. Qureshi, and J. J. Wright, "Hypocholesterolemic Activity of Synthetic and Natural Tocotrienols," *Journal of Medicinal Chemistry* 35, no. 20 (1992): 3595–3606.

14. *Ibid.*

15. A. Augustyniak et al., "Natural and Synthetic Antioxidants: An Updated Overview," *Free Radical Research* 44, no. 10 (2010): 1216–62.

16. E. B. Rimm, M. J. Stampfer, A. Ascherio, E. Giovannucci, G. A. Colditz, and W. C. Willett, "Vitamin E Consumption and the Risk of Coronary Heart Disease in Men," *New England Journal of Medicine* 328, no. 20 (May 20, 1993): 1450–56; M. J. Stampfer, C. H. Hennekens, J. E. Manson, G. A. Colditz, B. Rosner, and W. C. Willett, "Vitamin E Consumption and the Risk of Coronary Disease in Women," *New England Journal of Medicine* 328, no. 20 (May 20, 1993): 1444–49.

17. H. D. Sesso, J. E. Buring, W. G. Christen, T. Kurth, C. Belanger, J. MacFadyen, V. Bubes, J. E. Manson, R. J. Glynn, and J. M. Gaziano, "Vitamins E and C in the prevention of cardiovascular disease in men," *Journal of the American Medical Association* 300, no. 18 (2008): 2123–2133; "Vitamins E and C"; I. M. Lee, N. R. Cook, J. M. Gaziano, D. Gordon, P. M. Ridker, J. E. Manson, C. H. Hennekens, and J. E. Buring, "Vitamin E in the Primary Prevention of Cardiovascular Disease and Cancer: The Women's Health Study: A Randomized Controlled Trial," *Journal of the American Medical Association* 294, no. 1 (2005): 56–65; E. Lonn et al., "Effects of Long-Term Vitamin E Supplementation on Cardiovascular Events and Cancer: A Randomized Controlled Trial," *Journal of the American Medical Association* 293, no. 11 (2005): 1338–47; D. P. Vivekananthan, M. S. Penn, S. K. Sapp, A. Hsu, and E. J. Topol, "Use of Antioxidant Vitamins for the Prevention of Cardiovascular Disease: Meta-analysis of Randomised Trials," *Lancet* 361, no. 9374 (June 14, 2003): 2017–23.

18. I. M. Lee et al., "Vitamin E in the Primary Prevention"; E. Lonn et al., "Effects of Long-Term Vitamin E"; V. A. Kirsh et al., "Supplemental and Dietary Vitamin E, Beta-Carotene, and Vitamin C Intakes and Prostate Cancer Risk," *Journal of the National Cancer Institute* 98, no. 4 (February 15, 2006): 245–54; S. M. Lippman et al., "Effect of Selenium and Vitamin E on Risk of Prostate Cancer and Other Cancers: The Selenium and Vitamin E Cancer Prevention Trial (SELECT)," *Journal of the American Medical Association* 301, no. 1 (January 7, 2009): 39–51.

19. S. M. Lippman et al., "Effect of Selenium"; S. Liu, I. M. Lee, Y. Song, M. Van Denburgh, N. R. Cook, J. E. Manson, and J. E. Buring, "Vitamin E and Risk of Type 2 Diabetes in the Women's Health Study Randomized Controlled Trial," *Diabetes* 55, no. 10 (October 2006): 2856–62.

20. W. G. Christen, R. J. Glynn, H. D. Sesso, T. Kurth, J. MacFayden, V. Bubes, J. E. Buring, J. E. Manson, and J. M. Gaziano, "Age-Related Cataract in a Randomized Trial of Vitamins E and C in Men," *Archives of Ophthalmology* 128, no. 11 (November 2010): 1397–1405.

21. I. G. Tsiligianni and T. van der Molen, "A Systematic Review of the Role of Vitamin Insufficiencies and Supplementation in COPD," *Respiratory Research* 11 (December 6, 2010): 171.

22. G. Bjelakovic, D. Nikolova, L. L. Gluud, R. G. Simonetti, and C. Gluud, "Antioxidant Supplements for Prevention of Mortality in Healthy Participants and Patients with Various Diseases," *Cochrane Database of Systematic Reviews* 3 (March 14, 2012): CD007176. DOI: 10.

23. Y. Dotan, D. Lichtenberg, and I. Pinchuk, "No Evidence Supports Vitamin E Indiscriminate Supplementation," *Biofactors* 35, no. 6 (2009): 469–73; J. Blumberg and B. Frei, "Why Clinical Trials of Vitamin E and Cardiovascular Diseases May Be Fatally Flawed," *Free Radical Biology & Medicine* 43, no. 10 (2007): 1374–76.

24. Aggarwal et al., "Tocotrienols."

25. Farbstein et al., "Antioxidant Vitamins."

26. Lonn et al., "Effects of Long-Term Vitamin E."

27. Goran Bjelakovic, Dimitrinka Nikolova, Lise Lotte Gluud, Rosa G. Simonetti, and Christian Gluud. "Mortality in Randomized Trials," *Journal of the American Medical Association* 297, no. 8 (2007): 842–857; E.R. Miller, R. Pastor-Barriuso, D. Dalal, R. A. Riemersma, L. J. Appel, and E. Guallar, "Meta-analysis: High-dose Vitamin E Supplementation May Increase All-cause Mortality," *Annals of Internal Medicine* 142 (2005): 37–46.

28. S. O. Ebbesson et al., "Fatty Acid Consumption and Metabolic Syndrome Components: The GOCADAN Study," *Journal of the Cardiometabolic Syndrome* 2, no. 4 (2007): 244–49.

29. E. Lopez-Garcia, M. B. Schulze, J. E. Manson, J. B. Meigs, C. M. Albert, N. Rifai, W. C. Willett, F. B. Hu, "Consumption of (n-3) Fatty Acids Is Related to Plasma Biomarkers of Inflammation and Endothelial Activation in Women," *Journal of Nutrition* 134, no. 7 (2004): 1806–11; R. J. Deckelbaum, T. S. Worgall, and T. Seo, "n-3 Fatty Acids and Gene Expression," supplement, *American Journal of Clinical Nutrition* 83, no. 6 (2006): 1520S–25S.

30. S. V. Kaushik, D. Mozaffarian, D. Spiegelman, J. E. Manson, and W. Willett, "Long-Chain Omega-3 Fatty Acids, Fish Intake, and the Risk of Type 2 Diabetes Mellitus," *American Journal of Clinical Nutrition* 90, no. 3 (2009): 613–20.

31. L. Hooper et al., "Risks and Benefits of Omega 3 Fats for Mortality, Cardiovascular Disease, and Cancer: Systematic Review," *BMJ* 332, no. 7544 (2006): 752–60.

32. Kaushik et al., "Long-Chain Omega-3 Fatty Acids."

33. C. S. Foote, Y. C. Chang, and R. W. Denny, "Chemistry of Singlet Oxygen. X. Carotenoid Quenching Parallels Biological Protection," *Journal of the American Chemical Society* 92, no. 17 (1970): 5216–18; J. E. Packer, J. S. Mahood, V. O. Mora-Arellano, T. F. Slater, R. L. Willson, and B. S. Wolfenden, "Free Radicals and Singlet Oxygen Scavengers: Reaction of a Peroxy-radical with β-carotene, Diphenyl Furan and 1,4-diazobicyclo(2,2,2)-octane," *Biochemical and Biophysical Research Communications* 98, no. 4 (1981): 901–6.

34. R. Peto, R. Doll, and J. D. Buckley, "Can Dietary Beta-Carotene Materially Reduce Human Cancer Rates?" *Nature* 290, no. 5803 (1981): 201–8.
35. G. S. Omenn, "Chemoprevention of Lung Cancers: Lessons from CARET, the Beta-Carotene and Retinol Efficacy Trial, and Prospects for the Future," *European Journal of Cancer Prevention* 16, no. 3 (2007): 184–91.
36. G. S. Omenn et al, "Effects of a Combination of Beta Carotene and Vitamin A on Lung Cancer and Cardiovascular Disease," *New England Journal of Medicine* 334, no. 18 (1996): 1150–55.
37. Omenn, "Chemoprevention of Lung Cancers."
38. A. Saremi and R. Arora, "Vitamin E and Cardiovascular Disease," *American Journal of Therapeutics* 17, no. 3 (2010): e56–e65; Farbstein et al., "Antioxidant Vitamins."
39. Augustyniak et al., "Natural and Synthetic Antioxidants."
40. *Ibid.*; Farbstein et al., "Antioxidant Vitamins"; Aggarwal et al., "Tocotrienols"; Dotan et al., "No Evidence Supports Vitamin E"; A. R. Ndhlala, M. Moyo, and J. Van Staden, "Natural Antioxidants: Fascinating or Mythical Biomolecules?" *Molecules* 15, no. 10 (2010): 6905–30; E. M. Becker, L. R. Nissen, and L. H. Skibsted, "Antioxidant Evaluation Protocols: Food Quality or Health Effects," *European Food Research and Technology* 219, no. 6 (2004): 561–71.

CHAPTER 12

1. D. Pimentel et al., "Environmental and Economic Costs of Soil Erosion and Conservation Benefits," *Science* 267, no. 5201 (1995): 1117–23; R. Segelken, in Cornell University news release (Ithaca, NY: 1997); D. Pimentel in Canadian Society of Animal Science Meetings (Montreal, Canada: 1997).
2. Food and Agriculture Organization of the United Nations, "Deforestation Causes Global Warming," news release, September 4, 2006, http://www.fao.org/newsroom /en/news/2006/1000385/index.html.
3. H. Steinfeld, P. Gerber, T. Wassenaar, V. Castel, M. Rosales, and C. de Haan, *Livestock's Long Shadow: Environmental Issues and Options*, Food and Agriculture Organization of the United Nations: Rome (2006), ftp://ftp.fao.org/docrep/fao/010/a0701e /a0701e00.pdf.
4. *Ibid.*
5. R. Goodland, "Our choices to overcome the climate crisis," NGO Global Forum 14 (Gwangju, Korea, 2011).
6. I should point out that not all methods of cattle raising appear to contribute to global warming. There's evidence that well-managed pastured cows actually decrease carbon emissions by helping to build soil and improve grassland fertility. ("What's Your Beef?" National Trust, http://www.nationaltrust.org.uk/servlet/file/store5/item842742 /version1/What's%20your%20beef.pdf, 2012. While this paper's conclusions about the health effects of meat are uninformed, the carbon sequestration research it describes appears to be evidence-based.
7. David E. Kromm, "Ogallala Aquifer," *Water Encyclopedia*, accessed November 11, 2012, http://www.waterencyclopedia.com/Oc-Po/Ogallala-Aquifer.html; Manjula V. Guru and James E. Horne, *The Ogallala Aquifer* (Poteau, Oklahoma: The Kerr

Center for Sustainable Agriculture, 2000), http://www.kerrcenter.com/publications/ogallala_aquifer.pdf.

8. Manjula V. Guru and James E. Horne, *The Ogallala Aquifer.*

9. *Ibid.*

10. *Ibid.*

11. *Ibid.*

12. Neal D. Barnard, *Foods That Fight Pain: Revolutionary New Strategies for Maximum Pain Relief* (New York: Three Rivers Press, 1999): 368.

Part III

CHAPTER 14

1. G. L. Hildenbrand, L. C. Hildenbrand, K. Bradford, and S. W. Cavin, "Five-Year Survival Rates of Melanoma Patients Treated by Diet Therapy after the Manner of Gerson: A Retrospective Review," *Alternative Therapies in Health and Medicine* 1, no. 4 (1995): 29–37.

2. Dr. Max Gerson advocated a largely plant-based diet as a possible cancer cure beginning back in 1936, and was roundly condemned at a U.S. Senate hearing in the 1940s.

3. D. Kavanagh, A. D. Hill, B. Djikstra, R. Kennelly, E. M. McDermott, and N. J. O'Higgins, "Adjuvant Therapies in the Treatment of Stage II and III Malignant Melanoma," *Surgeon* 3, no. 4 (2005): 245–56.

4. D. J. Dewar, B. Newell, M. A. Green, A. P. Topping, B. W. Powell, and M. G. Cook, "The Microanatomic Location of Metastatic Melanoma in Sentinel Lymph Nodes Predicts Nonsentinel Lymph Node Involvement," *Journal of Clinical Oncology* 22, no. 16 (2004): 3345–49.

5. *Ibid.*

6. This rather crude estimate is based on one million total cancer diagnoses per year, a number derived from the approximately 500,000 cancer-related deaths per year and the estimated 50 percent mortality rate among all cancer patients.

7. D. W. Light and R. N. Warburton, "Extraordinary Claims Require Extraordinary Evidence," *Journal of Health Economics* 24 (2005): 1030–33.

8. D. W. Light and R. N. Warburton, "Drug R&D Costs Questioned: Widely Quoted Average Cost to Bring Drugs to Market Doesn't Appear to Hold Up to Scrutiny," *Genetic Engineering & Biotechnology News* 31, no. 13 (July 1, 2011), http://www.genengnews.com/gen-articles/drug-r-d-costs-questioned/3707/.

9. "Direct-to-Consumer Advertising," *Wikipedia*, last modified April 16, 2012, http://en.wikipedia.org/wiki/Direct-to-consumer_advertising.

10. "Big Pharma Spends More on Advertising Than Research and Development, Study Finds," *ScienceDaily* (blog), January 7, 2008, http://www.sciencedaily.com/releases/2008/01/080105140107.htm.

11. "Majority of Pharmaceutical Ads Do Not Adhere to FDA Guidelines, New Study Finds," *ScienceDaily*, August 18, 2011, http://www.sciencedaily.com/releases/2011/08/110818093052.htm.

12. "Big Pharma Spends More on Advertising than Research and Development, Study Finds," *ScienceDaily*, January 7, 2008, http://www.sciencedaily.com /releases/2008/01/080105140107.htm.

13. "Pharmaceutical Industry," *Wikipedia*, last modified October 30, 2012, http:// en.wikipedia.org/wiki/Pharmaceutical_Industry.

14. "List of countries by GDP (nominal)," *Wikipedia*, accessed December 2, 2012, http:// en.wikipedia.org/wiki/List_of_countries_by_GDP_(nominal).

15. S. Yusuf, "Two Decades of Progress in Preventing Vascular Disease," *Lancet* 360, no. 9326 (2002): 2–3; N. J. Wald and M. R. Law, "A Strategy to Reduce Cardiovascular Disease by More Than 80%," *BMJ* 326, no. 7404 (2003): 1419–24; E. Lonn, J. Bosch, K. K. Teo, D. Xavier, and S. Yusuf, "The Polypill in the Prevention of Cardiovascular Diseases: Key Concepts, Current Status, Challenges, and Future Directions," *Circulation* 122, no. 20 (2010): 2078–88.

16. Wald and Law, "A Strategy to Reduce."

17. Lonn et al., "The Polypill."

18. Wald and Law, "A Strategy to Reduce."

19. Combination Pharmacology and Public Health Research Working Group, "Combination Pharmacotherapy for Cardiovascular Disease," *Annals of Internal Medicine* 143, no. 8 (2005): 593–99; J. Wise, "Polypill Holds Promise for People with Chronic Disease," *Bulletin of the World Health Organization* 83, no. 12 (2005): 885–87.

20. Lonn et al., "The Polypill."

21. S. Ebrahim, A. Beswick, M. Burke, and S. G. Davey, "Multiple Risk Factor Interventions for Primary Prevention of Coronary Heart Disease," *Cochrane Database of Systemic Reviews* (October 18, 2006): CD001561.

22. Ebrahim et al., "Multiple risk factor interventions."

23. "Frequently Asked Questions August 2010: CODEX and Dietary Supplements," CodexFund.com, accessed November 11, 2012, http://www.codexfund.com/faq.htm.

24. Committee on Diet, Nutrition, and Cancer, *Diet, Nutrition, and Cancer* (Washington, DC: National Academies Press, 1982).

25. Thurston, "Dietary Supplements."

26. *Ibid.* Estimates of the size of the dietary supplement industry vary, depending on what types of products are considered. Nutrient supplements are only one part of this market.

CHAPTER 15

1. However, there has been increasing pressure in recent years for professors who wish to do research to also obtain enough funding to cover their salaries.

2. B. C. Martinson, M. S. Anderson, and R. de Vries, "Scientists Behaving Badly," *Nature* 435 (June 9, 2005): 737–38.

3. Almost all of the research funding for our laboratory research was provided by the U.S. National Cancer Institute of the NIH, with smaller amounts by the American Institute for Cancer Research, the American Cancer Society, and other public agencies.

4. Farbstein et al., "Antioxidant Vitamins."

5. Bjelakovic et al., "Mortality in Randomized Trials"; Miller et al., "Meta-analysis"; Lonn et al., "Effects of Long-Term Vitamin E."

6. Augustyniak et al., "Natural and Synthetic Antioxidants"; Farbstein et al., "Antioxidant Vitamins"; Aggarwal et al., "Tocotrienols."

CHAPTER 16

1. Richard Smith, "Medical Journals: A Gaggle of Golden Geese," *BMJ Group* (blog), July 3, 2012, http://blogs.bmj.com/bmj/2012/07/03/richard-smith-medical-journals-a-gaggle-of-golden-geese/.
2. A. Lundh, M. Barbateskovic, A. Hrobjartsson, and P. C. Gotzsche, "Conflicts of Interest at Medical Journals: The Influence of Industry-Supported Randomised Trials on Journal Impact Factors and Revenue—Cohort Study," *PLoS Medicine* 7 (2010): 1–7.
3. A. E. Handel, S. V. Patel, J. Pakpoor, G. G. Ebers, B. Goldacre, and S. V. Ramagopalan, "High Reprint Orders in Medical Journals and Pharmaceutical Industry Funding: Case-control Study," *British Medical Journal* 344 (June 28, 2012): e4214, doi:10.1136/bmj.e4212.
4. Jacob Goldstein, "Whole Foods CEO: 'We sell a bunch of junk,'" *Wall Street Journal Health Blog*, August 6, 2009, http://blogs.wsj.com/health/2009/08/05/whole-foods-ceo-we-sell-a-bunch-of-junk/.
5. A. Goldhamer, D. L. Lisle, B. Parpia, S. V. Anderson, and T. C. Campbell, "Medically Supervised Water-Only Fasting in the Treatment of Hypertension," *Journal of Manipulative and Physiological Therapeutics* 24, no. 5 (2001): 335–39; A. Goldhamer, D. L. Lisle, B. Parpia, S. V. Anderson, and T. C. Campbell, "Medically Supervised Water-Only Fasting in the Treatment of Borderline Hypertension," *Journal of Alternative and Complementary Medicine* 8, no. 5, (October 2002): 643–50.
6. C. D. Gardner, A. Kiazand, S. Alhassan, S. Kim, R. S. Stafford, R. R. Balise, H. C. Kraemer, and A. C. King, "Comparison of the Atkins, Zone, Ornish, and LEARN diets for Change in Weight and Related Risk Factors among Overweight Premenopausal Women. The A to Z Weight Loss Study: A Randomized Trial," *Journal of the American Medical Association* 297, no. 9 (2007): 969–77.
7. "Grants," The Dr. Robert C. and Veronica Atkins Foundation, accessed November 1, 2012, http://www.atkinsfoundation.org/grants.asp.
8. J. Lehrer. *The News Hour with Jim Lehrer*, January 20, 2007.
9. C. Emery and J. Rockoff, "Cancer Death Rate Falls," *News & Observer* (Raleigh, NC), January 18, 2007: 1A, 14A.
10. Associated Press, "Cancer Deaths Drop for 2nd Straight Year," MSNBC.com, January 17, 2007, http://www.msnbc.msn.com/id/16668688/ns/health-cancer/t/cancer-deaths-decline-nd-straight-year/.
11. *Ibid.*
12. National Cancer Institute, "NCI Budget Requests," last modified November 1, 2011, http://www.cancer.gov/aboutnci/servingpeople/nci-budget-information/requests.
13. "Obituary: Sidney Harman, 1918–2011," *BloombergBusinessweek*, April 14, 2011, http://www.businessweek.com/magazine/content/11_17/b4225024048922.htm.
14. "Alberto Ibargüen, President and CEO," John S. and James L. Knight Foundation, 2012, http://www.knightfoundation.org/staff/alberto-ibarguen/.
15. "Anna Spangler Nelson, Trustee," John S. and James L. Knight Foundation, 2012, http://www.knightfoundation.org/staff/anna-spangler-nelson/.

16. Lee Weisbecker, "Wakefield Group Joins VCs Going Invisible," *Triangle Business Journal*, July 6, 2009, http://www.bizjournals.com/triangle/stories/2009/07/06/story6 .html.

17. "Services," Aurora Diagnostics, 2011, http://www.auroradx.com/services/.

18. "Management," Powell Investment Advisors, 2011, http://www.powellinvestment advisors.com/index.php/management/.

19. ADM may be better known for its production of high fructose corn syrup, which some now blamed for rising obesity rates and for its protracted legal battles and fines, some of which were dramatized in the Matt Damon movie *The Informant*.

CHAPTER 17

1. "Top Interest Groups Giving to Members of Congress, 2012 Cycle," OpenSecrets .org, accessed November 9, 2012, http://www.opensecrets.org/industries/mems.php.

2. "Influence & Lobbying: Health Professionals," OpenSecrets.org, accessed November 1, 2012, http://www.opensecrets.org/industries/indus.php?Ind=H01.

3. "Elias Zerhouni," *Wikipedia*, last modified November 19, 2012, http://en.wikipedia .org/wiki/Elias_Zerhouni.

4. "Former NIH Director Elias Zerhouni Rejoins Johns Hopkins Medicine as Senior Advisor," Johns Hopkins Medicine, accessed December 2, 2012, http://www .hopkinsmedicine.org/news/media/releases/Former_Nih_Director_Elias_Zerhouni _Rejoins_Johns_Hopkins_Medicine_as_Senior_Advisor.

5. "Dr. Julie Gerberding Named President of Merck Vaccines," BusinessWire, December 21, 2009, http://www.businesswire.com/news/home/20091221005649/en /Dr.-Julie-Gerberding-Named-President-Merck-Vaccines.

6. John Stone, "Mr. Gates, Dr. Julie Gerberding Told Dr. Sanjay Gupta Vaccines Cause Autism, Did You Forget?" *Age of Autism*, February 7, 2011, http://www.ageofautism .com/2011/02/mr-gates-dr-julie-gerberding-told-dr-gupta-vaccines-cause-autism -did-you-forget.html.

7. U.S. Census Bureau, Statistical Abstract of the United States, "Table 134. National Health Expenditures—Summary: 1960 to 2009," accessed November 1, 2009, http:// www.census.gov/compendia/statab/2012/tables/12s0134.pdf.

8. Ali Frick, "GM CEO: Serious Health Care Reform 'Undoubtedly Would Help Level the Playing Field,'" *Think Progress*, December 5, 2008, http://thinkprogress.org /politics/2008/12/05/33286/gm-health-care-reform/?mobile=nc.

9. As discussed previously, RDI is a newer term for the older recommended dietary allowance, or RDA. For the purposes of this discussion, the two are interchangeable.

10. D. M. Hegsted, "Calcium and Osteoporosis," *Journal of Nutrition* 116 (1986): 2316–2319.

11. See *The China Study*, pp. 311–314.

12. T. C. Campell, T. Brun, J. Chen, Z. Feng & B. Parpia, "Questioning Riboflavin Recommendations on the Basis of a Survey in China," *American Journal of Clinical Nutrition* 51 (1990): 436-445.

13. The National Academies, "Report Offers New Eating and Physical Activity Targets to Reduce Chronic Disease Risk," September 5, 2002, http://www8.nationalacademies .org/onpinews/newsitem.aspx?RecordID=10490.

14. For more information, watch the brilliant series of lectures by Jeff Novick at http://
www.jeffnovick.com/RD/Should_I_Eat_That.html.
15. B. Starfield, "Is US Health Really the Best in the World?"
16. *Ibid.*
17. *Ibid.*
18. This attitude definitely got Broder somewhere, though. After he left the NCI in 1989,
he took up a research position at generic drug maker IVAX until he moved to his current post as chief medical officer at biotechnology giant Celera Corporation. "Ivax and
Teva on the Heels of Taxol and Zovirax," *The Pharma Letter*, April 7, 1997, http://www
.thepharmaletter.com/file/41937/ivax-and-teva-on-the-heels-of-taxol-and-zovirax
.html; "Samuel Broder," LinkedIn, accessed November 1, 2012, http://www.linkedin
.com/pub/samuel-broder/25/649/b31.
19. "Aflatoxin & Liver Cancer," The National Institute of Environmental Health Sciences,
last modified November 9, 2007, http://www.niehs.nih.gov/about/congress/impacts
/aflatoxin/index.cfm.
20. *Ibid.*
21. *Ibid.*
22. T. C. Campbell, J. Chen, C. Liu, J. Li, and B. Parpia, "Nonassociation of Aflatoxin
with Primary Liver Cancer in a Cross-Sectional Ecological Survey in the People's
Republic of China," *Cancer Research* 50 (1990): 6882–93.

CHAPTER 18

1. "About the Society," National Multiple Sclerosis Society, accessed November 1, 2012,
http://www.nationalmssociety.org/about-the-society/index.aspx.
2. "About the Academy of Nutrition and Dietetics," Academy of Nutrition and Dietetics,
2012, http://www.eatright.org/Media/content.aspx?id=6442467510.
3. Samuel S. Epstein, *National Cancer Institute and American Cancer Society: Criminal
Indifference to Cancer Prevention and Conflicts of Interest* (Bloomington, NY: Xlibris,
2011).
4. Cancer Prevention Coalition, "The American Cancer Society (ACS) 'More Interested
in Accumulating Wealth Than Saving Lives,' Warns Samuel S. Epstein, M.D.," PR
Newswire, accessed December 3, 2012, http://www.prnewswire.com/news-releases
/the-american-cancer-society-acs-more-interested-in-accumulating-wealth-than
-saving-lives-warns-samuel-s-epstein-md-117942029.html.
5. "Screening for Breast Cancer," U.S. Preventive Services Task Force, July 2010, http://
www.uspreventiveservicestaskforce.org/uspstf/uspsbrca.htm.
6. "Diet and Physical Activity: What's the Cancer Connection?" American Cancer
Society, last modified January 13, 2012, http://www.cancer.org/cancer/cancercauses
/dietandphysicalactivity/diet-and-physical-activity.
7. "Dairy Foods & Cancer Prevention," *Dairy Council Digest* 79, no. 1 (January/
February 2008): 6, http://www.nationaldairycouncil.org/SiteCollectionDocuments
/health_wellness/dairy_nutrients/dcd791.pdf.
8. William T. Jarvis, "Cancer Quackery," National Council Against Health Fraud, December 17, 2000, http://www.ncahf.org/articles/c-d/caquackery.html.

9. "Sources of Support," National Multiple Sclerosis Society, accessed December 2, 2012, http://www.nationalmssociety.org/about-the-society/sources-of-support/index.aspx.

10. "Women against MS Luncheon: Sponsorship Opportunities," Triangle WAMS Luncheon website, accessed November 1, 2012, http://www.trianglewams.org /event-details/sponsorship-opportunities.

11. See *The China Study*, pp. 194–98 for a review of the remarkable research of Dr. Roy Swank and his 34-year study of MS patients. See also R. L. Swank and B. B. Dugan, "Effect of Low Saturated Fat Diet in Early and Late Cases of Multiple Sclerosis," *Lancet* 336, no. 8706 (1990): 37–39.

12. "Nutrition and Diet," National Multiple Sclerosis Society, accessed November 1, 2012, http://www.nationalmssociety.org/living-with-multiple-sclerosis/healthy-living /nutrition-and-diet/index.aspx.

13. "The Academy's Annual Reports," Academy of Nutrition and Dietetics, 2012, http:// www.eatright.org/annualreport/.

14. Pamela Popper, *Solving America's Healthcare Crisis* (Worthington, OH: Bristol Woods Publishing, 2011), Kindle edition, Kindle location 4932.

15. Pamela Popper, email communication to author, October 15, 2012.

16. You can see the entire slide show at http://thechinastudy.com/and-slides.pdf. For more background and some smoking gun emails and internal AND documents, see Michael Ellberg's hard-hitting expose on Forbes.com, "Is the ADA Intentionally Using State Legislatures to Block Alternative Nutrition Providers?" http://www.forbes.com /sites/michaelellsberg/2012/07/10/american_dietetic_association_2/.

17. Pamela Popper, email communication to author, October 16, 2012.

18. "Commission on Dietetic Registration Continuing Professional Education Accredited Providers," Commission on Dietetic Registration, Academy of Nutrition and Dietetics, accessed November 1, 2012, http://www.cdrnet.org/whatsnew/accredited_providers .cfm.

19. "Benefits of Becoming a CPE Accredited Provider," Commission on Dietetic Registration, Academy of Nutrition and Dietetics, accessed November 1, 2012, http://www .cdrnet.org/pdrcenter/pabenefits.cfm.

20. J. Leonard Lichtenfeld, "During Breast Cancer Awareness Month We Must Not Only Celebrate Our Success But Also Understand Our Limitations," *Dr. Len's Blog*, American Cancer Society, October 3, 2012, http://www.cancer.org/aboutus /drlensblog/post/2012/10/03/during-breast-cancer-awareness-month-we-must -not-only-celebrate.aspx.

Index

A

Abbott Nutrition, 271, 274

Academy of Nutrition and Dietetics (AND), 180–182, 262–263, 271–276, *273, 274*

acne, 8

activism, 165–167

addictive foods, 165

advertisements, 155–156, 188, 193–194, 207–208, 211, 235, 237, 242–246

aflatoxin (AF), 61–64, 89–92, *101–103*, 128–130, 133–134, 258–261, 286–287

Agency for Healthcare Research and Quality, 255

Age of Genetics, 110, 117

aging, 9, 154

agricultural policies, 183, 193

agriculture, 81–82, 169

air, carcinogens and, 132, 137, 165–166

alternative health, 150

American Cancer Society (ACS), 180–182, 188, 205, 240, 241–242, 262–263, 264–269

American Diabetes Association, 205

American Egg Board, 277

American Heart Association, 205

American Institute for Cancer Research (AICR), 240, 268, 277

The American Journal of Cardiology, 232

American Medical Association, 248

American Society for Nutrition (ASN), 262, 276–278

Ames, Bruce, 136–137

Ames assay, 136–137

Amgen, 265

amino acids, 64, 99, 113–114, 118, 157

analogs, 157

anchovies, 159

anecdotal evidence, 20

Angell, Marcia, 233

angina, 18

Anhang, Jeff, 168

animal cruelty, 167, 170–172

animal products. *See also* dairy; meat

avoidance of, 7

cancer and, 30–34, 101, 130, 136, 143, 234–235, 288

diet choices and, 85

diet of, 129

environmental problems and, 166

enzyme activity and, 101–104

fossil fuels and, 166

global warming and, 167–168

harm of, 29–34

land and water resources and, 166

minimum daily requirements and consumption of, 253

muscle mass and, 81

production of, 189

studies on, 234

value of, 286

world hunger and production of, 173

animal research, 170

animal testing, 170–172

antihypertensive drugs, 143, 235

antioxidants, 10, 69–70, 152–154, 160–161

anti-privacy scenarios, 6

ApoCell, Inc., 244

appetite-suppressant shakes, 191

apple pesticides, 131

apples, 151–155

aquifer depletion, 166

Aramark, 271, 274

Archer Daniels Midlands (ADM), 246

Aristotle, 119
arthritis, 20, 159
artificial colors and flavors, 13, 31
asbestos, 133
Asimov, Isaac, 125
Aspergillus flavus. See aflatoxin (AF)
Astor, John Jacob, 19
AstraZeneca, 265, 278
Atkins Diet, 59, 235–236, 255
Aurora Diagnostics, LLC, 244
autism, 249

B
bacon, 194
bacterial infections, 148
bagels, 194
beans and legumes, 7, 70
beef
    water used to produce, 166, 169
beef industry, 268–269
Benyus, Janine, 81
benzene, 133, 134, 144
beta-carotene, 69–70, 158–161, 287
bias, 62–63, 168, 234, 238, 245–246
Big Bang, 76
Big Insurance, 248
Big Medicine, 248
Big Pharma, 203–209, 233–234, 248, 261
Big Promise, 108–109
Bike MS Project, 269
Bimbo Bakeries USA, 270
Binder, Gordon, 265
bioavailability, 68, 70
biochemistry, 78, 93–97, 114, 117, 184,
    218–219, 223–225
biodegradable items, 165
biodiversity, 189
bioflavonoids, 153
biomarkers, 162–163, 259
biomimicry, 81–82
Biomimicry (Benyus), 81
bladder cancer, 133–134
bleeding, 126
blind men story, 45–46, 54, 57, 141–142,
    146, 224–225
blood plasma, *72*

blood sugar, 63
blood tests, 110
bodily systems, 106
body chemistry, 106
body fat, 84, 86
bones, 193, 253
Boone, Daniel, 19
bottled water, 131
boundaries, lack of, 55
Boyer, Jeanelle, 153
breakfast cereals, 119, 194
"breakthrough discoveries," 15
breast cancer, 71, 80, 84–85, 240, 265–
    266, 278–280
Breast Cancer Awareness Month, 266
Breast Health Awareness Program, 266
Bristol-Myers Squibb, 265
British Medical Journal, 234
Broder, Sam, 257
Bush, George W., 240

C
cadmium, 144
calcium, 65, 67, 69–70, *72*, 188, 253, 267,
    270
California Institute of
    Telecommunications and
    Information Technology, 110
calories, 67, 136, 253–254
Campbell, Tom, 12, 212
cancer
    animal protein and, 30–34, 101–103,
        234–235
    bladder, 133–134
    breast, 71, 80, 84, 85, 240, 265, 266,
        278–279, 279–280
    carcinogens and, 91–92, 133
    chemotherapy and, 35, 143, 144
    cholesterol and protections from, 39
    colon, 38
    colorectal, 267
    cure for, 109
    development of, *128*–130, *129*, 136
    diagnosis of, 198–199
    diet and, 119–120, 129–130, 199–203,
        265

formation of, 61–64, *62*
future, 104
genes and, 126
incidence of mortality from, 80
liver, 30, 54, 61–64, 89–92, 104, 128–
130, 258–261, 287
lung, 76–77, 160, 240, 287
lymphatic system, 199–204
melanoma, 198–204
mortality rates and, 240–241
nutrient supplements and, 156
nutritional effects and, 136, 137,
234–235
oxidation and, 154
powerlessness of, 197–198
prevention of, 109, 154, 257
prostate, 230, 240
reducing the risk of, 131
reductionism and, 135
research of, 11, 201, 257, 265
reversal of, 154, 257
risk evaluation of, 132–135
screenings for, 265
smoking and, 120
survival from, 199–200, 203
treatment options of (*See*
chemotherapy; radiotherapy)
vitamin E supplements and, 157
WFPB diet and, 8, 9
Cancer Epidemiology, Biomarkers &
Prevention, 33
cancer minefield, 34–36
Cancer Research, 31, 232, 234–235
capitalism, 189, 216
carbohydrates, 7, 11, 64, 173, 194, 266,
289
carbon dioxide, 167–168
carcinogen bioassay program (CBP),
132–139
carcinogens
aflatoxin (AF), 61–64, 89–92, *101–*
103, 128–130, 133–134, 258–261,
286–287
animal protein, 21, 30–31, 39
asbestos, 133
benzene, 133, 134, 144

cadmium, 144
cancer occurance, 33
chemicals and, 131
cow's milk protein, 136
DDT (insecticide spray), 133
dioxin, 31, 132, 133, 139
exposure to, 131–132, 234
formaldehyde, 133, 144
lead, 144
mercury, 144
nitrosamines, 133
PCBs, 133
polycyclic aromatic hydrocarbons
(PAHs), 133, 134
testing for, 132
volatile organic compounds (VOCs),
144
carcinogogenic misdirection, 135
car crashes, 109
cardiovascular disease
nutrient supplements and, 156, 160
omega-3s and, 159
oxidation and, 154
pharmaceuticals and, 208–209
risk of, 16
vitamin E supplements and, 157
wholistic solution to, 191
carnivores, 82
carotenoids, 69–70
carrots, 65, 160, 237
car tires, 167
case-control studies, 83–86
casein, 37, 39, 62, 92, 136
cataracts, 157
catching a ball example, 73–74
catechin, 153
"Cattle Barons Ball," 268
cattle ranchers, 182
cause and effect, 191
CDC. *See* Centers for Disease Control
and Prevention (CDC)
cell phones, 131
cells, 93, 103–104, 114
Centers for Disease Control and
Prevention (CDC), 4, 249, 255
cereals. *See* breakfast cereals

Chase, Alston, 262
chemical reactions, 88, 95, 97–100
chemicals
  in apples, 152–154
  detoxification of, 101
  environmental, 130–131
  evaluation for mutagenicy, 136–137
  foreign, 101, 105, 149
  genetic mutations and, 126–127, 133, 138
  native, 105
chemistry, body, 106
chemotherapy, 35, 143–144, 197, 199, 202–203
Chen, Junshi, 245–246
chickens, 171–172
childhood nutrition programs, 89
children, 138–139, 159, 169–170
chili peppers, 160
China, 38–39, 80–81, 227–229, 242, 258
China Study, 38, 87, 136, 152, 245, 257, 288
The China Study (Campbell), 12, 14, 20, 22, 34, 80, 129, 212, 242, 246, 286, 289
Chinese medicine, 19, 54, 222
chiropractors, 156
chloride, 72
chlorogenic acid, 153
chlorophyllin, 258–259
cholesterol, 16, 37–39, 101, 154, 188, 209, 253
chromosomes, 112
chronic diseases, 4–6, 8, 108–109, 121, 127
chronic fatigue syndrome, 147
chronic musculoskeletal pain, 147
chronic pain, 8
A Civil Action, 131
classification systems, 54
ClimateCrisis.net, 167
Clinton, Bill, 12
clotting, 126
Coca-Cola, 266, 271, 274–275
codfish oil, 118
codons, 113

cohorts, 84
cold, 8
Collins, Francis, 116
colon cancer, 38
colorectal cancer, 267
The Complete Book of Running (Fixx), 109
Complete Genomics, 110
ConAgra Food Science Institute, 275
confined animal feeding operation (CAFO). *See* factory farms
conflicts of interest, 244
consumers, 183, 188
Cook, Martin, 201
cooking oils, 165
Copernicus, 27, 49
copper, 71, 72, 151
Cornell University, 21, 30–31, 61, 118, 136, 152, 166, 223, 245
coronary artery disease. *See* heart disease
Coro-Wise, 271
Corporation for Public Broadcasting, 232
corruption of research, 219–220
cosmetics, 131
cow manure, 172
cows. *See* livestock production
cranberries, 132
crops, 58, 169
CT scans, 108

D
daily minimum requirements, 59
dairy, 11, 13, 29, 31, 36, 89, 92, 171, 182, 188, 192–194, 253–254, 267, 270, 272, 275
da Vinci mode, 51–53
DDT (insecticide spray), 133
death, 5–6, 109, 114. *See also* mortality rates
deep-fried foods, 165
deforestation, 8, 165–166
Dentzer, Susan, 243, 246
deoxyribonucleic acid. *See* DNA
depression, 84, 85, 86
De Revolutionibus, 27
detergents, 131

diabetes
  coma from, 143
  genes and, 126
  omega-3s and, 159
  reductionism and, 63, 191
  type 2, 4, 8, 159–160
  vitamin E supplements and, 157
  WFPB diet and, 17
  wholistic solution to, 191
dialysis, 108
diet. *See* nutrition
dietary fat. *See* fat
Dietary Supplement Health and
    Education Act, 211
dietary supplements, 85, 150, 153, 258.
    See also medicinal herbs; nutrient
    supplements
dieticians, 271–276
"dieting," 25
digestive systems, 82
Digest of the National Dairy Council,
    267
dioxin, 31, 132, 139
disease
  advocacy for, 278
  cause of, 126–127, 147–148
  eating plant-based foods to reduce,
    182
  elimination of, 117
  management of, 140, *149*
  mutagen-initiated, 136–137
  nature *vs.* nurture and, 119–121
  plague of, 108
  prevention of, 24
  rate of, 79
  risk of, 80, 116, 234
  study of, 78
  susceptibility of, 116
  taxonomy of, 146–147
disease-care system, 4–6, 140, 141–146,
    149, 190
Disraeli, Benjamin, 214
DNA, 99, 102, 104, 107, 110, 111–115,
    258–259. *See also* genes
dogma, 56–57
Doll, Richard, 119

Douglass, James W., 26
drought, 169
drug responsiveness, 114
drugs. *See also* prescription drugs
  dosages of, 145–146
  money and, 216–217
  regulations of, 210
  relying on unnatural, 144–146
  side effects of, 145
  synthetic, 149
  treating specific ailments iwth, 144
  trials, 83, 87
"During Breast Cancer Awareness
    Month We Must Not Only
    Celebrate Our Success but Also
    Understand Our Limitations,"
    279–280

E
early humans, 81
eating habits, 84
Editorial Review Board, 33
education level, 86
eggs, 171–172, 194, 275
Einstein, Albert, 140, 231
electrolytes, 106
elephant story. *See* blind men story
Elliott, William L., 93
encephalomalacia, 286
energy, 93, 98
energy-efficient light bulbs, 165
Engel, Charlie, 89
environmentalism, 165–167, 209
environmental mutagens, 130–131, 148
environmental stimuli, 126
environmental toxins, 31, 132, 134, 265
enzymes
  chemical reactions and, 98
  cyclic ADP ribose hydrolase, *99*
  function of, 54–55, 70–71, 88
  homeostasis and, 106
  metabolism and, 97–100
  mixed function oxidase (MFO), 88,
    91–92, 91–92, 100–105, *101, 102,*
    103, 145, 287–288
  nutrients and, 100

enzymes (*Cont.*)
  nutrition and, 92
  reactions, *99*
epidemiology, 79, 86–87, 147
epigenics, 225
epoxides, 102, 105
Epstein, Samuel, 265, 266
erectile dysfunction, 8
Erin Brockovich, 131
Esselstyn, Caldwell, Jr., 18, 22–23, 236
evolution, 7, 127, 181
evolutionary biology, 82
Excalibur Donor roster, 265, 266
exercise, 84, 209

F
Facebook, 12–13, 173
factory farms, 8, 59, 170–173, 234
falsifiability, 56, 219–220
family farms, 172
farmland, 166
fasting, 235
fat, 7, 13, 37, 63, 71, 84, 86, 136, 254
fatalism, 238
fate, 137
fats, 64
fatty acids, 71, 150, 158–160
Federal Food, Drug, and Cosmetic Act,
  211–212
Federal Trade Commission (FTC), 211
Federation of American Societies for
  Experimental Biology, 276
Federation Proceedings, 134, 136
Fels Institute, 31
female hysteria, 146–147
fertilizer, 169–170, 173
fiber, 151, 237–238
fibromyalgia, 147
fish consumption, 159, 266
fish oil, 63, 159
Fixx, Jim, 109
flies, 171
flour, 11, 13, 289
flu, 8, 126, 249
food
  active agents of, 148

carcinogens and, 131, 132, 137
choices, 6–7, 129
deep-fried, 165
fortified, 194, 216
groups, 59, 192–194
intake of, 79
policy, 58
portion sizes of, 266
regulations of, 210
systems of, 59
Food Additive Amendment, 132
Food and Drug Act, 132
Food and Drug Administration (FDA),
  18, 59, 65–66, 90–91, 206–207, 211,
  258
Food and Nutrition Board of the
  National Academy of Sciences
  (FNB), 254
food labels, *65*, 266
food packaging, 59, 60–61, *65*, 252
food pyramid, 59, 245, 254
forests, 189
formaldehyde, 133, 144
for-profit research, 225, 229–230
fortified foods, 194, 216
fossil fuels, 166
fraud, 28
free markets, 189, 216, 225
free radicals, 9, 10, 160
free will, 76
french fries, 165
frequently asked questions, 10–11
fruits, 7, 58, 59, 84, 270
Fuller, Thomas, 3
funding for medical research, 217–230,
  262–281

G
Galileo, 49
garbage, 167
Garner, Colin, 102
Genentech, 265
General Mills, 271, 277
General Mills Bell Institute of Health and
  Nutrition, 275
General Motors, 252

genes. *See also* DNA
  damage to, 128
  disease and, 126
  expression of, 112, 114, 122–123
  faulty, 122
  health and, 126
  mutations of, 63, 126–127, 130, 148
  nutrition *vs.*, 121–124
gene sequencing, 110
gene therapy, 182
genetic determinism, *122*
genetic predispositons, 84
genetic research, 6, 36, 61–64, 108,
    110–115, 118, 143, 189
George, David Lloyd, 75
Gerberding, Julie, 249
Gerson Institute, 199–200
Gilenya, 269
ginseng, 19–20
GlaxoSmithKline, 265
global warming, 8, 167–169
glucose-metabolism network of
    reactions, 93, *94*, 95, *96*, *97*
gluten-free diets, 13
Gödel, Kurt, 51
Goethe, Johann Wolfgang von, 107
Gofman, John, 21–22
Golden Corral restaurant, 270
Goldhamer, Alan, 235
Golub, Robert, 235–236
Goodland, Robert, 168
Google, 12–13, 54
Gore, Al, 167
"Got Milk?" campaign, 193–194
government-subsidized food service
    programs, 66–67
grain, 166
Grand Rounds lecture, 34
grants, 257
Great Lakes, 169
Greece, 49
greenhouse gases. *See* carbon dioxide;
    methane
green leafy vegetables, 156, 160
grocery stores, 13
groundwater contamination, 8, 166

H
happiness, 85
Hart, Ron, 136
Hawking, Stephen, 78
health, 25, 88, 109, 142–143, 279–281
health-care system. *See also* disease-care
    system
  access to, 84
  corruption of, 195
  cost of, 116
  crisis, 116–117
  debate, 250–252
  improvement of, 141
  nutrition and, 25
  profits and, 190–192
  reductionism and, 150–151
  reform of, 248–249
  understanding the, 182–190
health interventions, 17–22
health issues, *190*, 191
health outcomes, 6
health policy, 248
health professionals, 248
health shops, 155
Healthy Eating, Healthy World, 167
heart attacks, 8–9, 109, 143, 191, 238
heart disease, 8, 18, 22–23, 80, 109, 126,
    143, 157, 197, 230
hemophilia, 126
herbal compounds, 162
herbicides, 173
herbivores, 82
hereditary conditions, 147
herring, 159
Hershey Center for Health & Nutrition,
    271
Hicks, J. Morris, 166
Higgs boson, 78
high blood pressure. *See* hypertension
high-dose to low-dose interpolation,
    133
high-fructose corn syrup, 66, 182
HMO (health maintenance
    organization), 251–252
Hoffmann, Frederick, 267
holism, 48, 53

Hollywood, 192
homeostasis, 105–106
hormones, 101, 165
hospital food guidelines, 66
hospitalizations, 114
hot dogs, 31, 162
human anatomy, 52
human body, 68–69
human genome, 110, 114
Human Genome Program, 114, 116
humanism, 50
hydrolyzed collagen, 269
hygiene, 109
hypertension, 4, 143, 209, 235
hypochondria, 147
hysteria, 146–147

I

Ibargüen, Alberto, 244
ice cream, 162
ideal human diet, 7
Iger, Bob, 181
illnesses, 125, 197
immune system, 70–71, 200
income, 84
An Inconvenient Truth (Gore), 167
industrial agriculture, 173
industry, 168, 248–250
industry leaders, 182
infection, 108, 148
information cycle, 184, 214–215
ingredients, 64–67
injuries, traumatic, 142–143
instinctual food choices, 81
insulin usage, 8, 191
insurance, 203, 250–252
integrity of research, 219–221
intellectual property protections, 216
International Statistical Classification
    of Diseases and Related Health
    Problems (ICD-10), 146
intestinal distress, 8
in-utero chemical exposure, 138–139
iodine, 67
iron, 67, 69–72

"Is It Safe to Play Yet?", 131
Italy, 245
It's a Wonderful Life, 192

J

jaw shape, 82
Jefferson, Thomas, 196
John S. and James L. Knight Foundation,
    244
Johns Hopkins University, 249,
    258–261
Johnson, Lyndon, 207
Johnson & Johnson, 243
Jones, T. H., 88
journalists, 181–182, 236
*Journal of the American Medical
    Association (JAMA)*, 5, 23, 232,
    235–236, 255

K

Katz, Jonathan, 107
Kellogg, 271
Kerr Center for Sustainable Agriculture
    in Oklahoma, 169
Kraft Foods Global, Inc., 275
Krebs cycle, 93, 95
Kubena, Karen, 70
Kurzweil, Ray, 54

L

laboratory animals, 21, 89, 101–102,
    118, 128–130, 133–134
Lake Huron, 169
laminated furniture, 131
land holders, 172
land resources, 166
lead, 144
Lehrer, Jim, 240, 244
lemon juice fasts, 85
Lichtenfeld, J. Leonard, 279–280
lifestyle, 83, 191, 209, 248–249
Light, Donald, 205–207
light bulbs, 165, 167
Linnaeus, Carl, 19
literal filters, 47

Liu, Rui Hai, 151–155, 221–222
liver cancer, 30, 54, 61–64, 89–92, 104,
    128–130, 258–261, 287
livestock production, 166, 168–173. *See
    also* agriculture
lobbyists, 249, 250
local growers, 59
low carb diets, 13, 85, 173
low-fat diets, 235–236, 238, 255
lung cancer, 76–77, 160, 240, 287
lung disease, 157
lycopene, 61, 237
lymphatic system cancer, 199–203

M
Mackey, John, 234
macrobiotic diet, 59
macronutrients, 64
mad cow disease, 58
Magee, Peter, 31, 234–235
magnesium, 70, 71, *72*, 151
makeup, 131
malnutrition, 8, 29, 72
maltitol powder, 269
mammography, 266
manganese, 70, 151
Manila Department of Health, 89
manufacturing plants, 90
marketplace, potential, 218–219
Mars, Incorporated, 271
Maslow, Abraham, 76
Massachussets Institute of Technology,
    258
Maté Factor Cafe, 285
Mavko, Kay, 272, 274
McCay, Clive, 117
McDonalds, 17, 83, 266
McDougall, John, 236
McGill Faculty of Medicine, 34
McMurray, David, 70
McNeil Nutritionals, 271
meal-replacement shakes, 85
meaningful significance, 23–24
meat, 13, 165, 168, 182, 251, 266, 270. *See
    also* animal products

media, 6, 14–16, 130–131, 153, 155–157,
    167, 181, 184, 187–188, 194,
    231–246
medical errors, 254–256
medical industry, 197–203, 204
medical records standardization, 147
medical research, 217–218, 226–227
medical school training, 24
medical system, 146
Medicare, 255
medication, 114
medication errors, 5, 255
medicinal herbs, 19
melanoma, 198–204
mental filters, 47
Merck, 265, 278
mercury, 144, 159
"Metabolic Pathology," 257
metabolism, 93, 95, 97–100, 106
metabolites, 93, 98, 101–103, 106
methane, 168
"The Microanatomic Location of
    Metastatic Melanoma in Sentinel
    Lymph Nodes Predicts Nonsentinel
    Lymph Node Involvement," 200
microwave ovens, 131
migraines, 8, 20
military, 193
milk. *See* dairy
milk proteins. *See* casein
Miller, Jim and Betty, 102
minerals, 64, 67, 68–69, 70, 212
mineral supplements, 150
minimum daily requirement (MDR), 253
misinterpretation by omission, 240–242,
    244–246
mixed function oxidase (MFO), 88,
    91–92, 100–105, *101*, *102*, *103*, 145,
    287–288
modern medicine, 108, 150
modern science, 54–55, 56–57
molds, 138
molecular genetics, 225
molybdenum, 71
mood, 84–85, 114

Morrison, Lester, 21–22
mortality rates, 4, 156, 158–159, 230
MRI scans, 108
Mulder, Gerardus, 31
multivitamins. *See* vitamins
muscle mass, 81
muscular dystrophy, 286
mutagen-initiated diseases, 136–137
myopic specialization, 223–225

N
National Academy of Sciences (NAS),
    65–66, 119, 162, 205, 210, 254, 267
National Cancer Institute, 228, 241, 257
*National Cancer Institute and
    American Cancer Society: Criminal
    Indifference to Cancer Prevention
    and Conflicts of Interest* (Epstein),
    265
National Cattlemen's Beef Association,
    271
National Dairy Council, 268, 271
National Health Insititute, 90
National Heart, Lung, and Blood
    Institute, 256
National Human Genome Research
    Institute, 116
National Institutes of Health (NIH), 11,
    24, 31, 205–206, 217–219, 227–228,
    237, 240, 249, 256–261
National Mammography Day, 266
National Multiple Sclerosis Society (MS
    Society), 262–263, 269–271
National Science Foundation, 218
National Toxicology Program (NTP), 136
Native Americans, 19
natural health community, 151
natural-living expos, 155
"natural medicine" community, 155
Nature, 153, 219, 232
nature *vs.* nurture, 119–122
Nelson, Anna Spangler, 244
Nestle HealthCare Nutrition, 275
neutraceutical industry, 210–212, 269
*New England Journal of Medicine
    (NEJM)*, 232, 234, 235

Newsweek, 242–244, 246
New World Encyclopedia, 100
New York Times, 110, 131, 245
niacin, 151
NIMBY (not in my backyard), 131
nitrates, 31, 169–170
nitrogen, 253
nitrosamines, 133
nonprofit agencies, 193
Novartis, 265, 269
nuclear facilities, 165
nurture, nature *vs.*, 119–122, 124
nutraceuticals, 150
nutrient composition, 37, 61, 67–68,
    70
nutrient consumption, 33, 69–70
nutrient micromanagement, 155
nutrients, 64
    deficiencies in, 67
    enzymes and, 100
    human body's utilization of, 68–69
    interactions between, 70–71, 95, 97
    mega-doses of, 71
    path of, 93
nutrient supplements, 67, 85, 155–163,
    210–212
nutrition, 83, 243, 251, 270
    beliefs in, 59
    biochemical basis of, 93–97
    cancer development and, 136, 137,
        234–235
    complexity of, 155
    decline of the age of, 117–119
    definition of, 60
    disease management *vs.*, *149*
    disease prevention and, 149
    disease treatment and prevention and,
        24, 119–120
    enzymes and, 92
    genes *vs.*, 121–124
    homeostasis and, 106
    ideal, 7
    improving health with, 248–249
    inputs of, 123
    poor, 149
    prevention of disease and, 130, 135

reversal study on heart disease and, 22–23
science of, 60–64
study of, 117, 204, 218–219
technical approach to, 216
wholism and, 152–153
nutritional database, 66–67, 252
nutritional determinism, 122–*123*
nutritional genomics, 225
nutritional labels, 59, 247
nutritional science, 60–64, 86–87, 221–222
nutritional therapy, 35
"Nutrition and Cancer," 257
nuts and seeds, 7, 159

O
oatmeal, 237–238
Obama, Barack, 248
obesity, 63, 84, 85, 182
odds of winning statistics, 121
Office of Technology Assessment, 119–120
Ogallala Aquifer, 169
Ohio Board of Dietetics, 272
oil, 7, 11, 289
omega-3 fats, 150, 158–161, 191, 212
One Flew Over the Cuckoo's Nest, 192
online petitions, 173
OpenSecrets.org, 248
oranges, 151
organizational funding, 264–281
organ transplants, 108
Ornish, Dean, 22, 235–236
osteoporosis, 188, 253
Oxford English Dictionary, 60
oxidation, 9–10, 154

P
p53, 259
Paleo Diet, 59
palm kernel oil, 269
Panax. *See* ginseng
particle physics, 78
patents, 216
pathology, 137–138

PBS, 239–242, 244–246
PBS NewsHour, 240–242, 244–246
PCBs, 133, 159
peaches, 69
peanut fungus, 61–64, 90, 141
peanuts
liver cancer and, 89–91
shelled, 90
peer-reviewed journals, 16, 31, 200, 220–222, 233–234
PepsiCo, 244, 271, 275
personal responsibility, 279–281
pesticides, 131, 171
Peto, Richard, 119
pH, 82, 106
pharmaceuticals. *See* prescription drugs
pharmaceuticals industry, 203–209, 217–218
Philippines, 30, 89, 90, 92
philosophy, 79
phlorizin, 153
phosphorus, 70, 151
physical activity, 114
physics, 78
physiology, 82
pigs, 172
Pimentel, David, 166
placebos, 83
plant-based foods
animal cruelty as reasoning to eat, 148–149, 170, 174
embracing, 182, 270, 286, 289
Eunutria example, 7
land and water resources and, 166
reasoning for, 9–10, 80
study of, 272
world hunger as reasoning to eat, 174
plant oils, 71
plant protein, fossil fuels and, 166
plants, healing effects of, 144–145
plastic cups and bottles, 131
plastic shopping bags, 165
policy makers, 130, 167, 181, 183, 184, 188, 194, 248–250
pollution laws, 183

polycyclic aromatic hydrocarbons
  (PAHs), 133, 134
polymath, 52
polypills, 208–209
polyunsaturated fats, 71, 157
Popper, Karl, 38
Popper, Pamela, 272–274
popular culture, 194
popular foods, 89
posture, 82
potassium, 70, *72*, 151
potatoes, 166
Potter, Henry F., 192
poultry feed, 132
Powell, Earl W., 244
Powell Gene Therapy Center, 244
power, subtle, 192–195, 246
power lines, 131
praying, 280
prebiotics, 150, 212
pregnancy, 159, 169–170
Prescription Drug Advertising
  Guidelines, 207–208
prescription drugs, 5–6, 16, 18, 24, 114,
  150–151
preservatives, 13
primates, 81
prisons, 193
Pritikin, Nathan, 22
probiotics, 150, 212
processed foods, 7, 11, 13, 81–82, 85,
  165, 182, 187, 209, 234, 269–270,
  275
profit-distorted information cycle, 186–
  187, 192–195, 196
propaganda, 236
prostate cancer, 230, 239
protein. *See also* animal products
  amino acids and, 114, 118
  blood tests and, *72*
  calories from, 9–10
  cancer and, 92, 101–103
  chemical reactions and, 71
  deficiency of, 29, 67
  diet and, 7
  DNA expression into active, *113*

enzymes, 98
harm of, 30–34
minimum daily requirements and, 253
mixed function oxidase (MFO) and, 92
muscle and bone growth and, 118
peanuts and, 89–90
quality of, 92
recommended daily intake of, 254–256
studies of, 136
subtle power and, 194
Proxmire, William, 210–211
Ptolemaic astronomy, 49
public education, 183
public insurance, 248
public nutrition, 66
public service announcements, 209
pumpkin, 160
Pure Protein, 269

Q
quantum theory, 78
quercetin, 153

R
"race for the cure," 3–4
radiotherapy, 35, 197, 199, 266
radon, 131
rainforests, 173
rainwater, 169
Ranexa, 18, 23
Ratched, Nurse, 192
reactivity, 141, 142–143
recommended daily allowances (RDAs),
  59, 66
recommended daily intakes (RDIs),
  66–67, 252–253, 257
reductionism. *See also* food packaging;
  nutrient supplements
  cancer research and, 135
  complexity of, 106
  dietary supplements and, 151
  environmental toxins and, 132–133
  funding for research and, 221–222
  genetic research and, 114, 118
  history of, 48–50
  inadequacy of, 88

intellectual cost of victory of, 56–57
limitations to, 285–286
media and, 236–240
medical industry and, 197
nutritional science and, 59, 60–64
paradigm, 288
pointlessness of, 71–73
problems with, 67–71, 173–174
profits and, 190–192, 288
quantum theory and, 78
science and causality, 76–78
studies promoting pharmaceuticals and, 234
study evidence of, 82–86
in the supermarket and the home, 64–67
treatments and, 144
underlying pathologies and, 147
understanding the universe and, 50–51
unpredictability and, 109
vs. genetics, 111
wholism *vs.*, 47–48
refrigeration, 81–82
research and development (R&D), 205
research funding, 194, 217–230
research journals, 232–236
Research Triangle Park (NC), 136
respirators, 108
restaurant critics, 58
restaurants, 13
retrocasuality, 78
rheumatoid arthritis, 159
riboflavin, 151, 253
ribonucleic acid. *See* RNA
river cleanup projects, 165
RNA, 112–115
Rohn, Jim, 67

S
saccharin, 133–134
salt, 7, 11, 289
Sanofi pharmaceutical company, 249
Sara Lee, 270
sardines, 159, 237
saturated fat, 37

Saturday Evening Post, 245
school lunch programs, 66, 182, 183, 192–194, 247, 254, 257, 272
science, impoverishment of, 215–217
scientific elitism, 225
scientific method, 26–29, 215
scientific paradigm, 27–29, 32, 37, 40, 46
scientific research, 183
"Scientists Behaving Badly," 219
scurvy, 67
seat belt enforcement, 183
Seattle, Chief, 164, 165–166
selenium, 67, 70, 71, 157
serum cholesterol, 154
Shaffer, Beth, 272
shampoo, 131
side effects, 142
Simon, Paul, 27
skin cancer. *See* melanoma
Smarr, Larry, 110
smiling, 85
Smith, Richard, 234, 243
smoking, 76, 77, 120, 160, 209, 251, 264, 265–266
Smuts, Jan, 53
social ostracism, 278
social policy, 164
socioeconomic standing, 86
Socrates, 247
Sodexo, 274
sodium, 70, 72
soft drinks, 251, 266, 272
soil loss, 166, 173
solar energy, 165
Solving America's Healthcare Crisis (Popper), 272
sorbitol, 269
Soyjoy, 271
"Special Edition on the Future of Medicine," 242–244
species-to-species extrapolation, 134
Stamps, E. Roe, IV, 244
Standard American Diet (SAD), 13, 143, 192, 245
Starfield, Barbara, 5
Star Wars, 192

statin drugs, 188
statistical significance, 23–24
Steinem, Gloria, 58
stents, 143
Stoloff, Len, 258
stomach stapling, 191
stroke, 8, 9, 80, 143
study design, funding influences and, 218–219
subatomic particles, 78
Subcommittee on Alternative and Complementary Methods of Cancer Management, 267
subsidized foods, 193
subsistence-farming, 174
substrates, 98, 100, 106
sucralose, 269
sugar, 7, 11, 13, 182, 289
suicide, 38
"Summer Bun Program," 270
Summit Group, 244
sunlight, 131, 138
supermarkets, 58–59, 64–67
superstition, 145
surgery, 24, 35, 189, 192, 197, 217, 255
symptoms, treating, 141–142, 143, 149, 191
Sysco, 274

T
tabula rasa, 119
Talmud, 45
tamoxifen, 278–279
taste buds, 11
taxpayer dollars, 162, 188, 205, 206–207, 260
t-bone steaks, 89
techno-biology, 216
technology, 82, 107, 110, 215–216
Technology, 215
teeth, 193, 253
teeth, shape and number of, 82
television, 236, 239–242
Temple University School of Medicine, 31
Texas A&M University, 70
theology, 49

thermostats, 167
Third World villagers, 67
Thomas, Lewis, 125
thrombolytic drugs, 18
tobacco, 76, 264, 265–266
tobacco companies, 76
tomatoes, 237
toxin exposure, 83, 84, 130–131, 165–166
traditional healers, 144
transportation, 168
traumatic injuries, 142–143
True North Health Center, 235
truth, goal of, 214
Truvia, 271
tuna, 159
TV commercials, 6
twin studies, 130

U
underground water resources, 167, 169–170
Underwood, Ann, 242–243
Unilever, 271
Unilever/Best Foods, 266
United Nations, 166
United Nations' Food and Agricultural Organization, 167–168
United Nations' World Health Organization, 146
United States, 38–39, 90, 245
universities, research funding and, 217–218, 221–222
University of California, Berkeley, 136
University of Georgia, 117
University of Medicine and Dentistry of New Jersey, 205
University of Miami, 244
University of Oxford, 120, 245
University of Victoria, Canada, 205
university professors, 217
unpredictability, 109
U.S. auto industry, 252
U.S. Department of Agriculture, 66, 245, 254

U.S. Department of Health and Human Services, 255
U.S. Dietary Guidelines Advisory Committee, 245
U.S. Federal Trade Commission, 162
U.S. Government, 5–6, 13, 66, 115–116, 132, 181–182, 187, 193, 247–250, 289
U.S. National Cancer Institute, 35
U.S. Preventative Services Task Force, 266
USAID, 89
USA Today, 245
US Foods, 275
uterus, misbehaving, 146–147

V
vaccines, 116, 249
Vader, Darth, 192
VA hospitals, 193
vegan diets, 11
vegetables, 7, 58, 59, 84, 251, 258–259, 270
vegetarian diets, 11, 194, 275
Venter, J. Craig, 116
victim blaming, 137
violence, 38
Virginia Tech, 30, 61, 89–91, 93, 95, 170
viruses, 131, 138, 148
visionary entrepreneurs, 182
vitamins
    A, 70, 71, 72, 118, 151, 158, 160, 237
    B2, 151, 253
    B6, 151
    B12, 118
    C, 67, 68, 70, 71, 151, 152–153
    classification as food and, 212
    coining of the word, 118
    D, 67, 70
    deficiency of, 67
    E, 70, 151, 156–158, 161, 230
    human body's utilization of, 68–69
    K, 151
    nutrient pairs and, 70
    reductionism and, 64–65
    supplements, 65, 85–86, 119, 150 (*See also* nutrient supplements)

volatile organic compounds (VOCs), 144
volunteering, 173

W
Wakefield Group, 244
Wallace, David Foster, 46
Wall Street Journal, 234
Warburton, Rebecca, 205–207
Warner, Margaret, 239
War on Cancer, 109, 130–132, 189, 237, 239–242, 278
water
    carcinogens and, 131, 137
    drinking, 193–194
    filters for, 131
    pollution of, 165–166, 169–170
    production of food and usage of, 166, 169
    resources of, 166
    underground resources of, 167, 169–170
WebMD website, 159
Webster's Dictionary, 60
weight, 8, 191, 209
Weight Watchers Diet, 59, 68
well-being of humans, 215
Wells, H. G., 14
Wendy's, 266
WFPB diet
    barriers to widespread adoption of the, 12–13, 14, 181
    criticisms of, 14–15
    description of, 11, 289
    effects of, 7–10
    health effects of, 20
    ingredients for, 13
    purity of diet and, 11
    scientific evidence for the, 12
    speed at which nutritional benefits appear and the, 17
wheat, 166
whole food concentrates, 150, 151, 212
whole foods, 211, 286
Whole Foods (store), 234
whole grains, 7
whole plant products, 85

wholism
  embracing, 286
  evidence for, 79–86
  free-markets and, 216–217
  nutrition and, 148–149
  reductionism *vs.*, 47–48, 77, 86
  research and, 234
  vitamin C potency and, 152–153
  the "whole" in, 53–56
wine, 237
Women, Infants, and Children program, 254
Women Against MS, 270
World Bank, 168

World Bank Group, 168
World Cancer Research Fund, 241
World Congress of Nutrition, 33
World Health Organization, 146, 249
world hunger, 166, 167, 172–174, 189

Y
yoga magazines, 155

Z
Zerhouni, Elias, 249
zinc, 71
Zone diet, 68

Ready to save your life? Hailed as one of the most important books ever written on health and nutrition, *The China Study* reveals life-changing truths everyone deserves to know . . .

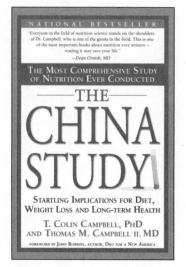

The China Study
The Most Comprehensive Study of Nutrition Ever Conducted and the Startling Implications for Diet, Weight Loss, and Long-term Health

By T. COLIN CAMPBELL, PhD
and THOMAS M. CAMPBELL II, MD

In *The China Study*, bestselling authors T. Colin Campbell, PhD, and Thomas M. Campbell II, MD, detail the connection between nutrition and cancer, diabetes, heart disease, and obesity. Additionally, the report examines the nutritional confusion produced by powerful lobbies, government entities, and opportunistic scientists. *The New York Times* has recognized the study as the "most comprehensive large study ever undertaken of the relationship between diet and the risk of developing disease." *The China Study* cuts through the haze of misinformation and delivers an insightful message to anyone living with cancer, diabetes, heart disease, obesity, and those concerned with the effects of aging.

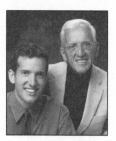

For more than 40 years, T. COLIN CAMPBELL, PhD, has been at the forefront of nutrition research. His legacy, the China Study, is the most comprehensive study of health and nutrition ever conducted. Dr. Campbell is the Jacob Gould Schurman Professor Emeritus of Nutritional Biochemistry at Cornell University. He has received more than 70 grant-years of peer-reviewed research funding and authored more than 300 research papers. The China Study was the culmination of a 20-year partnership of Cornell University, Oxford University, and the Chinese Academy of Preventive Medicine.

Visit THECHINASTUDY.COM to learn more and TCOLINCAMPBELL.ORG for updates on Colin's foundation!

"I have often been asked—a few hundred times, I think—what do my family and I eat? ... Now I am happy to say that there is a cookbook that comes about as close to the real deal for our family as I can imagine it. This is it."
—T. COLIN CAMPBELL, PhD, coauthor of *The China Study*

LeAnne Campbell, daughter of *The China Study*'s T. Colin Campbell, delivers easily prepared and delicious recipes that support optimal nutrition in ...

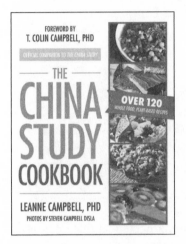

The China Study Cookbook

Over 120 Whole Food, Plant-Based Recipes

By LEANNE CAMPBELL, PhD

The China Study Cookbook takes the vital scientific findings from *The China Study* and puts the science into action. Written by LeAnne Campbell, PhD, daughter of *The China Study* coauthor T. Colin Campbell, PhD, and mother of two hungry teenagers, *The China Study Cookbook* features delicious, easily prepared plant-based recipes. From her Fabulous Sweet Potato Enchiladas to No-Bake Peanut Butter Bars, all of LeAnne's recipes have no added fat and minimal sugar and salt to promote optimal health. Filled with helpful tips on substitutions, keeping foods nutrient-rich, and transitioning to a plant-based diet, *The China Study Cookbook* shows how to transform individual health and the health of the entire family.

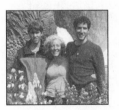

LEANNE CAMPBELL, PhD, has been preparing meals based on a whole food, plant-based diet for almost 20 years. Campbell has raised two sons—Steven and Nelson, now 18 and 17—on this diet. As a working mother, she has found ways to prepare quick and easy meals without using animal products or adding fat.

Visit **THECHINASTUDY.COM** and **THECHINASTUDYCOOKBOOK.COM** to learn more!

More than 100,000 copies sold in the series ...

The Happy Herbivore Series

By LINDSAY S. NIXON

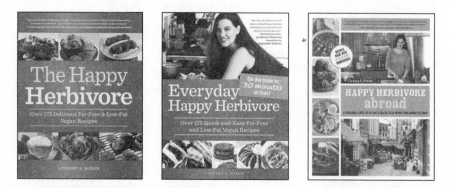

Lindsay S. Nixon's website, HappyHerbivore.com, topped over five million page views in 2012 alone with her sought-after, plant-based diet tips, delicious recipes, and cooking how-tos. True to her creed, Nixon's vegan dishes in her cookbooks are simple and refreshing for your palate.

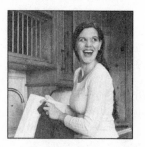

LINDSAY S. NIXON is author of the bestselling Happy Herbivore vegan cookbook series: *The Happy Herbivore Cookbook*, *Everyday Happy Herbivore*, and *Happy Herbivore Abroad*, which have sold more than 100,000 copies combined. Nixon has been featured on The Food Network and *Dr. Oz*, and she has spoken at Google. Her recipes have also been featured in *The New York Times*, *Vegetarian Times*, *Shape Magazine*, *Bust*, *Women's Health*, WebMD, and countless other online publications. A rising star in the culinary world, Nixon is praised for her ability to use everyday ingredients to create healthy, low-fat recipes that are easy to make and light on your wallet.

Visit HAPPYHERBIVORE.COM to learn more!

"It turns out that if we eat the way that promotes the best health for ourselves, we also promote the best health for the planet."

—T. COLIN CAMPBELL, PhD, coauthor of *The China Study*

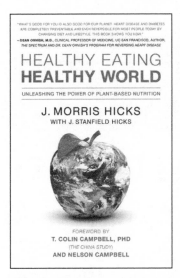

Healthy Eating, Healthy World
Unleashing the Power of Plant-Based Nutrition

By J. MORRIS HICKS
with J. STANFIELD HICKS

This powerful book explains exactly why a plant-based diet is the best choice you can make for yourself and for the planet. Simply incorporating more whole plant food and fewer animal products into your regular diet, you can enjoy vibrant health while greatly reducing your risk for ailments such as diabetes, cancer, and heart disease. And, if everyone adopted this diet, we would see improvement in poverty levels, health care costs, the energy crisis, and many environmental problems. While this sounds too good to be true, it's not. *Healthy Eating, Healthy World* arms you with the knowledge you need to make better food and lifestyle choices. It is a comprehensive yet accessible guide to incorporating healthy and delicious foods into your diet, so you can improve your life and your world.

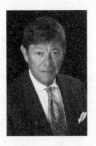

A former senior corporate executive with Ralph Lauren in New York, J. MORRIS HICKS has always focused on the "big picture" when analyzing any issue. In 2002, after becoming curious about our "optimal diet," he began an intensive study of what we eat from a global perspective. Leveraging his expertise in making complex things simple, he is now delivering his powerful message in his book, on his daily blog, and in public speaking engagements—embarking on his new career as a writer, speaker, blogger, and consultant—promoting health, hope, and harmony on planet Earth.

Visit THECHINASTUDY.COM to learn more!

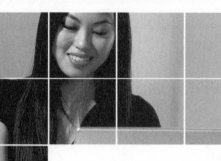

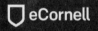
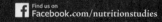

PLANT-BASED NUTRITION

Certificate offered through 🛡 **eCornell**

As a board-certified family practitioner with over 10 years clinical experience, I found the certificate program in Plant-Based Nutrition to be the most inspirational medical education I have ever taken. - Courtney E., MD

24/7 ACCESS

SELF-PACED

WORLDWIDE INTERACTION

Ready to take the next step?

The T. Colin Campbell Center for Nutrition Studies courses are currently offered through the highly rated eCornell platform. eCornell is a subsidiary of Cornell University and provides online professional and executive development to students around the world.

NO PRE-REQUISITES

CONTINUING EDUCATION

LIVE INSTRUCTORS

Earn up to 30 continuing education credits!

Who should enroll in this certificate program?

Individuals seeking to improve their own personal health, as well as medical, nutritional, and health education professionals who want to enhance their skills and education.

HEALTH PROFESSIONALS

DIETITIANS

HEALTH EDUCATORS

ATHLETES

GENERAL PUBLIC

PARENTS

How to enroll:
1-866-eCornell or (1-866-326-7635)
Outside of the USA:
1-607-330-3200
Email:
info@ecornell.com

T. COLIN
CAMPBELL
Center *for*
Nutrition Studies

nutritionstudies.org

JOIN OUR FAMILY AT WWW.WHOLEVANA.COM AND HELP TO LAUNCH A REVOLUTION!

The Wholevana℠ community is a group of people who have come together to support one another in their quest for better health and to spread the positive message of plant-based nutrition to others.

The theme of Wholevana℠ is simple: we foster human relationships around an idea that is deeply meaningful to everyone on the planet, and to the planet itself. Our web platform lets people everywhere participate in building a real community, one rooted in our workplaces, neighborhoods, and places of worship, and committed to the most empowering idea of our time.

A Bottom-Up Revolution

Many past efforts to promote plant-based nutrition have focused on celebrity personalities who build diet brands around themselves and push information out to the public.

Our goal is different. We are not interested in building ourselves up. This health message will spark a revolution fastest if anyone with a passion for health can become a hero, first in their own lives, then in the lives of others.

Plant-based nutrition is not a diet and it is not unique to any one of us—it is quite simply, Nature.

How did we come up with the name "Wholevana"?

In considering a domain name, our first impulse was to play off the title of this book. We like the concept of "whole" because we have built a social networking platform that fosters a community to support people as they embark on a journey toward better health.

Then, from this first impulse, we created the word "Wholevana." Not only does this word roll off the tongue well, there is relevant meaning behind it. "Vana" in ancient Sanskrit means "forest." So this word literally means "the whole forest."

When I was a kid growing up, the idiom my siblings and I heard from my father more than any other was his complaint that people tended "not to see the forest for the trees." Perhaps because he grew up a country boy spending many hours in the fields and forests, he loved this idiom about the forest and trees.

This "whole forest" concept is a good metaphor for what we are doing. Within the forest is much complexity and change, but there is also a connection that binds all the trees and their friends—the animals, soil, microorganisms, and air—into an unbroken whole. This bond is the essence of our community and health message.

Nelson Campbell
Founder and President of Campbell Wellness

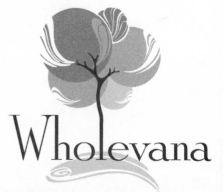